CONCEPTUAL FOUNDATIONS
of Occupational
Therapy

CONCEPTUAL FOUNDATIONS
of Occupational
Therapy

Second Edition

Gary Kielhofner, DrPH, OTR, FAOTA
Professor and Head
Department of Occupational Therapy
and
Associate Dean for Academic Affairs
College of Health and Human Development Sciences
and
Professor
School of Public Health
University of Illinois at Chicago
Chicago, Illinois
and
Foreign Adjunct Professor
Karolinska Institute
Stockholm, Sweden

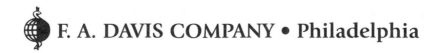 F. A. DAVIS COMPANY • Philadelphia

F. A. Davis Company
1915 Arch Street
Philadelphia, PA 19103

Printed in the United States of America
Last digit indicates print number: 10 9 8 7 6 5

Publisher, Allied Health: Jean-François Vilain
Senior Allied Health Editor: Lynn Borders Caldwell
Developmental Editor: Marianne Fithian
Production Editor: Jessica Howie Martin
Cover Designer: Louis J. Forgione

As new scientific information becomes available through basic and clinical research, recommended treatments and drug therapies undergo changes. The author and publisher have done everything possible to make this book accurate, up to date, and in accord with accepted standards at the time of publication. The author, editors, and publisher are not responsible for errors or omissions or for consequences from application of the book, and make no warranty, expressed or implied, in regard to the contents of the book. Any practice described in this book should be applied by the reader in accordance with professional standards of care used in regard to the unique circumstances that may apply in each situation. The reader is advised always to check product information (package inserts) for changes and new information regarding dose and contraindications before administering any drug. Caution is especially urged when using new or infrequently ordered drugs.

Library of Congress Cataloging-in-Publication Data
Kielhofner, Gary, 1949-
    Conceptual foundations of occupational therapy / Gary Kielhofner.
    —2nd ed.
        p.   cm.
    Includes bibliographical references and index.
    ISBN 0-8036-0256-1 (hardcover)
    1. Occupational therapy. I. Title.
RM735.K54   1997
616.8'515—dc21   97-4078
                                                                          CIP

For Beatrice D. Wade

In memory and gratitude for the legacies she left to
the profession and to the Department of Occupational
Therapy at the University of Illinois at Chicago

PREFACE

Throughout the writing of this book, both this and the first edition, I was constantly reminded of my own personal journey in occupational therapy. Twenty-five years ago I first entered an occupational therapy clinic as an aide, fulfilling the alternative service obligation of a conscientious objector. What originally promised to be a 2-year detour from a career in clinical psychology turned out to be an introduction to my life work. I was drawn to the combination of helping and practical action in occupational therapy, which seemed so much more cogent than the predominantly talk-oriented approaches used in psychology. At the end of a year, I matriculated into an occupational therapy program with the support of a supervisor who allowed a flexible work schedule to accommodate my classes.

The educational program was my first big disappointment in occupational therapy. Almost all I had seen in the clinics impressed me. But in the classroom I (along with my classmates) found a disconcerting lack of coherence. It was not so much that the specific facts and concepts offered in classes were not useful enough in and of themselves. Rather, it seemed that, although I was beginning to understand human anatomy, how the unconscious worked, and the intricacies of neuromuscular physiology, and although I had acquired a number of practical skills, something more basic was missing. Simply put, it seemed that I was not really learning about occupational therapy, that all the important knowledge in the curriculum came from other fields. The occupational therapy content was elusive at best. There was only a vague hope offered by several professors that everything would "come together" in clinical internships. I often wondered why the best was saved for last.

My misgivings were reinforced upon attending the American Occupational Therapy Association annual conference, where a number of presentations focused on the problem of *identity* in occupational therapy. It seemed as though members of the field shared a collective *identity crisis*. We all were, or were becoming, occupational therapists, but no one seemed altogether sure of what that meant. At that same conference, I was encouraged by a number of presentations in which therapists were proposing conceptual ways to explain occupational therapy on its own terms instead of resorting to other disciplines' theoretical constructs. This effort was particularly notable in the work of Dr. Mary Reilly and her students and colleagues at the University of Southern California (USC). The experience had an impact on me. I dropped out of my occupational therapy program at the end of the first year and began again at USC. There I had the opportunity to participate in the exciting enterprise of developing a more comprehensive conceptualization of the nature of occupational therapy.

As a result of this experience and my desire for a clearer conceptual articulation of occupational therapy, I begin writing immediately as a new therapist. In the beginning years, I presented my ideas as constituting, variously, a conceptual framework, a model, and a paradigm. It would be nice to say that I had some clear ideas at the outset about what these different terms meant, or, more to the point, that I had a clearly formulated idea about how knowledge gets generated and organized in a profession. However, that was not the case. Rather, I have struggled throughout my professional life with the problem of how we might properly think about the range of knowledge within occupational therapy. And I have pondered related questions about which knowledge is relevant, irrelevant, and most important. A tendency to be opinionated on the topic has provided me with a wealth of good, critical feedback, both in conversation and in the literature. Increasingly, I realize the debt I owe to those who cared enough about what I said to disagree with me.

This second edition represents my *current* thinking on the knowledge base of occupational therapy—my best attempt to decipher what exists and to speculate about what could and should be. In attempting to mirror the ideas and themes manifest in occupational therapy, I have, no doubt, interjected the perspective of my own grasp of these elements and a particular ideological position developed through a personal history of experiences in the field. In the end, that will be both the strength and weakness of the arguments contained herein.

Because I like to recognize order in the world, there is an admitted tendency in this text to perceive a systematic structure in the knowledge base where others might legitimately disagree, recognizing a more disorderly reality. However, I believe that my approach provides a valuable way of thinking about occupational therapy knowledge. It allows comparison of different ideas and concepts, and it recognizes the fact that we use knowledge in different ways and for different purposes. Thus, I offer it as one of a number of ways to view occupational therapy knowledge—a way that I hope will prove useful for those entering into occupational therapy and for those in the field who wish to step back and take a new look at their profession.

Part of the purpose of this text is rhetorical, that is, to persuade the reader to take a different view of occupational therapy. Nevertheless, the book will have best served the reader if it becomes a springboard for further serious thought about the field's knowledge and how it is used in practice. Similarly, the book will have best served the field if it stimulates further dialogue and critical thought about the nature of occupational therapy and the nature of the knowledge that defines and explains it. Finally, I look forward to critical feedback to help my own thoughts to continue to evolve.

Gary Kielhofner

ACKNOWLEDGMENTS

The arguments in this book have been in the making for some time. Along the way, many people have influenced, collaborated with, supported, and criticized me. Without their efforts, this volume could never have come to fruition.

I cannot write about occupational therapy without a debt of gratitude to Dr. Mary Reilly and her colleagues at the University of Southern California. The work they accomplished, well before my time there as a student, and Dr. Reilly's mentoring during my graduate studies irrevocably set the direction of my thinking. Also, Anne Moscy's contributions to the literature, her criticism of my work, and many hours of lively discussion have left their mark. The experience of analyzing the history of occupational therapy and working the model of human occupation with Janice Burke still echoes through this book. Roanne Barris and I together hashed out, in rudimentary form, some of the ideas about organization of knowledge represented herein.

My colleagues and students at the University of Illinois at Chicago have discussed these ideas extensively with me, piloted them in the classroom, and provided feedback on portions of the manuscript. In particular, I am grateful to the classes of graduate students who used drafts of both editions of this book as a "text" in my Theories of Occupational Therapy course and provided helpful discussion and criticism.

The occupational therapy program in Stockholm, Sweden, along with the Karolinska Institute, has sponsored courses organized around the content of this book. The experience of leading courses with occupational therapists and educators from several countries throughout Europe has been most stimulating and enhanced many of the ideas in this volume. I wish to express my sincerest appreciation for the exciting exchanges I have had with my European colleagues. I am particularly indebted to Lena Borell and Hans Jonsson, who organized the courses and provided unfailing personal and professional support. I hope I have repaid them in some small way by attempting to give this volume a more international character.

F. A. Davis provided me with a first-rate group of reviewers, who went above and beyond the call of duty to provide thoughtful criticism of the entire manuscript. I am grateful to the following people for reviewing this edition of the manuscript:

Anne E. Dickerson, PhD, OTR
Chair/Associate Professor
Occupational Therapy Department
East Carolina University
Greenville, NC

Jaime Phillip Muñoz, MS, OTR
Clinical Instructor
Department of Occupational Therapy
Duquesne University
Pittsburgh, PA

Louise R. Thibodaux, MA, OTR, FAOTA
Associate Professor
Division of Occupational Therapy
University of Alabama at Birmingham
Birmingham, AL

Janet H. Watts, MS, PhD, OTR
Associate Professor
Occupational Therapy Department
Virginia Commonwealth University
Medical College of Virginia
Richmond, VA

Additionally, I want to convey my gratitude to the following people who reviewed the first edition of this text:

Sally Hobbs Jackson, MS, OTR
Associate Professor
Occupational Therapy Department
Lenoir-Rhyne College
Hickory, NC

Elizabeth M. Kanny, PhD, OTR, FAOTA
Assistant Professor
Division of Occupational Therapy
Department of Rehabilitative Medicine
University of Washington
Seattle, WA

David L. Nelson, PhD, OTR, FAOTA
Professor
Department of Occupational Therapy
Medical College of Ohio School of Allied Health
Toledo, OH

Ann M. Neville-Jan, PhD, OTR, FAOTA
Associate Professor
Occupational Therapy Department
University of Southern California
Los Angeles, CA

Louise R. Thibodaux, MA, OTR, FAOTA
Associate Professor
Division of Occupational Therapy
University of Alabama at Birmingham
Birmingham, AL

I am indebted to Clare Hocking for providing a number of thought-provoking papers concerning values in occupational therapy, as well as for the contribution she and her New Zealand colleagues have made to the discourse about values in the field. I am also grateful to Susan Mann Dolce and her junior class, who provided thoughtful input to me concerning my discussion of values in the first edition of this book.

Laura Barrett and Trudy Mallinson have provided helpful comments and feedback on various sections of the text and tolerated my "thinking out loud" about a number of issues and passages in the book. Kirsty Forsyth and Shari Gilbert provided able and willing assistance in some of the work of producing the final manuscript. I am grateful for their support.

I would also like to thank my graduate students Carrie Crawford, Meika Nowak, and Matt Rigby for their help with editing, creating graphics, and compiling the glossary.

Dating back to the first edition, Jean-François Vilain and Lynn Borders Caldwell of F. A. Davis provided unfailing support of the project. I will always be grateful for their faith in me, their patience, and their persistence. As I produced the second edition, Lynn Borders Caldwell has been solicitous, cheerful, helpful, and understanding.

CONTENTS

CHAPTER 4

THE EMERGING PARADIGM   **53**

CHAPTER 5

CONCEPTUAL PRACTICE MODELS   **95**

CHAPTER 6

THE BIOMECHANICAL MODEL   109

CHAPTER 7

THE COGNITIVE DISABILITIES MODEL   127

CHAPTER 8

THE COGNITIVE-PERCEPTUAL MODEL   145

CHAPTER 1

INTRODUCTION

E arly in this century, Susan Tracy, one of the founders of occupational therapy in North America, sent a greeting card to another occupational therapist, Jennie K. Allen. The front of the card bore a nicely executed watercolor of a bluebird perched on a blooming tree branch (Fig. 1–1). On the reverse side of the card, Tracy wrote, "Done without help by a patient sent from the [psychiatrist] tagged 'not able to concentrate *at all!*' " Since she offered no further elaboration, Tracy apparently expected Allen to grasp straightaway the significance of the story she was relating.

When I first encountered this card, it occurred to me that I have heard other versions of this story told by occupational therapists. For example, Chin-Kai Lin, a therapist from Taiwan, recently told me the story of a woman with a severe head injury. Her formerly beautiful face, distorted through facial nerve palsy and the weight of her dark future, seemed fixed in a permanent frown. One day Chin-Kai convinced the patient to join in with a traditional Chinese choir. As she began to sing an ancient sacred poem, her face slowly lifted, transforming into a cheerful smile.

The same kind of story remains alive in the lore of occupational therapy across time and culture, suggesting that it evokes something that occupational therapists will recognize as deeply important about their practice.

Ultimately, Tracy's and Chin-Kai's stories, along with others of the same genre, are about the power of the field's therapeutic tool, occupation, to evoke capacity. These narratives typically contrast a patient's performance in therapy with how the patient was judged capable of performing by others, or with the patient's prior performance. The stories tell about a kind of therapeutic sorcery, in which nonapparent capacities, motives, or feelings are summoned by occupations.

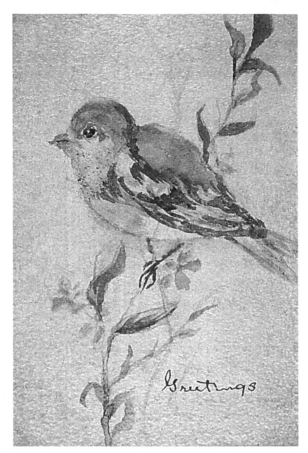

Figure 1–1. Watercolor produced by a patient of Susan Tracy, who sent it to Jennie K. Allen. Ms. Allen later passed it on to Beatrice D. Wade, who founded the occupational therapy program at the University of Illinois at Chicago. Ms. Wade left the watercolor to the department, and it is on permanent display in the department library.

Recently, Nelson[5] published a theoretical paper in which he introduced a new concept, "occupation form." Behind this concept is the idea that occupations (water coloring being one of an endless number of such occupations) have a shape or "form." This occupational form consists of the context, the objects used, the social definition and meaning of the thing to be done, and the ways of doing it that are "known" within a society or culture. Occupational form, Nelson and others now hypothesize, can exert an important influence on people, eliciting and shaping performance and experience.

Research by occupational therapists has provided some support for this hypothesis. For example, studies have shown that varying the occupational form can change how persons move their bodies, how much effort they use, what they experience, and even the degree of impairment they exhibit.[1,2,7,8]

Over the last 2 years, colleagues and I have developed and tested an interview to assess how work environments influenced the performance and well-being of disabled workers.[4] The design of this assessment is based, in part, on the concept of occupational form.

Tracy's and Chin-Kai's stories, the theoretical concept of occupational form, the research into how occupational forms influence performance and experience, and the incorporation of this concept into a practical assessment are interrelated aspects of occupational therapy's conceptual foundations.

The conceptual foundations of occupational therapy incorporate many elements: assumptions, ideals or values, viewpoints, concepts, theory, research, guidelines for practice, and a range of clinical strategies and tools. In this book I will show how and why all these elements belong to the conceptual foundations of the field, and I will underscore that they are interrelated in important ways. My main thesis is that these elements exist together as part of a complex unfolding conversation about the nature and practice of occupational therapy.

Oral traditions, including stories about occupational therapy's impact on patients, perpetuate certain views of the nature of occupational therapy. The introduction of theoretical concepts in publications provides a better understanding of phenomena that are part of the practice in the field. The development of practical tools based on concepts increases the technical expertise with which occupational therapists can complete their work. As in the examples I began with, these very different ways of considering or enacting occupational therapy give substance, depth, clarity, validity, and practicality to some aspect of occupational therapy. That they give different voices to a particular matter of concern enriches the field's appreciation of that matter. I strongly suspect that those elements that come to be most important in occupational therapy are the ones that ultimately find many forms of expression. To understand why this is so, it is helpful to consider what occupational therapists do when they practice.

Occupational Therapy Practice

A Columbian occupational therapist in Bogota screens children in kindergartens for developmental delays and develops an activity program to stimulate such children's normal development. A therapist working through the Red Cross in a rural district of Botswana assists a group of disabled adults to establish a small bakery that generates income for them. A community-based therapist in Linkoping, Sweden, works with a group of young persons who are mentally retarded, helping them manage finances, do laundry, and prepare meals so that they can live effectively in special apartments set aside within a community housing complex. A therapist in the United States goes into the home of a mother in Chicago who has been paralyzed from an automobile accident, helping her rearrange her kitchen and cooking routines so she can still prepare meals for her family. A Canadian therapist helps an oil derrick worker injured outside Calgary to regain his confidence and capacity for returning to the job. A Japanese therapist in Akita assists an elderly woman who has had a stroke to figure out how she can still conduct the tea ceremony with dignity.

In all these circumstances, occupational therapists provide services to persons whose impairments interfere with satisfying participation in their everyday occupations. Whether by helping a child to play and thus develop, a group to bake and sell bread, young adults to manage everyday responsibilities for apartment living, a mother to prepare a meal, a worker to operate equipment, or an elderly person to prepare and serve tea, occupational therapists assist persons to occupy themselves in keeping with their desires and circumstances.

These occupational therapists have specialized knowledge about such things as the importance of play to development, how limited ability for movement can be augmented through specialized equipment, environmental modifications that can maximize function from a wheelchair, the importance and consequence of a person's beliefs about personal ability, and how to identify which activities are most critical to a person's rebuilding life following a traumatic event.

These therapists also have in common a conviction that being meaningfully occupied is fundamental to well-being. They share a similar philosophical orientation that emphasizes respect for the unique desires and abilities of the individual.

These occupational therapists deliver their services in different cultures and health care systems, yet there is a striking similarity in their outlook and practices. Despite their different native tongues, cultures and sociopolitical systems, and local circumstances, occupational therapy always remains recognizably occupational therapy.

These occupational therapists share common views about what is important for their patients and clients and that they approach diverse problems along similar lines, suggesting that they have all partaken in some kind of common dialogue. One cannot but conclude that some kind of collective discourse has shaped their professional views and abilities. Another way of framing this is to say they share identity and competence.

Identity and Competence

Together, identity and competence give a unique stamp to any professional group. They are what members of a field such as occupational therapy hold in common, and they bind the members together.

Identity refers both to that which distinguishes a person and to the way that person sees things. For example, when persons refer to themselves as conservative or liberal, they are saying something about who they are and about a set of beliefs and perspectives they hold. Thus identity refers both to a recognizable characteristic or aspect of a person, and at the same time to the person's outlook. This is no less true of professional identity. It is professional identity that allows therapists to have a consistent view of the nature and meaning of their work and to present themselves to others as a particular type of professional.

Professional identity enables one to say, in effect, "As an occupational therapist, this is my perspective; these are things I consider important; these are the kinds of problems I address; and this is how I try to solve them." Moreover, this professional identity helps to make the collective field of occupational therapy a particular kind of profession (i.e., one that emphasizes or focuses on certain things, solves certain kinds of problems, and uses particular kinds of methods to solve those problems). This identity allows other professionals and lay persons to know something about what occupational therapists are and what they do.

One reason, then, that occupational therapists throughout the world appear quite similar is that they share a common professional identity. They have an understanding of the nature and purpose of their profession, and they share certain perspectives that, in their totality, are unique to occupational therapists. This shared understanding of occupational therapy and this outlook bind the world community of occupational therapists into a single professional community. In this sense, the profession transcends the national organizations, the unique educational institutions, and the particular variations of the profession in each country or culture.

Competence is the knowledge and abilities that therapists bring to bear on a particular problem of a specific patient or client. Competence involves being able to identify and understand certain problems that patients face. It also involves knowing how to address those problems (e.g., how to employ appropriate strategies, techniques, equipment, and other resources in the course of therapy to effectively solve problems).

In the same way that identity gives therapists worldwide a similar character and outlook, shared competence enables therapists worldwide to offer similar kinds of services in a variety of circumstances.

The Relationship of Conceptual Foundations to Identity and Competence

An important thesis in this book is that the identity and competence of the individual therapist come from the *conceptual foundations* of the field. As already noted, I use the term, conceptual foundations, to refer to the collection of beliefs, assumptions, values, concepts, and techniques that make up the collective wisdom and "know-how" of the field.

These conceptual foundations are shaped by the writing, practice, teaching, discussion, theorizing, research, and storytelling that collectively make up a complex and interwoven conversation. This conversation allows therapists to shape a common vision, clarify shared meanings, and sort out what their professional practices should be.

The conceptual foundations of a field are represented in books and articles, and they are developed and advanced through research. Just as importantly, these conceptual foundations find expression and are tested and refined through how therapists practice, think about their actions, and talk or write about their work. *Every occupational therapist, thus, participates in the conceptual foundations of the field.* Each therapist, in his or her own way, receives and carries the messages of the conceptual foundations.

In framing the argument this way, I am taking a particular point of view on how theory, common sense, action, ideology, and logistics should interact in everyday practice. For example, more than a few questions have been raised about the role that the "conceptual" has in the everyday practice of therapists. Some writers[3,6] have emphasized that therapists practice in ways that go beyond what theory can specify. Many practitioners bemoan that theory does not always keep pace with the changing demands of practice environments or speak to all the situations and problems encountered in practice. Consequently, in place of using theory to guide their practice, therapists often rely on experience and common sense. On the other hand, theorists and educators sometimes observe that practitioners do not keep pace with changes in theory or make use of research. Each of these claims has some validity. Concepts sometimes fail to inform practice, and practice sometimes falls short of what theory and research indicate is best.

Nevertheless, practice and theory have a great potential to augment each other. Therapists who consciously and reflectively work from a theoretical perspective gain more from their experience. Practical experience deepens a therapist's understanding of theory. When conceptual and practical concerns become part of the dialogue about occupational therapy, the field is more readily advanced.

This, then, is why I assert that discussion, writing, clinical decision making, and research should be seen as interactive conversations, influencing each other in ways that are not trivial. The concepts of a field can only provide a vision of what should be when yoked to a definite and intense conversation with practice.

The Plan of This Book

In this book, I aim to explain and describe the conceptual foundations of occupational therapy. I will begin by proposing a way to think about the conceptual foundations of occupational therapy. This view builds on the viewpoints I have already introduced and considers both what the profession is doing and what it could do to advance its knowledge and practice.

Trying to understand occupational therapy's conceptual foundations is a bit like trying to follow multiple conversations at an extended gathering of people. New themes sprout up out of a line of talk, some discussions die off, and others branch into separate lines of conversation. How and in what directions the talk goes depends on who is talking and responding, on the unique unfolding of a topic, and on what themes capture interests. When one examines the conceptual foundations of any field, it can be hard to see an explicit order in them. In part, sorting out elements of the field's conceptual foundations is difficult because, as knowledge develops, it does not assume a neatly organized form any more than do the multiple conversations of a large group of people.

Nonetheless, this lack of apparent order points out that some means of ordering the knowledge would be useful. To understand and use the field's knowledge, one must have a way of seeing how all its parts are related. One of the goals of this book, then, is to find and, to an extent, impart some order. Hence, in this text I present conceptual foundations of the field in a way that should allow the reader to identify, understand, compare, and critique parts of the field's knowledge.

Specifically, I will consider how the various beliefs, assumptions, values, concepts, and technology that make up the conceptual foundations are related to each other. I will also explore how all the elements that make up the conceptual foundation of the field have come into existence and have changed over time. Along with this, I will consider what kinds of processes (e.g., public discussion, theory development, research, application of ideas in practice) maintain and change the conceptual foundations of the field. Lastly, I will examine the current content of the conceptual foundations of occupational therapy, focusing on what kind of identity and competence they provide for modern occupational therapists.

The organization of this text is as follows. In the next chapter, I will outline a particular way of viewing the knowledge organization of occupational therapy, relating this organization to the concepts of identify and competence. Briefly stated, the next chapter proposes that occupational therapy's conceptual foundations consist of three concentric layers of knowledge. At the inner core is a paradigm, which provides the field and individual therapists with a sense of identity and a unique perspective. Surrounding this inner core is a band of conceptual practice models. These models provide the knowledge that gives occupational therapists their unique competence. The models incorporate theory that explains different phenomena occupational therapists address in practice; they also provide rationales, guidelines, and tools for carrying out therapy. The outermost layer is related knowledge. This knowledge is not unique to occupational therapy, but it supports therapists' competence, since it provides the information necessary to specific areas of practice. Hence it is taught, written about, and used as part of occupational therapy's conceptual foundations.

In Chapter 3 I analyze the history of development of the inner layer of occupational therapy's conceptual foundations, the paradigm. This history traces the emergence of occupational therapy knowledge as the profession developed in the first three-quarters of this century. Chapter 4 is devoted to a discussion of the field's contemporary paradigm. It examines the knowledge that provides occupational therapy with its current identity and outlook.

Chapter 5 begins the next section of the book by discussing in more detail what a conceptual model of practice is and how I identified the field's current models. The subsequent chapters, 6 through 13, present these eight conceptual models of practice. Each of these chapters uses the same format for presenting and critiquing the models. This should enable readers to compare and contrast models, and ultimately to decide how to interrelate and use models together in practice. At the end of each chapter, I also provide a list of the model's major concepts and their definitions. These chapters are designed to introduce the reader to the conceptual models of practice, and allow the models to be readily compared. However, my discussion of the models is general and, therefore, insufficient to provide the reader with the depth of knowledge necessary to understand the detailed theory and practical elements of each model. Hence, readers who wish to learn a particular model in depth should refer to the references at the end of each chapter and make use of these original sources.

The final section of this book reflects upon the conceptual foundations as a whole and looks toward the future of knowledge development and practice in occupational therapy. Chapter 14 considers the state of model development as a whole, considering the relationship of models to the paradigm and anticipating model development in the future. Chapter 15 considers how the conceptual foundations (both models and the paradigm) influence the identity and competence of occupational therapists. This chapter brings the discussion full circle to the view of the conceptual foundations I outlined earlier. Finally, Chapter 16 considers the arguments of this book in relationship to other viewpoints concerning the conceptual foundations of occupational therapy. This concluding chapter should serve to contextualize what I have argued.

Overall, the book should provide the reader a broad overview of the conceptual foundations of occupational therapy. From this perspective the reader should be able to see the field as a whole and recognize how the various parts of occupational therapy's conceptual foundations fit together. Additionally, the book should give a perspective on how the conceptual foundations have developed and where they might be headed in the future.

My hope is that each reader will finish the book with a more complete grasp of occupational therapy and with a sense of how to participate in its conceptual foundations. And, above all, I want readers to recognize that each new article they read in the profession's journal, each new concept they encounter in occupational therapy textbooks, each new technique or tool to which they are introduced, and every new clinical story told by another therapist represents a continuation and unfolding of the conceptual foundations of occupational therapy.

References

1. LaMore, KL, and Nelson, DL: The effects of options on performance of an art project in adults with mental disabilities. Am J Occup Ther 47:397–401, 1993.
2. Mathiowetz, V: Informational support and functional motor performance. Paper presented at the American Occupational Therapy Association National Conference, Boston, 1994.
3. Mattingly, C, and Flemming, M: Clinical Reasoning: Forms of Inquiry in a Therapeutic Practice. FA Davis, Philadelphia, 1994.
4. Moore-Corner, R, Kielhofner, G, and Fang-Ling, L: Construct validity of a work environment impact scale. Unpublished paper, University of Illinois at Chicago, 1996.
5. Nelson, D: Occupation: Form and performance. Am J Occup Ther 42:633–641, 1988.
6. Schon, D: The Reflective Practitioner: How professions think in action. Basic Books, New York, 1983.
7. Wu, CY, Trombly, C, and Lin, KC: The relationship between occupational form and occupational performance: A kinematic perspective. Am J Occup Ther 48:679–687, 1994.
8. Yoder, RM, Nelson, DL, and Smith DA: Added purpose versus rote exercise in female nursing home residents. Am J Occup Ther 43:581–586, 1989.

CHAPTER 2

THE ORGANIZATION AND USE OF KNOWLEDGE

T his chapter proposes a way of viewing the conceptual foundations of occupational therapy. This view has emerged over the past two decades and is influenced by the ideas of authors concerned with knowledge development in other fields, as well as contributors to the knowledge base of occupational therapy. In formulating this view of the field's conceptual foundations, my first goal was to create a valid characterization of how persons were viewing the conceptual foundations of occupational therapy and going about the work of building them. My second goal was to find coherence among the current collection of concepts, frameworks, and techniques in occupational therapy.

Sometimes it has seemed that these two goals were not compatible. In looking for purposes, process, and patterns in occupational therapy literature, one finds that authors have used different terms to refer to the knowledge they are discussing, developing, or applying. They describe their work as theory, science, conceptual frameworks, frames of reference, and so on. This is not merely a matter of semantics; persons genuinely differ in how they think about occupational therapy's conceptual foundations.* Thus, not only are many persons making contributions to the knowledge base of occupational therapy, they are doing it in somewhat different ways.

---

*I have not made an attempt to address all these different viewpoints on knowledge development. However, in this chapter I will acknowledge differences of opinion that are important for the present argument. Further, in Chapter 16, I will compare the viewpoint I take in this book with two important alternative views of knowledge development on occupational therapy.

I have sought to construct a useful way of thinking about occupational therapy's conceptual foundations and to use it as a means of organizing and interpreting existing knowledge. This way of viewing the conceptual foundations is partly descriptive (i.e., it explains how knowledge has developed) and partly prescriptive (i.e., it suggests how knowledge development might profitably proceed in the future). Arguably, my schema creates a partial fiction, identifying more coherence than may be available in the literature or intended by the authors. In defense of this approach, it allows for a necessary comparison and synthesis of a wide range of occupational therapy ideas.

The Relationship of Knowledge to Practice

In the previous chapter I argued that occupational therapy's conceptual foundations involve an intimate discourse between theory, research, and practice. Others in occupational therapy have also discussed the relationship of theory to practice. I will consider their viewpoints in order to clarify the point of view taken in this text.

Mosey[18] distinguishes between theory that provides an explanation of phenomena and the application of theory in practice. Arguing that occupational therapy's role is limited to theory application, she sees the work of developing and validating theory as belonging to academic disciplines whose concern is with basic knowledge and not application.* Hence, Mosey does not see theory development and practice as integrated activities of the profession.

I do not agree with her argument that the work of occupational therapy and other professions involves only the *application* of knowledge. Distinctions between basic and applied science reflect an outmoded view of how knowledge should develop. These distinctions are grounded, first of all, in a view that "intellectual progress should be dissociated from human or social progress, the former being a progress in knowledge, the latter being progress toward a good social world."[13] This distinction has traditionally been made in the interest of allowing scholarship to reveal *truth* without the encumbrance or bias of practical concerns. Interestingly, the distinction has also led to a hierarchical relationship in which the pure or basic sciences have traditionally been accorded a place of higher status, while applied work has occupied a lesser position.

My viewpoint is influenced by Maxwell's[13] argument that the separation of theory development and solving practical problems is irrational and results in much theory of questionable practical value, while many pressing human problems remain unsolved. He proposes a complete rethinking of the nature and purpose of science and scholarship, proposing that it should

*Academic disciplines refer to the traditional arts and sciences and include fields such as biology, history, physics, mathematics, and philosophy.

proceed in the interest of solving real problems: "We urgently need a new, more rational kind of academic inquiry which gives intellectual priority to the tasks of articulating our problems of living, proposing and critically assessing possible cooperative solutions, tackling problems of knowledge and technological know-how."[13] In a related vein, a recent Carnegie Foundation publication[1] calls for a rethinking of the old hierarchy of basic over applied research. Highlighting the need for relevance in research, it strongly emphasizes the value of a "scholarship of application" that achieves a meaningful dialogue between theory and its application.

These arguments reflect the growing recognition that it is no longer advisable to separate the search for knowledge from the search for solving problems. The idea of a division of labor, in which academic disciplines create theory and professions apply it, only perpetuates an unnecessary and unproductive division of theory and application.

Another important consideration is the constraint posed on a field that concentrates only on the application of existing theory. If all theoretical knowledge were to come from outside the field, occupational therapy would have little to say about what gets explained and how it is conceptualized. Instead, the decisions about what needs explaining in a practice profession should arise out of the conditions of practice.[3] Indeed, the unique problems and dilemmas of occupational therapy are rich grounds for theorizing. To wait for some other discipline to find interest in and create explanations of vexing practice puzzles would hamstring efforts to develop the conceptual foundations of the field.

McColl, Law, and Stewart[15] discuss the relationship of theory and practice at the level of the practitioner. They distinguish between theory that helps therapists to "analyze and understand" and that which enables the therapists to "know what to do." In so doing, they draw upon the classic distinction between *knowing about* and *knowing how* also emphasized by Mattingly and Fleming.[12] This is an important distinction since simply knowing about something is not the same as knowing how to use that knowledge. Indeed, as Schon[20] has pointed out, there has been an incorrect assumption that theoretical explanation is sufficient to guide practical application. Instead, theory (and related research) designed to explain phenomena often fall short of the complexity that persons must deal with in solving problems related to those phenomena.

Rather than accentuating the divide between theoretical explanation and practice, I want to underscore the need for better ways to connect theoretical explanation and practical action.* Making this connection involves organiz-

---

*The division between theoretical explanation and practical application can also result in an artificial divide between those persons involved in theory and research and those persons in practice. For example, Quiroga[19] argues that in the first three decades of occupational therapy in North America, theory development was largely left to a few leaders (mostly men), while matters of practical development of the profession's practice were left to others (mostly women).

ing and developing knowledge in ways that make explicit the relationship between theoretical explanation and practical action. Hence, the view I take in this text is calculated to bring into bold relief the problem of theory and action in the profession. This viewpoint hinges on three assumptions:

1. Theory development and theory application are *both* responsibilities of the profession.
2. The gap often found between theoretical explanation and practical action is, to a large extent, a function of how knowledge is developed and organized.
3. When knowledge is developed and organized in such a way as to emphasize and facilitate the dialogue between explanation and practical problem solving, the gap between theory and practice can be narrowed, if not eliminated.

These three beliefs have guided my attempts to unravel and describe the conceptual foundations of occupational therapy. I have sought to avoid unnecessary distinctions and separations between basic and applied work, and between the theoretical and the practical in occupational therapy, emphasizing instead their interaction and interdependence. Theory provides ways of understanding necessary to practice. Practice points to what we should know and, by applying theory to real life, enriches our understanding of theory. The theoretical and practical can and should be interwoven.

Conceptual Foundations as Concentric Layers of Knowledge

Chapter 1 argued that occupational therapy's conceptual foundations address professional identity and competence. Identity has to do with the nature of the service that occupational therapy provides and the outlook that therapists employ. Competence refers to what a therapist knows how to do in providing service. Practical application requires both knowledge that provides a general outlook or vision and knowledge that gives guidelines for doing.

To the degree that identity and competence are the two fundamental practical problems that a field must address, knowledge development should proceed along lines that address these problems. And, if one examines occupational therapy, there is considerable evidence that knowledge development resonates with these two issues.

First, occupational therapists generate knowledge aimed at defining and identifying what occupational therapy is and at providing therapists with a unique way of seeing their work. A second type of knowledge gives occupational therapists guidance in knowing how to understand specific patient or client problems and what to do about them. Members of the field have generated these two types of knowledge to make sense of those unique things that occupational therapists do.

These two areas of knowledge are not all that occupational therapists know and use. Therapists need a range of knowledge that provides necessary background for different areas of practice. Such knowledge is not generated in occupational therapy but is incorporated into the conceptual foundations.

The conceptual foundations of occupational therapy can be envisioned as three concentric layers of knowledge:

1. An innermost core or *paradigm*
2. A surrounding band of *conceptual practice models*
3. An outer sphere of *related knowledge* (Fig. 2–1)

I refer to the paradigm as the innermost core because it most directly addresses the identity and outlook of the field. Surrounding the paradigm, several conceptual practice models articulate more diverse concepts that are being generated, tested, and applied by practitioners and theorists. It is through these models that the field's theoretical concepts are developed and its treatment approaches are laid out. Conceptual practice models articulate theory that provides a rationale for therapy and guides therapists in practice. The related knowledge of the field is a collection of concepts, facts, and techniques from other fields that are used in occupational therapy practice.

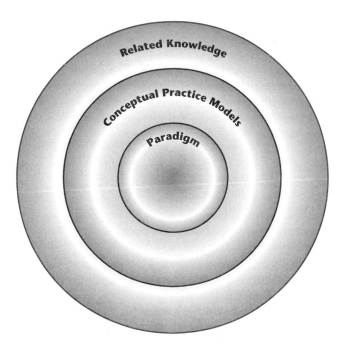

Figure 2–1. Concentric layers of knowledge in the conceptual foundations.

Table 2–1. Characteristics of the Layers of Knowledge

Layer	Content	Purpose
Paradigm	Broad assumptions and perspectives	• Unify the field • Define the nature and purpose of occupational therapy
Conceptual Practice Models	Diverse concepts organized into unique occupational therapy theory	• Develop theory • Provide rationale for and guide practice
Related Knowledge	Concepts, facts, and techniques borrowed from other disciplines	• Supplement unique knowledge of the field • Apply in practice

Unlike the paradigm and the models, this layer of knowledge is *not* unique to occupational therapy. Rather, it is gathered into the field because of its relevance to the kind of work done by therapists. Like every field, occupational therapy uses related knowledge to support and fill in gaps in its own unique knowledge (i.e., its paradigm and models). Table 2–1 summarizes the characteristics of these three layers of knowledge. In the following sections I will discuss each layer in more detail.

The Paradigm

In his examination of how knowledge developed in the physical sciences, Kuhn[8] observed that members of a discipline are bound together by a shared vision. Further, he argued that this collective vision was a set of ideals and constructs that constituted a unique perspective shared by members of the discipline. These shared ideals and constructs created a context for the work of the discipline. Kuhn referred to this common vision of members of a profession as its paradigm.*

---

*The concept of paradigm was first applied to occupational therapy in an analysis of the field's history.[5,6] That analysis emphasized how the paradigm influenced practice. Later, Christiansen[1] argued that a paradigm is also necessary for scientific inquiry in occupational therapy, to enable the field to correct, improve, and accumulate knowledge. He noted, after Lakatos,[9] that the assumptions of a paradigm are surrounded by a belt of auxiliary concepts and hypotheses that are subjected to scientific scrutiny. I would add that, in occupational therapy, these auxiliary concepts and hypothesis are stated and studied in the field's conceptual practice models.

Mosey[16] objects to the application of the paradigm concept to occupational therapy, arguing that paradigms exist in academic disciplines (e.g., physics and biology) but not in professions or applied sciences such as occupational therapy. This view is consistent with her distinction between the work of disciplines in creating theory and the work of professions in applying theory. In contrast to Mosey, Tornebohm[13,14] argued that paradigms *do* operate in practical disciplines, including occupational therapy.

The concept of the professional paradigm proposed here builds on the original work of Kuhn and on others who have critiqued and applied his ideas. In this book, I use the concept of paradigm in two interrelated ways. First, I define it as a *conceptual perspective*, made up of fundamentals articulated in the literature and discussed by those seeking to define the nature and purpose of the field. Secondly, I propose that the paradigm is the *cultural core* of the discipline.

Tornebohm[22,23] asserts that a paradigm is reflected in what members of the profession are concerned with and in how they view the world. He also argues that the paradigm defines the profession for its members and presents ideals about how to practice. Thus, he notes that the paradigm proposes a conceptual perspective that incorporates a definition of practice, a basic viewpoint, and ideals.

Macintyre[14] argues that to share a professional culture is to have common beliefs and perspectives that both make sense of and guide or regulate professional action. As the culture of the profession, the paradigm allows therapists to understand, in a very broad way, what they are doing when they practice; that is, it provides them with an understanding of the nature of their work, its primary concerns and methods, and its values. These elements of the paradigm provide the individual practitioner and the whole profession with a viewpoint and a self-image. In short, the paradigm provides professional identity.

Elements of a Professional Paradigm

The perspectives of Kuhn,[8] MacIntyre,[14] and Tornebohm[22,23] are useful for considering, in a general way, what a paradigm is. However, it is also necessary to think about the elements that make up a paradigm. Consequently, it is important to consider occupational therapy as a profession, asking what does its paradigm consist of, and why?

Inasmuch as the paradigm functions as an integrating culture, it contains core themes or ideas that members of the profession see as their basic concerns. I will refer to these elements of the paradigm as *core constructs*. Secondly, since the paradigm must provide a particular outlook or perspective, it also needs to contain a way of seeing the world, a basic orientation to the nature of things with which members are concerned. This aspect of the paradigm I call the *focal viewpoint*. Lastly, any integrating culture provides ideas and a vision of what matters most to members of the group. In this same way, the paradigm's third element is *integrating values*. Hence, I propose that the paradigm of occupational therapy contains core constructs, a focal viewpoint, and integrating values (Fig. 2–2).

Core Constructs. As a practice profession, occupational therapy must address essential questions about the service it provides: What human need does the service address? What kinds of problems does it solve? What is the

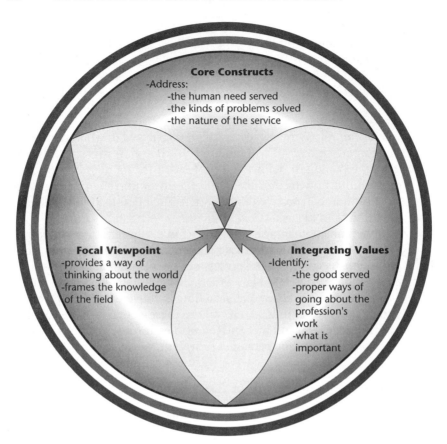

Figure 2–2. Elements of the paradigm.

nature of its service (i.e., how does it solve those problems)? These are the questions to which the core constructs of the paradigm are addressed. By identifying the aspect of human well-being for which occupational therapists take responsibility, the kinds of problems they solve, and the methods they use to solve those problems, the field defines itself. These three elements (the human need addressed, the problems solved, and the problem-solving methods) are explicated in a collection of themes or ideas that together are the field's core constructs.*

---

*The concept of core constructs refers to those constructs that are global to the field as a whole and therefore part of the paradigm. These are different from the concepts that are used as part of the theoretical arguments within models of practice. Core constructs do influence the kinds of concepts that appear in the theoretical arguments of models of practice, but they "transcend" these specific models and represent a more universal way of thinking in the field. In fact, when similar concepts are found in several models of practice, it is likely that these concepts reflect or derive form a core construct in the paradigm.

To illustrate the idea of core constructs, let us consider the profession of medicine. Physicians address the human need for biological well-being and survival. These medical practitioners solve problems (diseases and traumas) that threaten survival and well-being. They do this by repairing damage and by slowing, minimizing, or eradicating disease. Knowledge of what is normal (e.g., blood pressure, temperature, composition of body fluids) provides a picture of the how the body works. The problems medicine addresses are disturbances to this normal state of affairs. Medicine defines and categorizes these problems through a diagnostic system. Moreover, physicians seek to resolve these problems through therapies that include medication and surgery.

For medicine this vision of its practice is articulated through such core constructs as disease, diagnosis, and medication. Not everything that physicians do fits neatly into such core constructs, but they do give medicine a general identity. In later chapters, we will look to occupational therapy, asking what themes and ideas make up its core constructs. These themes and ideas are distinct from those of medicine and help to differentiate occupational therapy from medicine. For example, while medicine focuses on disease and diagnosis, occupational therapy focuses on how persons' occupational lives are disrupted by disease and other factors. Such differences of perspective are essential elements of the paradigm that gives each profession a distinct identity.

Focal Viewpoint. Professions require more than concepts to identify what human need they address and what they do. Because they develop and use knowledge, they need a viewpoint that organizes their knowledge and gives them a way of thinking about the world.[10] Medicine's viewpoint sees the body as a complex machine made up of parts and processes.[11,21] Medicine is predicated on being able to "see inside" this human machine; this is made possible by such things as physical exams, x-rays, laboratory tests, and biopsies.

Also basic to medicine's viewpoint is the idea of causation. Medicine sees the body as being made up of component parts that operate according to discoverable laws. Understanding diseases or traumas means understanding how they cause disruptions to normal structure and function. This concept of causation also guides medicine's use of biochemical and other physical interventions to cause changes that counter the effects of disease or trauma. Thus, medicine is made intelligible by a viewpoint that (a) emphasizes the machine-like nature of the human body, (b) looks for the causal links between structures and functions in the body, (c) understands the causes of conditions that threaten the body, and (d) applies treatments designed to cause a restoration of order.

In contrast to medicine, occupational therapy's viewpoint is oriented to understanding complex connections between the person and the environment and how these are influenced by disease and trauma. Hence, for example, occupational therapists seek to restore order in the relationship between the person and the environment, even when the disruption in this relationship is due to permanent damage to the body.

Professional paradigms all contain this focal viewpoint, which "frames" the situation, identifying what the specific facts of a field will mean. The focal viewpoint allows the profession to attend to and interpret the world in its own way. This viewpoint also influences what kind of knowledge the field will consider relevant to its work. For example, medicine is not centrally interested in the concept of culture since culture is not considered to figure strongly in the causation or treatment of disease. Occupational therapy, on the other hand, must consider culture as an essential element of the environment in which the person functions.

Integrating Values. Finally, because professions are engaged in practical action, they require ideas about the "good" they serve and about "proper" ways of going about what they do. Hence, each profession has its own unique values, which emphasize what is important from its point of view. In medicine the preservation of life operates as an important value. Physicians see their work as fundamentally good because it preserves and extends life. In occupational therapy, the quality of life as attained in one's everyday occupations is an important consideration.

Expression of the Field's Paradigm

When speaking about a paradigm I am not referring to a "thing" that can be readily located. As Kuhn[8] points out, the paradigm is largely implicit. It is often taught and reinforced through the use of *exemplars* in which the paradigm is illustrated in a particularly salient way. Exemplars are succinct demonstrations of how the work of the discipline could and should be done. Stories about practice in occupational therapy, which reveal something essential to occupational therapy, are exemplars for the field's paradigm.

Recall the example of Susan Tracy's story about the psychiatric patient who was able to produce a fine watercolor despite the physician's judgment that he could not concentrate. This story illustrated how occupational therapy's paradigm was different from medicine's. Tracy's story suggested a view of the patient different from that of a machine. Moreover, the story did not tell about how something was done to modify the patient from within. Rather, it suggested that when environmental circumstances are right, behavior can be elicited from the patient. It emphasized getting the patient to do something rather than what could be done to the patient. In this story are implied certain core concepts, a viewpoint, and values, as we will see in the next chapter. Stories about practice always mirror some aspect of the paradigm.

Of course, the paradigm is articulated and exemplified in other ways as well. Theoretical articles, books, and professional presentations that introduce or expand the core constructs or focal viewpoint of the field are important contributions to the paradigm. Official documents and professional publications that outline and discuss and debate values of occupational therapy are significant expressions of the field's integrating values. Moreover, the paradigm is taught, reinforced, and reshaped in education and in practice as persons learn about, experience, and put into action the identity and perspective of occupational therapy.

The Paradigm: Summary

The paradigm of a field functions as a conceptual perspective and as a culture. It consists of core constructs, a viewpoint, and values. These elements of a paradigm are what define and give coherence or wholeness to the entire profession and thus unify the field.* Together, they reveal what the discipline takes to be its fundamental nature and purpose, how it envisions the phenomena it addresses in practice, and what it considers important in practice.

The core constructs are interrelated themes that underlie the entire field. They can be found in the literature of the field and in what members fundamentally know and believe about the field and about their practice. These concepts ordinarily answer three fundamental questions: (1) What human need does this field serve? (2) What problems does it address? and (3) How does it solve these problems? The focal viewpoint of the field may be defined as the commonly shared view of the phenomena in which members of the field are interested. It is how therapists collectively envision that aspect of the world with which they are concerned. It serves as a "map of the

---

*Discussions of occupational therapy's conceptual foundations have sparked an ongoing debate over the relative merits of unity versus diversity in the body of knowledge. I have argued, along with others, that occupational therapy requires a unified body of unique knowledge for its own coherence and to sustain societal support.[4,24,25] Additionally, proponents of a unified body of knowledge point to the needs to *articulate an identity for the field, to unite practice across specialty areas, and to facilitate cumulative knowledge development* in the field.[2,7,24]

In contrast to these arguments, others have raised concern that a unified theory of occupational therapy would be too confining, would block creativity, and would negate ideas that did not fit neatly within it.[9,17] This counterargument asserts that the field cannot afford to become too single-minded or narrow in its orientation.

Consequently, there appears to be a conflict between the need to achieve a coherent and unified conceptual foundation and the need to maintain openness, creativity, and originality. I do not believe, however, that this conflict is real. Both diversity and unification can and must be accommodated in the conceptual foundations of a practice profession. In fact, the two tendencies—one toward unification and the other toward diversification—can be complementary forces that keep each other in check as the knowledge base develops; that is, the field's conceptual foundation must consist of both a defining, unifying core and a surrounding, related collection of diverse knowledge.

territory," providing therapists a perspective on how their universe of concern is put together. The integrating values are the deeply held convictions of the discipline concerning the value of the profession and how it should carry out its business. These values identify why practice matters and what ought to be done in practice.

Members of the profession contribute to, assimilate, and give expression to the paradigm in their action. The paradigm, in turn, gives members a distinctive professional identity. In this sense, the paradigm is a culture through which members, individually and collectively, make sense of their profession.

Conceptual Practice Models

While the paradigm provides a common understanding of what it means to be an occupational therapist, it does not provide specific prescriptions for practice. Such prescription is the purpose of the conceptual practice models that make up the second layer of knowledge in the conceptual foundations of occupational therapy.

A conceptual practice model presents and organizes a number of theoretical concepts used by therapists in their work. In occupational therapy, each model addresses some specific phenomenon or area of human function. For example, one model addresses the biomechanics (i.e., structures and functions of the musculoskeletal system) underlying movement. Other models address the phenomena of sensory processing, perception and cognition, and motivation. Each model explains an area of functioning and specifies the interventions pertaining to particular kinds of problems. Because each model focuses on specific areas, the field will require more than one model to address occupational therapy's range of concerns. I will discuss eight conceptual practice models in this book.

Components of a Conceptual Practice Model

Models can be thought of as having the following components:

1. An interdisciplinary conceptual base.
2. Theoretical arguments* about order (i.e., organization and function) in the area of concern; disorder (i.e., dysfunction) in the area

---

*A distinction could be made between facts (i.e., knowledge about a phenomenon that is empirically verified beyond reasonable doubt, such as the gross anatomy of the musculoskeletal system) and theory, which is intelligent speculation about the workings of some phenomena. However, all knowledge systems have their more or less factual territory, at the fringes of which exist theories about further properties and processes. Thus, to avoid burdensome distinctions, I use the term "theory" to refer to both empirically demonstrated knowledge and that which seeks to explain in the absence of complete verification.

of concern; and therapeutic intervention (i.e., planned preservation and/or change of the order of the phenomena with which the model is concerned).

3. Technology for application (e.g., assessment protocols and instruments and treatment methods).

4. Empirical scrutiny of the model (i.e., research that tests theoretical arguments and demonstrates how the model works in practice).

These components are parts of a dynamic and ongoing process of knowledge development (Fig. 2–3).

Let us examine in more detail how this process occurs. Authors of conceptual practice models build on knowledge from other disciplines as well as from concepts inside the field. For example, sensory integration (discussed in Chapter 12) is a conceptual practice model concerned with the brain's processing of sensory information for motor action; it builds on knowledge from neurology and neuropsychology, and on sensorimotor treatment concepts developed in occupational therapy. The model of human occupation (Chapter 10) synthesizes knowledge from systems theory, psychology, social psychology, sociology, and anthropology, while building on previous occupational therapy knowledge, to explain the motivation for and patterning of occupational behavior. The interdisciplinary conceptual foundation on which a model is built includes both theories and the research supporting those theories.

The authors of conceptual practice models create theory to explain the organization and function (order) of some aspect of human behavior or performance on which the model focuses. Similarly, the models provide theoretical arguments about disorder or dysfunction. Finally, they provide theoretical explanations of how therapy can be used to maintain or alter function (i.e., theoretical arguments about preservation and change). The theoretical arguments concerning order, disorder, and therapeutic interven-

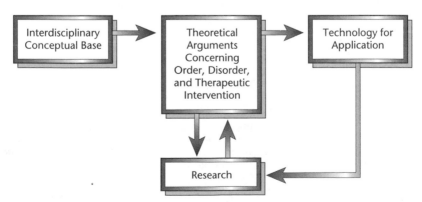

Figure 2–3. Components of a conceptual model of practice.

tion in conceptual practice models are the primary theoretical activity of occupational therapy. A mature conceptual practice model organizes concepts from within and outside the field into *unique theoretical arguments* that reflect the paradigm of the profession. In this way, models are much more than mere structures to guide application of theory.* The theoretical arguments of each model give logic and coherence to the clinical applications that the model provides.

As models develop, their technology for clinical application is constantly expanded and refined. Theorists and practitioners create clinical assessments, accumulate case examples, write guidelines or protocols for application, and develop programs based on the model. Dissemination of these clinical applications in journals, textbooks, and presentations make the model more useful in clinical practice. Similarly, problems and insights encountered in practice may lead to changes in the model.

Research allows empirical scrutiny of the practice model. Studies test the accuracy of the theoretical arguments as they relate to the phenomena they seek to explain. Research also produces descriptive data helpful in elaborating the theory. Further, research tests the effectiveness of the technology for application based on the theory. Practice models provide a context for both applied and basic research. *Basic research* examines the model's theoretical arguments about organization and dysfunction. *Applied research* tests arguments about preservation and change and the usefulness of clinical applications. The two types of research are complementary, and both are necessary.

The number and relevance of applications that the practice model offers influence how widely it is adopted in the field, but only empirical support of the model will ensure its survival. Practitioners understandably concern themselves with how readily a practice model will provide them useful guidelines for application. Eventually, when pressed to justify or demonstrate the effectiveness of services, occupational therapy must offer empirical support for the truth and utility of its conceptual practice models.

As I noted earlier, each conceptual practice model represents a dynamic process in which knowledge is developed and used through theorizing, application, empirical scrutiny, and revision (see Fig. 2–3). The theory of the model provides explanations of phenomena with which it is concerned; these explanations can be verified, disproved, or refined through research.

---

*Although this definition of models of practice shares attributes of Mosey's frames of reference, a critical difference is that the models express theory unique to occupational therapy.[11] Mosey views frames of reference as organizing theoretical concepts for practice. In many cases, a frame of reference (e.g., the developmental, acquisitional, and "analytical" object relations frames of reference) borrows a theory from another discipline and applies it to occupational therapy practice without formulating unique occupational therapy theory. Such a frame of reference does not qualify as a model of practice (as defined here). I would consider such a frame of reference as related knowledge. This point is elaborated in Chapter 16.

The theory also explains and directs clinical application. Basic and applied research provide feedback to the model, allowing theory to be corrected and elaborated as scientific evidence is accumulated. Similarly, applications in practice can provide critical feedback leading to changes and elaborations of the theory. This dynamic process of input from the interdisciplinary base and the feedback loops from practice and research are necessary to keep a model vital. Finally, the theoretical and empirical work done within the model may make contributions to the interdisciplinary areas from which the model's underlying concepts came.

The conceptual practice models are part of the "know-how" of members of the field. When therapists use the field's knowledge, they engage in an active process of clinical reasoning using conceptual practice models. The models provide special professional lenses through which the therapist sees the patient or client, develops plans, and solves problems.

Related Knowledge

Although conceptual models provide much of the basic knowledge that guides practice, therapists routinely need additional knowledge. For instance, practice may require the use of some concepts and skills not unique to occupational therapy and not contained in occupational therapy's conceptual practice models. For example, all helping professions involve a therapeutic use of self (i.e., the use of one's personality to interact with the patient). Consequently, therapists may employ, as related knowledge, theory and techniques concerning therapeutic use of self. Related knowledge may also include information that belongs to another profession, yet is also useful and necessary to occupational therapy practice. For example, medicine's knowledge of disease processes is critical to occupational therapy practice, even though occupational therapy is very different from medicine. Another example, from the field of psychology, is the theory of behavior modification, whose principles and techniques are sometimes useful in occupational therapy practice. In these instances, occupational therapists use related knowledge to supplement the knowledge that defines and guides the main elements of occupational therapy practice. Related knowledge is also applicable in research, administration, politics, and other activities of the field (e.g., knowledge about how to conduct scientific inquiry and information about the workings of the health care system).

Related knowledge is necessary to support practice, research, and other activities of the field. Although theorists and other writers use such knowledge in discussing occupational therapy concerns, it is not knowledge developed by the field. Related knowledge is not unique to occupational therapy. It is important that the field distinguish between the related knowledge it employs and its own unique knowledge.

Dynamics of the Conceptual Foundations of Occupational Therapy

The paradigm, conceptual practice models, and related knowledge, together constitute the conceptual foundations of occupational therapy. The paradigm and the models of practice constitute the field's unique knowledge.

The relationship between the paradigm and the models is one of mutual influence (Fig. 2–4). The paradigm is a global vision, and the models are practical attempts to implement that vision in practice. The core constructs, focal viewpoint, and integrating values of the paradigm are part of the perspective of those who develop and refine conceptual practice models. Additionally, as new models are developed and used, they may challenge and shape the paradigm. Experience in developing and using practice models may point to ways that the paradigm might be questioned, refined, and/or elaborated on.

Although the paradigm is the most stable element of a discipline, its elements may change gradually over time as it is elaborated and modified. Occasionally paradigm change involves a radical transformation, which Kuhn[8] called revolution. This occurs when the core constructs, viewpoint, and values undergo a major redefinition. Such overall paradigm change

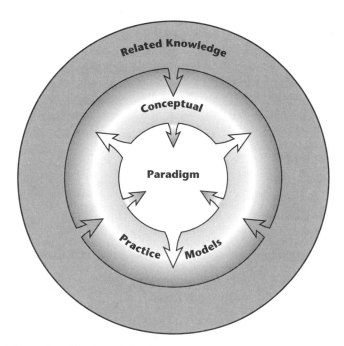

Figure 2–4. Dynamics of the knowledge base.

means a transformation in the deep culture of the profession—that is, changes in the beliefs, perspectives, and values of members of the profession. In the following chapter, I will discuss how such radical transformation has been part of the history of occupational therapy.

While the paradigm is relatively stable, conceptual models of practice constantly change. Application of the model in practice and research provides feedback that results in constant alteration of the model. Models need to change more rapidly than the paradigm to respond to changing patient/client populations, changing health care delivery circumstances, research findings, and other practical demands emanating from therapeutic work.

The paradigm allows the field to maintain stability in the midst of this change; that is, the field can sustain its most important character while developing new concepts and extending its technology. New knowledge can develop and ideas can change within the larger, more stable culture of the paradigm. In this way the paradigm and models together moderate change in the discipline. The core culture of the field is relatively constant while its models are always changing.

Conclusion

In this chapter I argued that three different types of knowledge are relevant to occupational therapy, each used for a different purpose. The occupational therapy paradigm is the fundamental vision of the field. It constitutes a professional culture that is revealed in the assumptions, viewpoints, and values that members of the profession share. Conceptual practice models lay out theory and guide practice. The paradigm is a force for unity, whereas the various models, which address a range of phenomena, provide diversity. The paradigm and models influence each other. The paradigm provides stability and constancy; it changes much more slowly than the models, which are constantly revised as information from research and practice becomes available. Related knowledge supplements the field's unique paradigmatic and model-based knowledge.

In the next chapter I will chronicle the history of the field's paradigm development, thereby telling the story of the profession from its beginnings. Chapter 4 looks at the way the paradigm is evolving. Subsequent chapters explain and critique several conceptual models of practice. The organization of knowledge described in this chapter will be used as a framework throughout these discussions.

References

1. Boyer, EL: Scholarship Reconsidered: Priorities of the Professoriate. The Carnegie Foundation for the Advancement of Teaching, Princeton, 1990.

2. Christiansen, C: Toward resolution of crisis: Research requisites in occupational therapy. Occupational Therapy Journal of Research 1:115, 1981.
3. Dickoff, J, James, P, and Wiedenbach, E: Theory in a practice discipline. Nursing Research 17, 415–435, 1968.
4. Fleming, MN et al: Occupational Therapy: Directions for the Future. The American Occupational Therapy Association, Rockville, MD, 1987.
5. Kielhofner, G, and Barris, R: Organization of knowledge in occupational therapy: A proposal and a survey of the literature. Occupational Therapy Journal of Research 6:67, 1986.
6. Kielhofner, G, and Burke, JP: Occupational therapy after 60 years: An account of changing identity and knowledge. Am J Occup Ther 31:675, 1977.
7. Kielhofner, G, and Gillette, N: The impact of specialization on the professionalization or the survival of occupational therapy. Am J Occup Ther 33:20, 1979.
8. Kuhn, T: The Structure of Scientific Revolutions, ed 2. University of Chicago Press, Chicago, 1970.
9. Labovitz, DR, and Miller, RJ: Commentary: Organization of knowledge in occupational therapy: A proposal and a survey of the literature. Occupational Therapy Journal of Research 6:85, 1986.
10. Lakatos, I: Falsification and the methodology of scientific research programmes. In Lakatos, I, and Musgrave, A (eds): Criticism and the Growth of Knowledge. Cambridge University Press, Cambridge, UK, 1970.
11. Leder, D: The Absent Body. Chicago, University of Chicago Press, 1990.
12. Mattingly, C, and Fleming, MH: Clinical Reasoning: Forms of Inquiry in a Therapeutic Practice. FA Davis, Philadelphia, 1994.
13. Maxwell, N: What kind of inquiry can best help us create a good world? Science, Technology, and Human Values 17, 205–227, 1992.
14. Macintyre, A: Epistemological crises, dramatic narrative, and the philosophy of science. In Gutting, G (ed): Paradigms and Revolutions, University of Notre Dame Press, Notre Dame, IN, 1980.
15. McColl, MA, Law, M, and Stewart, D: Theoretical basis of occupational therapy. Slack, Thorofare, NJ, 1993.
16. Mosey, AC: Occupational Therapy: Configuration of a Profession. Raven Press, New York, 1981.
17. Mosey, AC: Eleanor Clarke Slagle Lecture: A monistic or a pluralistic approach to professional identity? Am J Occup Ther 39:504, 1985.
18. Mosey, AC: Applied Scientific Inquiry in Health Professions. American Occupational Therapy Association, Rockville, MD 1992.
19. Quiroga, VAM: Occupational Therapy: The First 30 Years—1900 to 1930. American Occupational Therapy Association, Rockville, MD, 1995.
20. Schön, DA: The reflective practitioner: How Professionals Think in Action. Basic Books, New York, 1983.
21. Toombs, SK: The Meaning of Illness: A phenomenological Account of the Different Perspectives of Physician and Patient. Kluwer Academic Publishers, Boston, 1993.
22. Tornebohm, H: Reflections on Practice-Oriented Research. University of Goteborg, Goteborg, 1985.
23. Tornebohm, H: Caring, Knowing and Paradigms. University of Goteborg, Goteborg, 1986.
24. West, W: A reaffirmed philosophy and practice of occupational therapy for the 1980s. Am J Occup Ther 38:15, 1984.
25. Wiemer, R: Traditional and nontraditional practice arenas. In Occupational Therapy: 2001. American Occupational Therapy Association, Rockville, MD, 1979.

CHAPTER 3

THE DEVELOPMENT OF OCCUPATIONAL THERAPY KNOWLEDGE

I n 1917 a small group of individuals gathered to form the National Association for the Promotion of Occupational Therapy. This event is generally viewed as the formal beginning of occupational therapy in North America. In fact, this meeting was preceded by a number of other significant accomplishments. Training of occupational therapists had already begun. Several books and numerous articles about occupational therapy had been written. It was this development, organization, and formal sharing of knowledge that made possible the beginning of the professional association. Moreover, a powerful unifying idea brought together the people of diverse backgrounds who were the first occupational therapists. These fundamental ideas underlying occupational therapy were articulated in many ways in the field's early literature. A 1915 book entitled *The Work of Our Hands* neatly set forth the early occupational therapy vision:

> When [the patient] gets down to honest work with her hands she makes discoveries. She finds her way along new pathways. She learns something of the dignity and satisfaction of work and gets an altogether simpler and more wholesome notion of living. This in itself is good, but better still, the open mind is apt to see new visions, new hope and faith. There is something about simple, effective work with the hands that makes [humans] . . . creators in a very real sense makes them kin with the great creative forces of the world. From such a basis of dignity and simplicity anything is possible. Many a poor starved nature becomes rich and full. All this is aside from the actual physical gains that may come from new muscular activities.[33]

The occupational therapy vision and its realization in early practice gave an important *identity* to the fledgling profession. It reflected a new and unique way of viewing and dealing with the problems of persons whose capacities were impaired. Further, it allowed the field to define itself as a useful service and thereby find a place in the health care system. What occupational therapy had achieved was the construction of its first paradigm.

This chapter explores the development of this early paradigm of occupational therapy and shows how the paradigm of the field has evolved. In tracing the development of the paradigm since early this century, I will tell the story of the emergence and shifts of mainstream ideas of occupational therapy theory and practice. As we will see, this is a story of shifting identity.

Paradigm Development

The members of emerging fields do not set out to create paradigms. Rather, they seek to put into operation a fundamental idea, to persuade others to their point of view, to explain the worth of what they are doing, to gain support, and to impart to others what they know how to do. Nonetheless, paradigm construction is what results when people accomplish the aforementioned tasks.

From his examination of physical science, Kuhn[41] concluded that paradigms develop in identifiable stages (Fig. 3–1). During a *preparadigm* period, the initial ideas that instigate the formation of a field first emerge. The paradigm is later formed as members of a discipline articulate and subscribe to a common set of ideas.

In Chapter 2, I argued that the paradigm of a practice-based profession such as occupational therapy consists of core constructs, a focal viewpoint, and integrating values. The core constructions reflect the basic

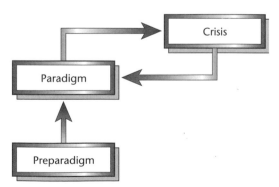

Figure 3–1. Stages of paradigm development.

themes of the field. The focal viewpoint is the way in which members of the field conceptualize the phenomena with which they are concerned. The integrating values specify what is important in practice. Together, these elements form the basic conceptual perspective and professional culture that give identity to the field and bind members together into a shared vision of their work.

Over time, paradigms may change. According to Kuhn,[41] the transition from one paradigm to another involves an intermediate state of *crisis*, wherein discipline members reject the guiding principles of the old paradigm. Rejection of a previous paradigm can occur for such reasons as criticism of a field's paradigm by powerful outsiders, or the inability of the paradigm to deal with new problems with which the field is faced. Since the paradigm is a field's basic culture and conceptual viewpoint, members find it unsettling to abandon the ways of thinking and doing that the paradigm provides. In the language of the common idiom, we might say that a paradigm shift represents both a "change of mind" and a "change of heart." This is why the transition is referred to as a crisis.

Crisis terminates when a new paradigm is articulated and accepted. When the paradigm changes, the world that is "out there" to be acted on appears fundamentally different to practitioners. Importantly, paradigm shifts in a profession alter the sense of identity and the vision of practice that members share. Kuhn[41] calls this conceptual shift *revolution*, a term intended to convey the dramatic conceptual restructuring that takes place. As we will see, occupational therapy has had its own revolutions.

Kuhn's[41] thesis concerning paradigm change challenges the idea that science or knowledge develops slowly and incrementally and new facts are added to the stockpile of already existing knowledge. Rather, a field can and does go through periods of radical change in its most fundamental views. When this happens, the field must reinterpret previous knowledge. This means that what members of a field thought was the correct and proper way to see and do things is recognized as somehow flawed. The change from an old to a new paradigm requires members of the field to make a leap of faith, undergoing, as it were, conversion to a new point of view. Macintyre[45] points out that this change from an old to a new viewpoint is narratively structured. That is, when members of a discipline abandon one fundamental way of seeing things for another, it is because they understand how it was possible to have seen the world in the old way and, at the same time, see the new way as superior. Consequently, to understand the sequence of paradigms in a field, one must grasp the story of the profession's changing view of its nature, purpose, practical concerns, and values. Occupational therapy's history of changing paradigms is, then, the basic story of the profession. Within the story of its paradigm development, the identity of occupational therapy may be found. Hence, this history traces the essence of occupational therapy.

The Moral Treatment Preparadigm

In the eighteenth and nineteenth centuries, there arose, first in Europe and then in North America, an approach to the care of mentally ill persons referred to as moral treatment. This approach was inspired by the humanitarian philosophy of the time.[46] A central premise of moral treatment was that participation in the various tasks and events of everyday life could restore persons to more normal functioning. Occupational therapy's most important roots are found in moral treatment.[9,11,19,43] Early occupational therapists derived their fundamental concepts from the moral treatment writings, and the early practice of occupational therapy reflects its therapeutic concepts and practices. We can consider moral treatment the preparadigm of occupational therapy.

Moral treaters believed that people became mentally ill because they succumbed to external pressures by adopting faulty habits of living, which disengaged them from the mainstream of life. Moreover, they believed society had an obligation to help those with mental illness return to a normal life pattern. The treatment approach was predicated on the assumptions that the mentally ill person still retained a measure of self-command and that improvement depended largely on the patient's own conduct. Thus "employment in various occupations was expected as a way for the patient to maintain control over his or her disorder."[9] Moral treatment was an environmental therapy; physical, temporal, and social environments were engineered to correct the patient's faulty habits of living, which were believed to be the core of mental illness. Participation in such occupations as education, daily living tasks, work, and play was used to normalize disorganized behavior.[11]

In the midnineteenth century, several forces worked together to end the practice of moral treatment in the United States. Rapid population growth combined with large waves of immigration led to overcrowding in state hospitals. Social Darwinism and its "survival of the fittest" ethic, coupled with prejudice toward those in mental hospitals, eroded the social commitment to treat mentally ill persons. Within the consequently congested and underfunded facilities, moral treatment declined and gave way to a custodial model in which patients were primarily warehoused.[11,46]

The Paradigm of Occupation

At the beginning of the twentieth century a diverse group of practitioners (e.g., physicians, nurses, architects, craft persons) began to reapply moral treatment in several areas of caring for ill and disabled persons. They generated a new therapy that came to be known as *occupational therapy*.

Several writers were influential in forming the early occupational therapy vision. Adolph Meyer was a physician who first sought explanations for mental illness in brain pathology. Later he abandoned this approach and saw mental illness as a breakdown of normal habits of living. Meyer's theory heavily influenced the early occupational therapists. Eleanor Clarke Slagle is generally considered the primary founder of occupational therapy. A colleague of Jane Addams, she began a training program for occupational therapists in Chicago. Slagle's writings helped shape the vision of occupational therapy. Her clinical programs were based on the concept of habit training, an approach built on Meyer's idea of mental illness as a disturbance of habits of living. William Rush Dunton, another physician, was a descendent of Benjamin Rush, a moral treatment physician. Dunton was responsible for bringing many of the moral treatment concepts into occupational therapy. Dunton, himself, later became a registered occupational therapist. His books were some of the most important in early occupational therapy. Thomas Kidner was a Canadian architect who designed hospitals. He became interested in the problem of long convalescence, which was part of the process of recovering from tuberculosis. Kidner observed that both physical capacities and the habits of living were eroded during the long convalescence. In his writings, he emphasized how programs of occupation would restore both physical capacity and reorganize the person's life pattern. Herbert Hall was a psychiatrist especially interested in the use of crafts to restore interest and self-confidence in persons with mental illness. Susan Tracy was a nurse by training. Her influential book emphasized the motivational aspects of therapy, explaining how it was necessary and possible to capture the patient's interest in meaningful occupations and thereby draw the patient away from the illness and back toward participation in life activities.

As early leaders in the field described the principles of using occupation to influence recovery from illness and adjustment to disability, they generated the elements that made up the first paradigm. The first four decades of occupational therapy literature show a remarkable degree of consensus concerning the core constructs, focal viewpoint, and integrating values of the field. Writers articulated a paradigm of occupation that surely must have found its expression in practice and formed a divergent group of people into a new discipline.

Core Constructs

In different contexts, several writers expressed core assumptions of this first paradigm. In 1922, in the inaugural issue of the field's formal journal, *Archives of Occupational Therapy*, Meyer set forth the following core construct. It concerned the role of occupation in human life:

> Our conception of man is that of an organism that maintains and balances itself in the world of reality and actuality by being in active life

and active use, i.e., using and living and acting its time in harmony with its own nature and the nature about it. It is the use that we make of ourselves that gives the ultimate stamp to our every organ.[50]

This first construct linked health to being occupied.

Meyer and Dunton articulated the second construct: Occupation consists of an alternation between modes of existing, thinking, and acting.[20,50] They postulated that a balance between creativity, leisurely diversion, aesthetic interests, celebration, and serious work was essential to health.[20,36,50] This meant that health was reflected in the habits that organized the everyday use of time.[50] Habits controlled the basic rhythm and balance of life. These habits were, in turn, maintained through ongoing engagement in everyday occupations.

A third construct was the unity of mind and body, which were seen as inextricably linked, with the mind governing the body. Morale and will were two fundamental traits of the mind. Morale, a concept borrowed from the moral treatment era, referred to the ability to see the present and future with a sense of interest and commitment. Will referred to the ability to make decisions based on a clear sense of value and desire.[6,73] Morale and will were maintained by engagement in the occupations of everyday life, which provided a sense of interest, value, accomplishment, and challenge.[20,50] The concept of mind-body unity was interwoven with the observation that occupation was a particularly powerful force in maintaining well-being. While individuals employed their bodies in occupations, their attention was also directed to the creative and practical dimensions of the task at hand. Occupation created a synergy of body and mind that maintained the integrity of each.

The fourth construct concerned what occurred when participation in occupation was interrupted. Since it was human nature to be engaged in occupation, and since occupation maintained the mind and body, "enforced idleness . . . [could] do damage to the mind and to the body of the ill person."[65] Idleness (or lack of occupation) resulted in demoralization, breakdown of habits, and physical deterioration, with the concomitant loss of ability to perform competently in daily life.[32,76] The ill effects of idleness were assumed to infuse the individual:

> In every functional disturbance, in addition to disorders of the central nervous system, there is a mental reaction. Pain, anemia, impairment of circulation, and sense impressions and emotions, such as anxiety and depression, are all communicated to the brain. . . . In ennui the tonicity of the muscles is affected so that they actually contract less strongly and develop less force. In melancholia the general physique, and especially the heart, is acted on. . . . Morbid introspection produces a particularly vicious cycle of thinking, since continued attention focused on any particular part of the body may actually increase its morbid condition.[73]

According to the fourth construct, the negative effects of idleness infiltrated both body and mind, while each magnified the disorder in the other.

The final construct was that since occupation maintained the body and mind, it was suited to regenerate lost function. Occupation was recognized as a successful organizing force because it required an exercise of function in which mind and body were united.[20,36,73] The following illustrates this view:

> Let our minds be engaged with the spirit of fun and competitive play and leave our muscles, nerves and organs to carry on their functions without conscious thought—then our physical exercise will be correspondingly more beneficial and we can readily picture the effect exerted on the mood of the sullen, morose patient by the genial glow which suffuses the body following active exercise.[65]

Occupation was also seen to provide a diversion from physical and psychic pain that encouraged the individual to use his or her mental and physical capacities.

Focal Viewpoint

The focal viewpoint of early occupational therapy centered on three phenomena and their interrelationships: mind, body, and environment. The mind was the pivotal area of concern. Motivating the person, influencing attitudes and morale, and eliciting physical activity through mental engagement were primary themes. The following proposal for motivating a patient typifies discussions of the time:

> It is easier to find something that the patient can do than to find something he will do. One needs to be resourceful, with a large variety of appeals, for it goes without saying that even in health what appeals to one person will not to another. The difference is even more marked among the insane. Appeals may be made through praise, competition, rewards; to the sense of the beautiful or to the useful; through affection for relatives, home needs, gifts to friends, or more diffuse altruism, as helping other patients, making preparations for special entertainments, such as Christmas gifts and decorations, or work for children. . . .[72]

To early occupational therapists, motivation was seen not only as a problem of how to engage the patient in therapeutic occupations, but also as a necessary component of recovery. For example, the caveat "Remember that restoration of physical capacity without the will to do is a futile thing. Good medical practice demands healing of the mind as well as of body or organ. . . ."[65] Therefore, the aim of therapy was to "create a wholesome interest in something outside the patient's morbid interest in himself and his symptoms . . . [and] to prepare his mental attitude so that he may adjust himself to normal demands and environment after the hospital discharge."[73]

The human body was viewed as a dynamic entity, integrated into the larger pattern of everyday occupation:

> Our body is not merely so many pounds of flesh and bone figuring as a machine, with an abstract mind or soul added to it. It is throughout a live organism pulsating with its rhythm of rest and activity. . . .[52]

This focus meant that the therapist tried to understand not only how the body was used in various tasks but also how it required regular rhythms of work, rest, recreation, and sleep.

When the body was compromised through illness or injury, the immediate concern was to prevent further degeneration by engaging the body in occupations in whatever way possible. Therapists recognized that tasks had to be graded according to individuals' remaining capacity.[36]

Like the proponents of moral treatment, early occupational therapists believed that the environment was an important element of the therapeutic process. They saw the environment as composed of:

- Social attitudes concerning involvement in occupations (e.g., the ideas of craftsmanship and sportsmanship, the value of work)
- Occupations in which persons participated in normal life

Occupational therapy was viewed as a regulated environment in which patients could explore potentials and learn how to live effectively. To this end the social and task environments were carefully managed.

Therapists sought to provide a normal environment in the hospital. Natural rhythms of time use were seen as essential to the regeneration of habits in patients.[50,64,65] Such an environment conveyed to the patients the manner in which they would be able to lead meaningful and more normal lives. To be therapeutic, the occupational therapy environment required the presence of creative and challenging opportunities and of persons (usually therapists) who demonstrated interest and a high level of competency in these occupations:

> Much importance was placed on the occupation room, wherein opportunity was provided for various forms of interesting and useful work. Weaving rugs and finer fabrics, basket work, bookbinding and clay modeling were employed at the start. Fortunately there was secured an excellent leader, trained in teaching, conversant with the work taken up and interested in it. The room was open at definite hours each day, but at other times those who wished could work without the presence of the teacher if their condition permitted. . . . The atmosphere of interested activity prevailed. The work became the source of new purposes, of changed avenues of thought and of stimulated ambitions.[27]

In some cases the environment was highly regulated in an effort to imprint an orderly pattern of living on highly disorganized patients—that is, to develop healthy habits. Such habit training programs for severely mentally ill patients employed strict schedules of self-care and normal occupation.

The environment was also seen as a context for meeting a variety of patient needs. Simple games, music, and a colorful atmosphere were used to stimulate the senses of regressed individuals. As persons progressed, thera-pists directed them to more demanding occupations, which emphasized sportsmanship and craftsmanship.[21,32] Industrial therapy, the final phase of therapy, prepared the advanced patient for the world of work.[13,47] Patients worked in various hospital industries (e.g., laundry, building and grounds maintenance, kitchen) engaging in real-life tasks under conditions that mir-rored work outside the institution.

In sum, therapists saw the individual as a whole person (body and mind) in interaction with life tasks in the environment. Although the ther-apists realized that physical capacity was necessary to function, they put less emphasis on the detailed workings of the body than on environmental and mental matters. This is not to suggest that therapists did not consider how occupation could be used to achieve specific motor improvement. Rather, the therapists' fundamental vision was of occupation as the dynamic force that, by employing body and mind in interaction with the environment, maintained normal functioning. This focal viewpoint was both holistic and dynamic.

Integrative Values

Early occupational therapy inherited from moral treatment a belief in the essential worth of individuals and in their right to humane care. Interwoven with this idea was the dignity that the individual achieved in performance. To these early theorists, the worth of human life was realized in productive achievements and in creative and aesthetic pursuits.

Occupation was valued for its essential role in human life and for its ability to influence health. Early therapists saw the importance of culturally meaningful occupation as opposed to mere activity. Crafts, sports, recre-ation, and work were all valued because they embodied something impor-tant about the human spirit as reflected in the workmanship, sportsmanship, and craftsmanship that guided participation in such occupations. Finally, therapists valued holism, recognizing the connection between mind and body[65] and seeing the person as a participant in life's activities.[33] Recognition that humans were fundamentally doers and creators required that they be seen in the context of engaging in occupations.

Paradigm of Occupation: Summary

Occupational therapy's early paradigm centered on occupation, its role in human life and in health, and its potential as a restorative measure. I have identified the core constructs, focal viewpoint, and integrative values of this paradigm (Table 3–1) as reflected in discussions of the nature and process of occupational therapy practice, and of the ideas and principles basic to practice. Taken as a whole, this literature described a practice that

Table 3–1. The Paradigm of Occupation

Core Constructs	• Occupation plays an essential role in human life and influences each person's state of health. • Occupation consists of alternation between modes of existing, thinking, and acting, and requires a balance of these in daily life. • Mind and body are inextricably linked. • Idleness (lack of occupation) can result in damage to body and mind. • Occupation can be used to regenerate lost function.
Focal Viewpoint	• Environment, mind, and body, with a focus on motivation and environmental factors in performance.
Integrated Values	• Human dignity as realized in performance. • Importance of occupation for health. • Holistic viewpoint.

viewed people largely in terms of their motivations and environmental influences. The literature also emphasized the importance of the therapeutic media (e.g., crafts, dance, music, games, sports, and work activities) as representations of occupation in human life and as therapeutic agents.

As a result of this early paradigm, occupational therapy's identity was as a field that appreciated the importance of occupation in human life and used occupation as a restorative force. This vision of occupational therapy was sufficiently powerful to attract strong supporters who developed both the ideas and practice of the field.* It was also persuasive enough to secure a place for occupational therapy in health care.

Crisis in Occupational Therapy

In the late 1940s and the 1950s, occupational therapists came under pressure to establish a more "scientific" rationale for the field. Physicians criticized occupational therapy for lacking science;[42] for example:

---

*Since the purpose of this chapter is to trace paradigm development, I am not discussing models of practice. However, it is worth noting that during this first paradigm, conceptual practice models (as defined in this text) did not exist. That is not to suggest that the field lacked well-thought-out approaches to practice. Rather, these approaches (Slagle's habit training[64,65] being one good example) were structured applications of the constructs, viewpoint, and values of the paradigm. Only later, during the mechanistic paradigm, when the importation of interdisciplinary concepts and concerns for research grew, did the forerunners of current conceptual practice models emerge. In this regard, models are a more recent phenomena in the history of the field, reflecting the growing maturity of both theory and its application within occupational therapy.

No one who has seen a good occupational therapy program in action can doubt that it seems to result in great help for some patients, and some help for many. There appears, however, to be no rigorous and comprehensive theory which will explain who is helped, how, by what, or why; and there is little objective evidence that occupational therapy is actually effective.[51]

The biomedical perspective dominated the health care system, so these criticisms had to be taken seriously. Occupational therapists began to take to heart medicine's complaints and to seriously question their paradigm. Faced with a demand to think more like physicians, occupational therapists eventually forged a closer alliance with medicine.[57] This brought the occupational therapy's paradigm into a confrontation with the concepts of reductionism in medicine.

Reductionism in Medicine

In the twentieth century, medicine became increasingly scientific in its orientation.[58] Physicians embraced the highly successful reductionist scientific approach of the physical sciences. Reductionism is a complex scientific attitude; its fundamental assumption is that the world is a vast mechanism in which laws of cause and effect govern the interrelationships of its parts.[8] Scientists seek explanation by *reducing* phenomena to measurable units whose relationship to other units can be specified.[76] This approach is also characterized by the overall belief that any phenomenon can best be understood by dissecting and examining it, in the same way that a machine can be understood by taking it apart. Thus, for example, living organisms could be reduced to organs, organs to tissues, tissues to cells, and cells to the molecular structures of which they are composed. Hence the scientific attitude embraced by medicine sought to peer deeper and deeper inside to find explanations of illness.

Reductionist medicine focused almost exclusively on the inner mechanisms of body and mind. This reductionism also led physicians to view disease and its cure in mechanistic terms. A healthy person was seen as analogous to the "well-working" machine. Illness was viewed as the equivalent of damage or malalignment in a machine's parts.[8,14] Medical intervention in such a framework aims at identifying and repairing the broken or maladjusted part or parts. Repairs, replacements, and adjustments are made through surgery, chemotherapy, psychotherapy, and so on.

Given its reductionistic and mechanistic perspective, medicine found fault with and criticized occupational therapy's knowledge base. Occupational therapy's holistic view of body, mind, and environment appeared to lack a scientific base from the vantage point of scientific reductionism. While medicine focused on the medical practitioner as an external agent repairing the person, occupational therapy's viewpoint of *self-repair* through active agency of the patient (i.e., using occupation as a means of self-regeneration) did not make sense. Consequently, the core knowledge of occupational therapy was dismissed as unscientific.

With criticism of occupational therapy's knowledge base came recommendations for replacing it with medicine's concepts. For example, it was proposed that psychodynamic concepts were more important to mental health practice than traditional occupational therapy concepts:

> According to our point of view, occupation is neither the aim nor the mechanism operating in this field which uses the media now in operation in an occupational therapy situation. Hence, occupational therapy taken as such is undefinable if the framework within which it seeks theoretical clarification is psychodynamics.[5]

From the psychoanalytic perspective, the concept of occupation as an organizing force in therapy was too vague. Rather, these critics proposed that the true therapeutic impact of occupation was in its potential as a vehicle for expressing unconscious feeling. Similarly, critics writing from the physical disabilities perspective called for a refocusing to a neuromuscular perspective:

> A commonly accepted justification of the use of crafts and games as therapeutic media is the emotional value to the patient of an interesting and creative experience. The reasoning is accepted as a basic and important assumption empirically but not scientifically demonstrated. While the interest and pleasure of a creative activity are important, they do not provide the most fundamental and vital concept underlying occupational therapy of physical disabilities. . . . Realization of the importance of neurophysiological mechanisms in the treatment of the motor system is increasing. A study of them increases understanding of how the neuromuscular system operates in terms of purposeful function.[1]

These criticisms created a crisis of confidence in the first paradigm. In response, some leading occupational therapists called for a fundamental reorientation in the discipline's view of the therapeutic process. They proposed that occupational therapy needed to understand function and dysfunction in terms of underlying neurological, anatomical, and intrapsychic dynamics. They also argued that these underlying mechanisms were the factors that could be influenced in therapy. In sum, occupational therapy was urged to focus on the inner mechanisms that influenced human performance.

Although the transition to a focus on inner mechanisms was gradual and subtle, by the end of the 1950s it had revolutionized occupational therapy. This revolution resulted in the emergence of a new paradigm, a new professional culture. One writer presaged the new paradigm of occupational therapy in the following words:

> As we talk of techniques let us think of underlying principles and build procedure on scientific fact. The clues lie in the basic concepts of psychology, physiology and anatomy.[49]

The Mechanistic Paradigm

The new paradigm promised to bring occupational therapy recognition as an efficacious service with an accepted rationale.[2,22,60] The field was more able to articulate discrete, tangible objectives for modifying dysfunctional parts. Occupational therapy gained some measure of scientific respectability by adopting a perspective that paralleled that of biomedicine. In order to achieve these ends, occupational therapists reformulated their former viewpoint as well as their assumptions and values. In short, they accepted a new paradigm.

Focal Viewpoint

The internal intrapsychic, neurological, and kinesiological workings of the person became the focal viewpoint of the new paradigm. Although concerned with different phenomena, these perspectives became part of an accepted framework that looked inward to the mechanisms underlying function and dysfunction. The following quote illustrates the new viewpoint:

> Much of the time both the sensory and the psychotherapeutic situation are dealing with semi- or non-conscious experiences. The psychotherapist thinks in terms of subconscious psychological complexes and dynamics; the sensory integrative therapist includes many subcortical integrative mechanisms in his thinking and treatment planning. While one therapist is considering the Oedipus complex, the other is considering brain stem integrating processes. In both cases the *underlying mechanisms* are recognized, their effect on behavior analyzed, and methods of dealing with them contemplated.[3] [Italics added.]

Core Constructs

As the focal viewpoint refocused on inner mechanisms, the core constructs of the paradigm similarly shifted. This reorientation provided by the new paradigm is characterized in the following constructs:

1. All ability to perform was directly determined by the degree of integrity of the nervous, musculoskeletal, and intrapsychic systems.
2. Dysfunction could be traced to damage or abnormal development in one or more of these systems.
3. Functional performance could be restored by using activity to improve the internal systems and/or by adapting equipment, tasks, or environments to compensate for permanent limitations in these systems.

The first construct directed attention to the neurological, musculoskeletal, and intrapsychic system's underlying function. Recognizing that function requires coordinated movement, knowledge of the neurological and musculoskeletal principles of movement was considered essential.[66] The new paradigm, consequently, emphasized detailed analysis of the neuromuscular features of task performance. For example:

> Synergistic muscles may be used to prevent an unwanted movement, thus assisting in the performance of a task. Forcefully gripping a tool is used to illustrate this concept; the long finger flexors cross more than one joint and have the potential to act on each joint they cross. Forceful gripping of a tool would cause the wrist to flex if the wrist extensors did not contract synergistically to prevent this unwanted motion.[66]

As the quote illustrates, occupational therapy amassed substantial information about what movement patterns were used in tasks.

The psychodynamic perspective stressed the relationship of unconscious processes to performance and the development of this relationship in the course of maturation.[5,24,25] From this perspective, therapists saw activities as opportunities for individuals to achieve need satisfaction and as vehicles to express unconscious emotions.

Emphasis on understanding the underlying disordered mechanism led to increasing efforts to analyze and describe the disorder and its relationship to functional incapacitation. Precision in determining which neurological structures and processes were involved in a given problem was important, so that the therapist could attack the problem in therapy. Similarly, it was considered important to know how deficits in movement (e.g., limitations of range of motion, strength, and endurance) disallowed performance of daily activities. Therapists analyzed activities to determine the particular movements they required so that they could identify and bridge any gaps between a person's capacity and those demands.

From the psychodynamic perspective, dysfunctional behavior was seen as a result of internal tension (i.e., anxiety) or early blocked needs that prevented maturation of the ego.[5,24,77] Therapists sought to determine the underlying conflicts or unfulfilled needs that interfered with functioning since these were the mechanisms to be altered in therapy. The therapists often used activities to diagnose the patient's hidden feelings and unconscious motives. Therapists also interpreted the unconscious meaning of colors, themes, and other characteristics of patients' creations.[44,77]

The common theme in intervention was to identify the specific cause or problem underlying the inability to function and to change and/or compensate for it. In cases of neurological disorders, new treatment methods stressed identification of abnormal movement patterns and techniques to inhibit them and facilitate normal movement.[10,60,69] Other approaches used activities and specialized equipment to stimulate the malfunctioning nervous system in order to elicit normal responses.[3,4] Therapists tried to provide a therapeutic rationale for every activity used in therapy, and the rationale had to be in terms of the impact on underlying mechanisms affecting movement. For example:

> Sensory stimulus is developed through adapted cutaneous contact with tools, the beater of the loom, or the handle of a sander. . . . Gross motor reaching and throwing activities stimulate proprioception and kinesthetic awareness. . . . Use of a skateboard attached to the forearm for directed range of motion activities stimulates upper arm active movements.[68]

As illustrated in this quote, therapists sought, through understanding the nervous system and its various components, to influence the inner mechanisms that determined everyday functioning.

The new paradigm led to the development of new treatment methods for musculoskeletal dysfunction, including splinting and positioning for optimal performance, passive and active range of motion, and exercises to develop muscle strength. Therapists analyzed activities to determine the movements needed in crafts and other activities. Therapists made or prescribed adaptive devices to bridge the gap between patients' limited motion and the tasks they had to perform. Therapists also taught patients compensatory techniques of self-care, dressing, and other functional performances.

Occupational therapy in psychiatry was predicated on the belief that if a patient could learn to fulfill needs and could recapitulate and satisfy blocked childhood needs, the intrapsychic conflict could be removed and the patient would return to healthy functioning.[23,44,77] Activities were used to enable patients to achieve need satisfaction. Another aim of psychiatric occupational therapy was to guide the patient in regression to developmental stages that had not been completed. For instance:

> For the individual who needs to obtain satisfactions at an infantile level the occupational therapist structures and manipulates situations which make possible actual or symbolic gratification of oral or anal needs, dependency needs, infantile aggression, destruction or control and infantile play. For example, some activities which may offer satisfaction for oral and anal needs are those involving eating, preparation of food, blowing musical instruments, singing, et cetera, and those which use excretory substitutes such as smearing or building with clay or paints, preparations of soil, collecting garbage or trash, and others.[22]

Overall, psychiatric occupational therapists conceptualized treatment as a means to act out or sublimate feelings.[25]

In a related approach, therapists used activities to establish a therapeutic relationship that would permit the patient to develop healthy means of resolving intrapsychic conflict and fulfilling deeds. In this approach, activities themselves were less important than the therapist's therapeutic use of self:

> The effective therapeutic approach in occupational therapy today and in the future is one in which the therapist utilized the tools of his trade as an *avenue of introduction*. From then on his personality takes over.[16] [Italics added.]

In this approach the relationship with the therapist was the therapeutic mechanism; the activity served only as an occasion for therapist and patient to interact.

Across the three mechanistic approaches to treatment (intrapsychic, neurological, kinesiological), the common denominator was the attempt to isolate particular effects that the activity was meant to have on the neurological, musculoskeletal, or psychodynamic mechanisms. This approach resulted in more specificity in intended effects of therapy.

Integrative Values

The values of the paradigm reflected a new focus on a scientific approach. Therapists came to appreciate the value of objectivity and precision in problem identification and measurement. The value of scientific precision was predicated upon the belief that the therapist who better understood the components of the disability was more useful to the patient. Therapists came to appreciate how dysfunction of inner systems translated into limitations of capacity and how reduction of the dysfunction allowed persons to become more functional.

Therapists also changed their value orientation toward therapeutic media. Previously therapists valued media's relationship to occupation in life and media's usefulness in motivating patient participation. Now therapists began to appreciate the opportunities for muscle strengthening, expression of unconscious desires, and so on that media could provide. Occupational therapy began to see the use of media as a powerful therapeutic agent that first needed to be analyzed and then applied with precision.

Mechanistic Paradigm: Summary

In the 1960s occupational therapy's professional culture changed in important ways. New patterns of thinking and practice in occupational therapy constituted a new paradigm of inner mechanisms (Table 3–2). This mechanistic paradigm resulted in important advances in the field. Among the gains was a substantially increased technology for remediating specific dysfunctions. Occupational therapy's potential to modify patients' pathological conditions was made more clear. The paradigm also resulted in a deeper understanding of how bodily structures and processes facilitated or limited performance. The technology for adapting devices and environments to the needs of persons with motor impairment improved greatly. The psychodynamic perspective increased understanding of how emotional pathology might interfere with competent performance and elaborated the role of emotions in behavior.

The changes in occupational therapy's professional culture occurred gradually, throughout practice. The transition from the paradigm of occu-

Table 3–2. *Mechanistic Paradigm*

Core Constructs	• The ability to perform depends on the integrity of the nervous, musculoskeletal, and intrapsychic systems. • Damage or abnormal development in the inner systems can result in incapacity. • Functional performance can be restored by improving/compensating for limitations in inner systems.
Focal Viewpoint	• Internal mechanism, that is, internal intrapsychic, neurological, and kinesiological workings.
Integrated Values	• Precise knowledge and understanding of the inner workings. • Value of inner workings to function. • Value of media as a means to reduce incapacity.

pation to the mechanistic paradigm is manifest in important changes in thinking about occupational therapy practice and in the nature of practice itself. Such transformations of deep professional culture are never neat and precise. Rather, some ideas and practices from the first paradigm were still preserved in aspects of practice and occasionally expressed as part of the philosophy of the field. However, their cogency for practice was eroded. A new culture of occupational therapy had made its way into the thoughts, attitudes, and practice of therapists.

The Second Crisis

While the mechanistic paradigm achieved much of its promise, it also had some unforeseen consequences for the field. Occupational therapy's fundamental perspective toward human beings had been radically altered. The early appreciation of the occupational nature of human beings, mind-body unity, self-maintenance through occupation, and the dynamic rhythm and balance of organized behavior, was replaced with a new, in-depth perspective. Holistic thinking was replaced by a reductionist emphasis on the internal workings of the human psyche and body. In the same way, the therapeutic rationale drastically changed. The earlier rationale of therapy, which had recourse to such concepts as morale building, habit regeneration, and stimulation of interest, was replaced by psychodynamic, neurophysiological, and kinesiological rationales that emphasized pathology reduction.

Practice also began to change. In some cases occupational therapists completely dropped the participation in meaningful occupation from their therapeutic programs. This should not be surprising. It was a short distance from arguing that activity was merely a convenient method for therapeutic interaction to concluding that activity is not really necessary at all. Similarly, when the primary focus of an activity was to achieve greater strength, there was little reason to recommend it over pure exercise.

In other cases, the trappings of occupations were retained, but without the underlying rationale provided by the first paradigm. Sometimes this change was taken to such an extreme that patients were placed in rather absurd circumstances. For example, some clinics maintained the use of activities such as sanding or pushing looms, but these activities were disembodied. Patients sanded boards that were never used in woodworking projects;[67] they pushed the beaters of looms that were not strung for weaving. In parallel fashion, patients in mental health settings painted and did other creative activities, but their art work was not recognized or appreciated as art. Rather, its value was as a medium for revealing unconscious feelings. In such cases the pale form of occupations was retained in practice, but there was no appreciation of the occupation as a therapeutic force in its own right. Rather, occupation was a mere vehicle for "exercise" or "insight."

Therapists also came to have less appreciation of the patient's experience of the process of engaging in occupations. As therapists focused on the impact of activity on underlying mechanisms, they tended to lose sight of the meaning of the activity to the patient. The concept of "purpose" was substituted for the concept of meaning. Purpose referred to goal-directed activity, but it implied no obligation to consider either the personal or cultural relevance of the activity. The profession had strayed far from the original idea that meaning in occupations came from the fact that they were an essential part of the fabric of life and that they represented a fundamental mind-body experience for those who engaged in them.

Therapists operating under the first paradigm considered the patient's experience within the therapeutic occupation to be critical. Under the mechanistic paradigm, therapists lost concern for the patient's experience within occupations used as treatment, just as they lost appreciation of the nature and role of occupation in human life.

As the field took on a new *identity* closely aligned with the medical model, there was an uncomfortable misfit between the old practices still retained and the new concepts used to explain them. When the concern for occupations shrank to a more narrow concern for function and therapeutic occupations became media-directed toward reduction of pathological states, therapists were left with a more shallow notion of their work and without a unique professional identity. The misuse of occupation (as illustrated above) and the growing embarrassment over the ordinariness of crafts, daily living tasks, and other therapeutic activities were symptomatic of the discomfort of lacking a clear and compelling identity.

In addition to its own uneasiness with the new explanations for practice, occupational therapy was also influenced by new interdisciplinary thinking that challenged the reductionist view of the world underlying the medical model and the mechanistic paradigm. Biologists and behavioral scientists pointed out that reductionism was an inadequate scientific framework.[7] Many writers called for ways of thinking about and doing science besides reductionism.[12,40,76] They criticized reductionism for creating a passive and mechanistic version of human behavior.[8] They argued that humans must be recognized as conscious, striving, and complex beings whose organization involves many interrelated dimensions.

The call to move beyond reductionism created an intellectual climate in which occupational therapy's reductionist-based paradigm of inner mechanisms now appeared incomplete. Theorists within the field argued that occupational therapy had achieved too narrow a perspective. These critics pointed out that the paradigm's mechanistic concepts provided insufficient explanations for the effects of occupation on patients.[56]

The reductionist medical model especially failed to address the full range of problems of chronically disabled persons. These problems extended beyond deficits of internal mechanisms and included the struggle to achieve meaningful lives and to thrive within society.[17,61] In occupational therapy recognition was growing of the limitations for practice of such an approach. Knowledge of the nervous and musculoskeletal systems and emotional pathology was necessary but not adequate for occupational therapy.[54]

During the 1970s, the recognition grew that occupational therapy lacked a unifying identity.[29,35,53,78] Conflict grew within the field, which was becoming too diverse and fractionalized[71] and lacked unity across specialty groups.[30,39] Writers argued that the alliance with medicine resulted in an orientation to specific disease categories without recognizing underlying occupational therapy principles;[53,63] in diversion of the field from its original mission;[63] and in a loss of its most seminal idea, the importance of occupation as a health-restoring measure.[57]

Finally, one observer warned that occupational therapy was jeopardizing its existence by abandoning the "insights of perennial value" that engendered the profession and on which the social contract of occupational therapy is built.[63]

The Call for a New Paradigm

In the 1960s and 1970s, Reilly and others developed a cluster of concepts aimed at recapturing elements of the field's first paradigm. This school of thought, called occupational behavior, embodied the following tenets: a return to the central focus on occupation;[52,54,59,62,70,71] recognition of the human motivation for occupation;[15,26] study of the human sense of time, purpose, and personal responsibility for adaptation;[37,74,80] examination of the organizing influence of occupational roles on behavior;[34,48] the importance of the environment in supporting or impeding adaptation;[18,31,55,74] and the integration of interdisciplinary knowledge needed for this perspective under a holistic framework.[34,38,48,56,59]

While this tradition was originally confined largely to colleagues and students of Reilly, the theme of resurrecting occupational therapy's original concepts and ideals began to be echoed by others.[28,71,75,79] Over the last decade, these efforts have made contributions toward building a new paradigm. The nature of this paradigm is the topic of the next chapter.

Conclusion

In this chapter I have attempted to tell the story of the genesis and transformation of occupational therapy's professional culture as represented in a series of paradigms (Fig. 3–2). Occupational therapy emerged in the beginning of this century, drawing on principles and perspectives of moral treatment. The field originally embraced a paradigm of occupation, which incorporated a holistic outlook focused on mind-body and person-environment unity. This paradigm recognized the power of participation in everyday occupations to influence mental and physical well-being. It envi-

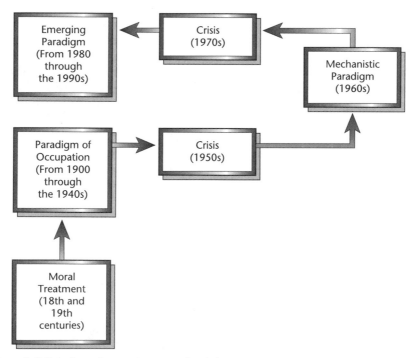

Figure 3–2. Paradigm changes in occupational therapy.

sioned therapy as participation in meaningful occupations that would have broad restorative effects, especially the regeneration of the will for life and reconnection to the environment.

Beset by criticism from the medical profession, occupational therapy began to question its original orientation and identity. This crisis resulted in the field adopting the reductionist viewpoint of the medical model. The result was a transformation in occupational therapy's view of humans, practice, and the field itself. The new mechanistic paradigm stressed recognition of the inner mechanisms (musculoskeletal, neurological, and intrapsychic) underlying the capacity for performance. It envisioned practice as the application of activities to reduce pathological states in these inner mechanisms. Although this new professional vision resulted in advances in certain knowledge, it also created confusion about professional identity and a loss of respect for and confidence in the therapeutic impact of occupation.

Consequently, occupational therapy has begun to return to many of its original themes to recapture its identity and a more holistic orientation. The work of many individuals now converges on a set of themes that I will refer to as the emerging paradigm of occupational therapy. A new professional culture is seeking to capture the best of both previous paradigms, achieving a strong sense of professional identity, balancing holism with precise knowledge, and integrating themes spanning the body, the mind, and the environment. These tasks are being done within the context of a recommitment to the field's focus on occupation.

References

1. Ayres, AJ: Basic concepts of clinical practice in physical disabilities. Am J Occup Ther 12:300, 1958.
2. Ayres, AJ: The development of perceptual motor abilities: A theoretical basis for treatment of dysfunction. Am J Occup Ther 17:221, 1963.
3. Ayres, AJ: Sensory Integration and Learning Disorders. Western Psychological Services, Los Angeles, 1972, p 266.
4. Ayres, AJ: The Development of Sensory Integrative Theory and Practice. Kendal & Hunt, Dubuque, IA, 1974.
5. Azima, H, and Azima, F: Outline of a dynamic theory of occupational therapy. Am J Occup Ther 13:215, 1959.
6. Barton, G: Teaching the Sick: A Manual of Occupational Therapy and Reeducation. WB Saunders, Philadelphia, 1919.
7. von Bertalanffy, L: General Systems Theory and Psychiatry. In Arieti, S (ed): American Handbook of Psychiatry, Vol 3. Basic Books, New York, 1966.
8. von Bertalanffy, L: General Systems Theory. George Braziller, New York, 1968, p 193.
9. Bing, R: Occupational therapy revisited: A paraphrastic journey. Am J Occup Ther 35:499, 1981.
10. Bobath, K, and Bobath, B: The facilitation of normal postural reactions and movements in the treatment of cerebral palsy. Physiotherapy 50:246, 1964.
11. Bockoven, JS: Moral Treatment in Community Mental Health. Springer, New York, 1972.
12. Boulding, K: General systems theory—the skeleton of science. In Buckeley, W (ed): Modern Systems Research for the Behavioral Scientist. Aldine, Chicago, 1968.
13. Bryan, W: Administrative Psychiatry. WW Norton, New York, 1936.
14. Buhler, C: Values in Psychotherapy. Free Press, New York, 1962.

15. Burke, J: A clinical perspective on motivation: Pawn versus origin. Am J Occup Ther 31:254, 1977.
16. Conte, W: The occupational therapist as a therapist. Am J Occup Ther 14:1, 1960.
17. Dubos, R: Mirage of Health. Harper & Row, New York, 1959.
18. Dunning, H: Environmental occupational therapy. Am J Occup Ther 26:292, 1972.
19. Dunton, WR: Occupational Therapy: A Manual for Nurses. WB Saunders, Philadelphia, 1915.
20. Dunton, WR: Reconstruction Therapy. WB Saunders, Philadelphia, 1919.
21. Dunton, WR: The educational possibilities of occupational therapy in state hospitals. Archives of Occupational Therapy 1:403, 1922.
22. Fidler, G: Some unique contributions of occupational therapy in treatment of the schizophrenic. Am J Occup Ther 12:9, 1958.
23. Fidler, G: The task-oriented group as a context for treatment. Am J Occup Ther 23:43, 1969.
24. Fidler, G, and Fidler, J: Introduction to Psychiatric Occupational Therapy. Macmillan, New York, 1958.
25. Fidler, G, and Fidler, J: Occupational Therapy: A Communication Process in Psychiatry. Macmillan, New York, 1963.
26. Florey, L: Intrinsic motivation: The dynamics of occupational therapy theory. Am J Occup Ther 23:319, 1969.
27. Fuller, D: The need of instruction for nurses in occupations for the sick. In Tracy, S (ed): Studies in Invalid Occupation. Whitcomb and Barrows, Boston, 1912.
28. Gilfoyle, EM: Eleanor Clarke Slagle Lectureship, 1984: Transformation of a Profession. Am J Occup Ther 38:575, 1984.
29. Gillette, N: Changing methods in the treatment of psychosocial dysfunction. Am J Occup Ther 21:230, 1967.
30. Gillette, N, and Kielhofner, G: The impact of specialization on the professionalization and survival of occupational therapy. Am J Occup Ther 33:30, 1979.
31. Gray, M: Effects of hospitalization on work-play behavior. Am J Occup Ther 26:180, 1972.
32. Hass, L: Practical Occupational Therapy. Bruce, Milwaukee, 1944.
33. Hall, H, and Buck, MMC: The Work of Our Hands: A Study of Occupations for Invalids. Moffat, Yard & Co., New York, 1915.
34. Heard, C: Occupational role acquisition: A perspective on the chronically disabled. Am J Occup Ther 31:243, 1977.
35. Johnson, J: Occupational therapy: A model for the future. Am J Occup Ther 27:1, 1973.
36. Kidner, TB: Occupational Therapy. The Science of Prescribed Work for Invalids. W Kohlhammer, Stuttgart, 1930.
37. Kielhofner, G: Temporal adaptation: A conceptual framework for occupational therapy. Am J Occup Ther 31:235, 1977.
38. Kielhofner, G: General systems theory: Implications for theory and action in occupational therapy. Am J Occup Ther 32:637, 1978.
39. King, LJ: Toward a science of adaptive responses. Am J Occup Ther 32:429, 1978.
40. Koestler, A: Beyond atomism and holism—the concept of the holon. In Koestler, A, and Smythies, JR (eds): Beyond Reductionism. Beacon Press, Boston, 1969.
41. Kuhn, T: The Structure of Scientific Revolutions, ed 2. University of Chicago Press, Chicago, 1970.
42. Licht, S: Modern trends in occupational therapy. Occupational Therapy and Rehabilitation 26:455, 1947.
43. Licht, S: Occupational Therapy Sourcebook. Williams & Wilkins, Baltimore, 1948.
44. Llorens, LA, and Young, GG: Fingerpainting for the hostile child. Am J Occup Ther 14:306, 1960.
45. Macintyre, A: Epistemological crises, dramatic narrative, and the philosophy of science. In Gutting, G (ed): Paradigms and Revolutions. University of Notre Dame Press, Notre Dame, IN, 1980.
46. Magaro, P, Gripp, R, and McDowell, D: The Mental Health Industry: A Cultural Phenomenon. John Wiley & Sons, New York, 1978.
47. Marsh, C: Borzoi: Suggestions for a new rallying of occupational therapy. Archives of Occupational Therapy 11:169, 1932.

48. Matsutsuyu, J: Occupational behavior—a perspective on work and play. Am J Occup Ther 25:291, 1971.
49. McNary, H: A look at occupational therapy. Am J Occup Ther 12:203, 1958.
50. Meyer, A: The philosophy of occupational therapy. Archives of Occupational Therapy 1:1, 1922.
51. Meyerson, L: Some observations on the psychological roles of the occupational therapist. Am J Occup Ther 11:131, 1957.
52. Michelman, S: The importance of creative play. Am J Occup Ther 25:285, 1971.
53. Mosey, A: Involvement in the rehabilitation movement—1942–1960. Am J Occup Ther 25:234, 1971.
54. Reilly, M: Occupational therapy can be one of the great ideas of 20th century medicine. Am J Occup Ther 16:1, 1962.
55. Reilly, M: A psychiatric occupational therapy program as a teaching model. Am J Occup Ther 20:61, 1966.
56. Reilly, M (ed): Play as Exploratory Learning. Sage, Beverly Hills, CA, 1974.
57. Rerek, M: The depression years 1929 to 1941. Am J Occup Ther 25:231, 1971.
58. Riley, JN: Western medicine's attempt to become more scientific: Examples from the United States and Thailand. Soc Sci Med 11:549, 1977.
59. Robinson, A: Play: The arena for acquisition of rules for competent behavior. Am J Occup Ther 31:248, 1977.
60. Rood, M: Everyone counts. Am J Occup Ther 12:326, 1958.
61. Safilios-Rothschild, C: The Sociology and Social Psychology of Disability and Rehabilitation. Random House, New York, 1970.
62. Shannon, P: Work-play theory and the occupational therapy process. Am J Occup Ther 26:169, 1972.
63. Shannon, P: The derailment of occupational therapy. Am J Occup Ther 31:229, 1977.
64. Slagle, EC: Training aides for mental patients. Archives of Occupational Therapy 1:11, 1922.
65. Slagle, EC, and Robeson, H: Syllabus for Training of Nurses in Occupational Therapy, ed 2. State Hospitals Press, Utica, NY, 1941.
66. Smith, HB: Scientific and medical bases. In Hopkins, HL, and Smith, ND (eds): Willard and Spackman's Occupational Therapy, ed 5. JB Lippincott, Philadelphia, 1978.
67. Spackman, C: A history of the practice of occupational therapy for restoration of physical function: 1917–1967. Am J Occup Ther 22:67, 1968.
68. Spencer, EA: Functional restoration. In Hopkins, HL, and Smith, ND (eds): Willard and Spackman's Occupational Therapy, ed 5. JB Lippincott, Philadelphia, 1978, p 355.
69. Stockmeyer, SA: A sensorimotor approach to treatment. In Pearson, P, and Williams, C (eds): Physical Therapy Services in the Developmental Disabilities. Charles C Thomas, Springfield, IL, 1972.
70. Takata, N: The play history. Am J Occup Ther 23:314, 1969.
71. Task Force on Target Populations. Am J Occup Ther 28:158, 1974.
72. Tracy, S: Studies in Invalid Occupation. Whitcomb & Barrows, Boston, 1912.
73. Training of Teachers for Occupational Therapy for the Rehabilitation of Disabled Soldiers and Sailors. Government Printing Office, Washington, DC, 1918.
74. Watanabe, S: Four concepts basic to the occupational therapy process. Am J Occup Ther 22:439, 1968.
75. Wiemer, R: Traditional and nontraditional practice arenas. In Occupational Therapy: 2001. American Occupational Therapy Association, Rockville, MD, 1979, p 43.
76. Weiss, P: Living nature and the knowledge gap. Saturday Review, November 29, 1969.
77. West, W (ed): Psychiatric Occupational Therapy. American Occupational Therapy Association, New York, 1959.
78. West, W: Professional responsibility in times of change. Am J Occup Ther 22:9, 1968.
79. West, W: A reaffirmed philosophy and practice of occupational therapy. Am J Occup Ther 38:15, 1984.
80. Woodside, H: Dimensions of the occupational behavior model. Canadian Journal of Occupational Therapy 43:11, 1976.

CHAPTER 4

THE EMERGING PARADIGM

The current paradigm status* of occupational therapy can be characterized in the following way: During the field's crisis, dialogue about occupational therapy's identity and perspective went in different directions, with
no agreement about the topic of conversation. For example, there were a
number of proposals concerning what should be the core constructs of
occupational therapy. Different writers proposed adaptation,[58] development,[61] and occupation[51,82] as alternative foci for the field. In recent years,
the topic of paradigmatic conversation has converged on the theme of occupation. Now, the discourse is about how we should view this phenomena
and what it means about practice. Hence, the emergence of a paradigm sig-

---

*The title for this chapter suggests that occupational therapy is still constructing a new para-
digm. Given the kinds of rapid paradigm shifts I described in the previous chapter, one might
ask why the current paradigm building is taking so long. The response is that occupational
therapy's previous paradigms were less sophisticated than the paradigm that is currently being
fashioned. The emerging paradigm represents a much more intense and complex conversation
than those which characterized these prior paradigms. This is due both to the increase in persons who do scholarly work in the field and to the exponential growth of knowledge from
other disciplines that influences occupational therapy's paradigmatic discourse. Christiansen[20]
has proposed something quite like this in another form. He has made a justifiable argument
that occupational therapy's history can be viewed as a pre-paradigmatic period and that the
field is, just now, in the business of building its paradigm. Christiansen's point is well taken,
and he correctly points out the increased level of theory development that needs to and is taking place in order for occupational therapy to build a robust paradigm. I originally characterized and continue to characterize the history of the profession through paradigm shifts because
I believe this way of viewing its history underscores the importance of the paradigmatic view
for the identity and practice of the field. That is, by seeing how occupational therapy's overall
way of understanding itself has shifted, we get a better grasp of why this aspect of our conceptual foundations is important.

nals not the end of dialogue about the field's identity and viewpoint, but rather the focusing of that dialogue to specific topics.

The aim of this chapter is to characterize how this emerging paradigm is being discussed and what is being said about it. I have sought not only to give the reader a bird's eye view of the dialogue, but also to get out ahead of it a bit, anticipating where things might be headed. Judgments had to be made about what are important themes and trends in this multifaceted discourse. This involved examining both the strength of arguments in the field and the directions toward which interdisciplinary literature will likely nudge the field. In characterizing the emerging paradigm, I have added my own voice (sometimes emphatically) to the discourse.

As I previously proposed, the occupational therapy paradigm can be identified and analyzed as constituting three elements:

1. Core constructs
2. A focal viewpoint
3. Integrating values

The *core constructs* elucidate occupational therapy's view of humans, identify the problems that occupational therapists solve, and present the global rationale underlying therapy. By addressing these three issues, the core constructs help to identify and justify the kind of services that occupational therapists provide. Moreover, these constructs provide the field with a vision of its own nature, by identifying what it is concerned with and what it does.

The *focal viewpoint* of occupational therapy identifies how the field collectively thinks about things. The *integrative values* express what is important in the practice of occupational therapy; that is, they exemplify what occupational therapists most care about. Furthermore, these values express the moral importance of occupational therapy, that is, why it is worth doing and how it should be done. The core constructs, focal viewpoint, and integrative values interweave, forming a conceptual perspective and a professional culture through which occupational therapists see their practice and their profession.

Core Constructs

A great deal of discussion concerning what constitutes the core of occupational therapy has taken place over the past two decades. Weimer[106] has provided one of the most direct articulations of where the discourse has converged:

> Ours is, and must be, the basic knowledge of occupation. It is that knowledge which permits the occupational therapist to look at an activity of daily living in a unique way, and so determine best how to facilitate the

patient's or client's goal achievement. Our exclusive domain is occupation. We must refine, research, and systematize it so that it becomes evident, definable, defensible and salable. The "impact of occupation upon human beings" was spelled out as our sole claim to professionalism by our founders in 1917. It is our latent power if we will but keep it as our focus and direction.

Weimer made this assertion about the centrality of occupation to the field nearly 20 years ago, when the idea of organizing the field's core constructs around the theme of occupation was still controversial.

Today, discourse in occupational therapy clearly demonstrates what Polatajko[81] calls "a discipline focused on occupation." I characterize these constructs as reflecting three broad themes:

1. Humans' occupational nature
2. Occupational dysfunction as a problem focus
3. Occupation and the dynamics of therapy

In the following sections we will examine the constructs that make up each of these themes.

The Occupational Nature of Humans

A number of writers have offered a definition or characterization of occupation.[1,15,71,91,112] Definitions tend to evoke the constructs that are most common in the field. Collectively, these definitions point out that occupation:

- Comprises work, play/leisure, and daily living activities
- Arises as a response to and fulfills a specific motive or need
- Involves doing or performance that calls upon specific capacities
- Entails completion of a specific form
- Interrelates with the sociocultural context
- Provides meaning
- Interweaves with the developmental process

These are the most recurrent ideas that concern the occupational nature of humans. In the sections that follow we will briefly examine each.

The Composition of Occupation. Occupational therapists recognize that occupation refers to a wide range of behaviors, which are ordinarily viewed as consisting of three areas: play/leisure, daily living tasks, and work. Play is developmentally the earliest form of occupational behavior, and it persists throughout life.[83,85,105] Exploration, fantasy, imagination, games, sport, and creative activities are all part of play. Play is recognized as both an attitude toward one's activity and as a form of behavior that is relatively free from the serious pressures or demands of life. Childhood play initiates the young into the adult life of the social group.[83,85] In play and games children imitate the requirements and roles of adult life and practice the values, belief systems, norms, and skills of the culture. This process of socialization enables the young to become participating members of the sociocultural world. The apparently nonserious activity of play significantly contributes to the continuity of society and culture.[83,85,105]

Adult play (also referred to as leisure) serves a complementary purpose. It reaffirms meanings and values.[43,105] Adult players and spectators may become intensively involved in the emotion and meaning of games, ranging from local team events to Olympic competitions. Organizational festivities (e.g., office parties and company picnics), holiday celebrations associated with national and religious holidays, social rituals (e.g., parades, picnics, fairs, graduation ceremonies), and cultural events (e.g., art exhibits, concerts, and plays) connect participants to a broader context of social and cultural meanings. Commitment to a way of life is solidified through such forms of play.

Daily living tasks are activities that serve to maintain one's self and lifestyle. They include self-care, ordering one's life space (e.g., cleaning and paying bills), and getting to resources (e.g., travel and shopping).[54] Daily living tasks (sometimes referred to as activities of daily living) are generally private and personal. They compose much of the routine of daily life; one recent text refers quite appropriately to this domain of occupation as "ways of living."[22]

Work is productive activity that contributes some service or commodity to others.[19,38,90] The various products of work include utilitarian or artistic objects, ideas, knowledge, help, information sharing, and protection. Work is linked closely to the most basic survival needs of humans, and it is through work that most persons attain access to the resources they require and desire for living. Related to work are those activities aimed at improving one's abilities to produce—that is, studying, practicing, and apprenticing. Even in societies with complex economic systems, only a portion of work is remunerated in the marketplace. Many forms of work involve the informal exchange of help and assistance. Examples of this type include taking care of the young, old, and infirm, and volunteer work. Moreover, the work of learning and apprenticing, while not immediately productive for societies, is important for their maintenance, since it enables its members to competently perform within society. Thus, the activities a person performs as a student, paid employee, volunteer, parent, serious hobbyist, and amateur are considered work in its broadest sense.

While play, daily living tasks, and work are disparate in form, they are considered to belong to a single domain of behavior by virtue of their interrelationships in everyday life and across the life span.[65,90] For example, play is considered to provide learning opportunities that are necessary for competence in adult work. Play in adult life maintains and restores morale and renews the individual for work. Workers earn the right to the leisure of old age. Daily living activities are necessary to prepare oneself (e.g., grooming and dressing) for work. Their variety gives texture and variety to life. Moreover, these occupational behaviors are the means by which individuals fill their time, create the circumstances of their everyday existence, and make their place in the world.

An important idea related to the interrelationship and interdependence of work, play, and daily living tasks is balance. The concept of balance suggests that there needs to be a dynamic alternation between modes of activity (e.g., between more serious and more playful modes). Sometimes this has been referred to as the balance of work and play, but as Christiansen[23] notes, the idea of simply partitioning time into so much work or play oversimplifies the concept of balance. A more sophisticated view suggests that balance refers to a complex organization of behaviors in which short-term and long-term orientation, playfulness and seriousness, private and public nature, along with other dimensions, are maintained in relation to each other.[23,50] As Wood[107] argues, the various forms of occupation are woven together into a kind of tapestry of daily life.

The Need and Motive for Occupation. A basic occupational therapy premise is that humans require creative, productive, and playful pursuits and flourish by engaging in them.[24,34,45,54,65,82] This argument views the human need for occupation as both biologically and psychologically based. The biological need is predicated on observations that occupational activity has diverse impacts such as maintaining physical (e.g., cardiorespiratory and musculoskeletal) fitness, developing the nervous system, and generating motor competence.[13,76,87] The psychological need is variously referred to as the requirement that persons engage in activity, discover and create, exercise capacity, or realize a degree of competence in occupations.[27,33,54,82,87,93,106,109,112] Participation in occupations provides individuals with satisfaction, development of capacities that are exercised, and self-actualization. Hence both biological and psychological welfare is dependent on participation in occupations.

Closely related to the idea of a need for occupation is the concept that humans desire or have a motive for occupation. Variously described, this occupational motive entails an urge to engage in and to experience oneself as competent in activity.[23,31,56,82] It is also recognized that, while there may be a global motive to engage in occupations, there are also important cultural influences and individual variations in motives for engaging in particular occupations.[56]

Occupational Performance and Capacity. Occupation involves doing or performance that requires the individual to have competence.[21,30,85] Occupational therapy's work with persons who have limitations of capacity has led the field to pay particular attention to the underlying abilities that are called upon and required in occupational performance. These are often referred to as occupational performance components.

Different categories of performance components can be found in occupational therapy literature. For example, Mosey[70] identified the following performance components: motor function, sensory integration, visual perception, cognitive function, psychological function, and social interaction. More recently, Christiansen[21] offered pharmacologic, physiological, sensory, neuromotor, cognitive, and psychosocial factors as a taxonomy of performance components. Although writers have proposed different taxonomies, the identification and understanding of performance components that impact on how persons function as occupational beings is an important aspect of occupational therapy's view of humans.

Importantly, the conceptualization of how these components affect actual performance is changing. Earlier views assumed a direct correlation between the intact performance components and competent behavior. However, it is now recognized that there is not a linear relationship between these components and performance.[64,102] Rather they are seen as contributing, along with the context and the occupation being performed, to the organization of actual performance.[28,56,64,96,102]

This changing view of the role of performance components will be a recurrent theme in this chapter and in later discussions of conceptual models of practice. Since several of these models focus specifically on performance components, the changing view of their role in occupational performance will alter how models conceptualize underlying performance components.

Occupational Form. A new construct, *occupational form*, focuses on *that which is being done* and how it influences performance. According to Nelson:[71]

> *Occupational form* is the preexisting structure that elicits, guides, or structures subsequent human performance; *occupational performance* consists of the human actions taken in response to an occupational form. . . . *occupation* can be thought of as the relationship between occupational form and occupational performance. As used in the framework presented here, the term *occupation* always refers to the occupational performance of an occupational form (i.e., the doing of something or the engaging in something).

Nelson goes on to point out that the occupational form refers to conditions external to the person. These include the constraints that the form itself imposes on performance (e.g., time constants and objects to be used) and the social context that defines the occupational form (i.e., specifies how it should be done and what is its social purpose and meaning).

Occupational forms arise as inventions of culture in response to adaptational requirements and as part of the way of life that members of the culture have invented.[56] Hence, occupational forms in all cultures include ways of obtaining, maintaining, and using food, clothing, and shelter. They also include culturally unique forms that represent how the social group has elaborated its way of life. Hence, square dancing, the twist, folk dancing, break dancing, and disco are different occupational forms of the same genre; each is related to a specific cultural and temporal context.

As one readily recognizes, each occupational form calls upon the performer to engage in a specific set of related behaviors, to have a particular attitude, and even to dress in particular ways. Hence the music, dress, movements, and settings of the different forms of dance noted above all differ, and represent the unique configuration of contextual elements that make up the occupational form. When an individual engages in an occupation or *performs*, he or she goes through the form, which is the original meaning of the Latin term, "perform." To perform a particular occupation means to enact a way of doing things that the form represents.

Occupational forms invite and organize performance. When, for example, I sit before the computer keyboard working on this chapter, I engage in certain movements necessary to type the words onto the page. I also engage in certain cognitive and creative processes to attempt to weave together ideas into arguments and illustrations. I am guided by my tacit understanding of the "occupational form" of professional writing, which is not my invention, but rather something that scholars over decades of writing articles and books have shaped into a way of presenting arguments. Indeed, many other books I have read have served as exemplars or models for how a book can be written, and they hover about my thoughts as I seek to compose a book. In my immediate environment are the articles and books of occupational therapists whom I consult in order to do the writing. They reveal to me not only the content of their concepts and arguments, but also a way of fashioning language toward a type of discourse. Hence, when I write, my performance is deeply embedded in the *form* of writing through which I am moving.

Although relatively new, the construct of occupational form has already been incorporated in occupational therapy in a number of ways. For example, some researchers who wish to understand the influence that occupation has on actual performance have incorporated the construct into investigations. These studies have shown that there is a qualitative difference in performance when persons are performing real occupations as opposed to merely executing a movement.[64,108]

The idea of occupational form has rapidly become a construct in the emerging paradigm of occupational therapy, since it offers a way of conceptualizing how the occupation that is being performed influences the performance of the person doing the occupation. Its incorporation into models of practice[64] is further evidence of its emergence as a core construct.*

---

*Nelson,[71] who introduced the concept of occupational form, discusses the environment as part of the occupational form. In contrast, I have discussed occupational form as part of the environment.[56] These two discussions view the same phenomena from different vantage points, but their overall conceptualization of occupational form is similar. Nonetheless, readers should be aware that different authors discuss this concept from different perspectives and, consequently, will relate the concept of occupational form to other concepts of the environment in different ways. In this chapter, I have emphasized what is similar, rather than what is different in these viewpoints, treating occupational form and environment as separate core constructs.

Occupation and the Environment/Context. As noted in the previous chapter, the environment has been considered an important construct since the time of the field's first paradigm. Discussions of the environment as "a critical factor in human performance" are recurrent in modern occupational therapy literature,[28] and changing views about the role of performance components (noted above) are correlated with an increasing emphasis on the role of the environment in occupational behavior.

Discussions of the environment emphasize both that the person must adapt to an environment that presents challenges to or demands on the person, and that the environment shapes and influences performance.[56,89,94] Said another way, the environment both demands certain things of the performer and provides conditions that are necessary to support performance.

The construct of environment or context has been conceptualized to include the physical domain (e.g., objects, materials, tools, architecture), social domain (e.g., social norms, cultural influences), and the temporal context (e.g., available time for performance, short-term versus long-term occupations).[56,89,94] Discussions of the environment increasingly emphasize that occupation can never be understood independent of the sociocultural, physical, and temporal context in which it takes place. Occupational behavior is always environmental behavior.

Occupation and Meaning. Another recurring theme in occupational therapy literature is meaning. Occupation is recognized as having a basic role in creating, affirming, and experiencing meaning in life.[92,109] The meaning experienced in occupations emanates from a variety of sources, including the purpose and process of performing the occupation, a personal history of experiences and associations with the occupation, the actual experience of performing the occupation, and the sociocultural definition of the occupation.

Performance of occupations requires attention to various goals, necessary operations, and occasions for problem solving. Focusing one's attention on these inherent requirements of the task creates one kind of meaning that is pragmatic and oriented to the "this-is-what-this-is" aspect of any performance. This kind of meaning in performance may account for why ordinary occupations can be so useful in relieving us of unpleasant thoughts and feelings. For example, most people can name one or more occupations in which they can engage when they are feeling anxious or depressed. These occupations, by requiring attention to their immediate features, transport one to a new realm of meaning, providing at once distraction and comfort.

Another source of meaning in occupations comes from the social and cultural milieu.[71] This meaning is associated with the occupation by virtue of its place within the larger sociocultural group. Some occupational forms only belong to particular cultures and, hence, have meanings unique to that group. Other occupational forms may vary in their particular meanings (e.g., the status associated with them) across cultures and groups. For example, hunting is a highly valued activity in some groups but is perceived quite negatively by others. Groups of persons who engage in fly-fishing look down upon those who use baited hooks. Moreover, the meaning of an activity may vary greatly, depending on who within the society is performing it and to what end. Professional fishing for a living certainly has a different context of meaning than fishing for sport.

More recently, a new idea has given more depth to the construct of meaning in occupation as it pertains to the individual experience of meaning. This is the concept of narrative or story. The fundamental argument is that persons experience meaning through stories that "emplot" or impart a framework for making sense of and understanding a series of events from life.[14,25,40,46,63,66] Stories link together past, present, and future into a coherent whole, and thus allow individuals to experience separate events and future possibilities as part of a meaningful whole.

The concept of narrative is linked to occupation in three important ways. First, the stories that are of interest to the field are those about one's occupational self, that is, they are occupational stories about one's work, play/leisure, and daily living experiences.[25,40] Occupational narratives weave together the events and actions of occupational life into a meaningful whole. Secondly, stories are linked to occupation because telling and doing are often interchangeable.[40,57] Narrative is not merely a literary or oral form, it is a mode of doing as well. It means that people engage in their occupations so as to locate themselves in an unfolding story and to achieve a particular direction or outcome in that story. Occupational behaviors have narrative meaning when they implicitly or explicitly express unfolding events relevant to a story in progress. The third link of stories to occupation is that stories motivate actions,[40,56] that is, stories are not only about what has been or is going on, they are about what might be, could be, or will be. Stories anticipate possible, desired, or dreaded outcomes and, therefore, lead persons to act. All people engage in occupational behavior so as to achieve certain outcomes and avoid others. Hence, we study for exams to achieve good grades, we engage in regular exercise to avoid becoming out of shape, and we nurture our children so that they will grow up to lead happy lives. Thus, it can be said that stories generate occupational behavior; that is, they envision futures, providing a context within which goal-oriented occupations make sense. For example, Clark[25] discusses how Penny, a professor recovering from a cerebral aneurysm, formulated a future story in which she imagined herself a British intellectual. Drawing on the power of this narrative, she soon chose a number of activities that enacted the story, such as shopping for a proper cane and attire, attending the opera, and cooking gourmet food.

While the theme of narrative is relatively new in occupational therapy, it has struck an important cord and has become a consistent theme in the literature. In particular, it has added a new dimension to understanding how individuals interpret and find meaning in their occupations, and how they choose occupations on the basis of narrative meanings.

Occupation and Development. Another core construct in the emerging paradigm is that individual human development and occupation are closely interwoven. Occupation cannot be completely understood without an appreciation of its developmental nature.[26,61] The developmental perspective stresses the unfolding of skills, motives, and life roles as shaped by biological, psychological, and environmental factors.[12] Yerxa[110] notes that "occupation emerges in a predictable developmental sequence, including the acquisition and use of play, self-maintenance, work, and other role-related behaviors." While this sequence is not invariant, occupational behavior takes on different forms at different life stages.

Occupational therapists have identified several developmental processes that are especially important to occupational therapy. They include:

1. The development of motor and cognitive capacities used in occupational performance
2. The development of emotional and social maturity
3. Socialization into occupational roles
4. The occupational choice process, which influences the acquisition of occupational roles across the life span

The course of occupational development has been described as the *occupational career.*[10] It involves a series of stages through which an individual moves. The human infant enters into a long period of play in which he or she acquires a vast array of capacities.[83,85] Through childhood participation in family life and its associated chores, each individual begins the socialization toward work.[10] Gradually, the player role gives over to the student role, which more directly prepares persons for the kinds of tasks required in adult work. As the adult enters into the work of the society, play takes on a new function, recreation.[83] Finally, work gives over to the leisure role. Some roles, such as family member, are lifelong, although their nature changes across the life span. For instance, the individual moves from child and sibling to spouse and parent. Other roles, such as that of friend, may continue throughout life. The process of role development occurs through socialization, in which individuals learn what roles they are expected to assume and what they should do in these roles.[39]

Occupational therapy writers also recognize occupation as an important force in human development.[3,106] Specific developmental outcomes result from participation in various occupations. For example, creative play has a positive impact on later adult problem-solving skills.

Bruce and Borg[12] summarize the importance of the developmental perspective:

> In looking at the entire life span developmentally, one is given an excellent basis not only for conceptualizing the changing role that activities serve as the individual grows and matures, but also for appreciating the ever-changing strengths and limitations that need to be considered in relation to skill building.

Stated another way, occupation is seen as both a facilitator and a product of development.

Summary. In this section, I identified and discussed (Table 4–1) core constructs related to the occupational nature of humans. These constructs give meaning to the concept of occupation and provide an orientation to its importance and nature. Appreciation of the dimensions of occupation is important for the identity of the field and serves as a framework influencing the concerns taken up by conceptual practice models.

Occupational Dysfunction

The emerging paradigm of occupational therapists provides a unique way of viewing human problems. The field describes these problems as occupational dysfunction, which refers to failure or difficulty engaging in healthy patterns of occupation.[86] Hence, the primary concern in the emerging paradigm is not with the specific limitations of cognition, movement, strength, sensation, or motivation per se, but rather with the breakdowns in occupational behavior that are associated with these problems. An occupational dysfunction is considered to exist when there is interruption or interference of those specific occupations a person wants to do and must do. Thus, occupational dysfunction is person-specific. It focuses on the impact of disease or trauma in a person's everyday occupational life.

The following are constructs that relate to the theme of occupational dysfunction:

- Personal impact of occupational dysfunction
- Multidimensional nature of occupational dysfunction
- Consequences of occupational dysfunction
- Social cost of occupational dysfunction

In the sections below we will briefly examine each of these constructs.

The Personal Impact of Occupational Dysfunction. Earlier, we identified occupation as a basic human need. When persons are denied access to or have restrictions in their occupations, they experience a reduction in quality of life. As Englehardt[29] points out persons' experiences of health are tied to the "activities open to them or denied to them." Further, when persons experience a disease or trauma that produces a limitation in performance, their primary questions concern possible restrictions on their previous

Table 4–1. **Core Constructs Related to Humans' Occupational Nature**

The Composition of Occupation	Occupation consists of: • Play—exploration, fantasy, imagination, games, sport, and creative activities • Daily living tasks—activities that serve to maintain one's self and lifestyle • Work—productive activity that contributes some service or commodity to society Work, play, and daily living tasks are interrelated and interdependent.
The Need and Motive for Occupation	• Humans have a biological and psychological need for occupation. • Participation in occupations provides satisfaction, development of capacities, and self-actualization. • The occupational motive is an urge to engage in activity and to experience oneself as competent in it.
Occupational Performance and Capacity	Occupation involves doing or performance that requires the individual to have competence.
Occupational Form	• The preexisting structure that elicits, guides, or structures subsequent human performance • The constraints that the form itself imposes on performance and the social context that defines the occupational form Occupational performance consists of the human actions taken in response to an occupational form.

Occupation and the Environment/Context	Environment (i.e., context) is a critical factor in human performance:
	• The person must adapt to an environment or context.
	• The environment shapes and influences performance.
	• Environment or context includes:
	  ○ The physical domain
	  ○ The social domain (e.g., social norms, cultural influences)
	  ○ The temporal context

Occupation and Meaning	• Occupation has a role in creating, affirming, and experiencing meaning in life.
	• Sources of meaning experienced in occupations:
	  ○ The purpose and process of performing the occupation
	  ○ A personal history of experiences and associations
	  ○ The emerging experience of performing the occupation
	  ○ The sociocultural definition of the occupation
	• Stories help to weave together the events and actions of occupational life into a meaningful whole.
	• People engage in their occupations so as to locate themselves in an unfolding story.
	• Stories motivate actions.

Occupation and Development	• Occupation is both a facilitator and a product of development.

activities.[22] Such questions reflect the fact that a lack of ability or opportunity for occupational performance creates human suffering.[18]

The personal consequences of being unable to perform ordinary occupations are multiple.[56] Persons may lose or fail to achieve identities that go along with the performance of occupational roles. They may be left with vast amounts of time that cannot be meaningfully filled. They may lose a sense of competence and self-worth.

Additionally, occupational dysfunction disrupts the life story.[25,40] The continuity and overall meaning of life and the ways in which an individual expected his/her life to unfold all come under threat with the onset of an occupational dysfunction.

Consequences of Occupational Dysfunction. Occupational dysfunction is not only a consequence of disease and trauma. It can also be a source of other dysfunctions. In some cases it can produce secondary problems that follow the disruption of occupation by disease. As the Fidlers[30] note, "A reduction in doing generates pathology." In other cases, a maladaptive pattern of occupational behavior can produce trauma.

A lack or disruption of participation in occupation may result in reductions of capacity.[106] From the atrophy of disused muscles to the loss of unpracticed skills, occupational therapists have observed that a host of secondary losses may occur when occupation is disturbed. Deprivation of satisfying engagement in occupation can be the source of depression, substance abuse, and other maladaptive psychological reactions.

Maladaptive patterns of occupational performance also may generate other problems. For example, children deprived of normal play opportunities may fail to develop necessary language, cognitive, and motor skills.[53] People working under physical or mental stress may become susceptible to such problems as repetitive motion injuries and cardiac illness.[36,51] In these and other ways, maladaptive patterns of occupational behavior may place individuals at risk of developing various physical and psychological disorders.

Multidimensional Nature of Occupational Dysfunction. Occupational dysfunctions are multidimensional problems resulting from the interplay of biological, psychological, and ecological factors.[56,69] Disruption of motor, cognitive, emotional, and other performance components can affect the ability to perform occupations, but seldom is an occupational dysfunction due to a single factor. For example, a limitation of physical capacity rarely represents the full extent of an occupational dysfunction. Limited physical capacity may lead to a breakdown of confidence and hope, to encounters with physical and social barriers, and to a disturbance of social roles and relations.

This concept of multifactorial dysfunction is also linked to the idea that performance is not related only to underlying capacity. The corollary is that problems in performance also are not directly related to restrictions in capacity.[28,56,102] Rather, limitations of capacity interact with conditions in the environment and with the occupational form being performed to influence how a person performs. Occupational dysfunction is linked, then, not only to restrictions in the emotional, cognitive, motor, motivation, and other elements within the person, but also to the factors outside the person. When a person is having difficulty performing, it is the relationship between these elements that must be examined.[55,100]

In sum, occupational therapists recognize that impairments are rarely limited to a single domain of one's being, but rather resonate throughout the biological and psychological domains of the person. Moreover, occupational performance dysfunctions are linked to a complex relationship between restrictions in capacity, environmental conditions, and the occupation being performed.

The Social Cost of Occupational Dysfunction. When individuals cannot adequately perform their occupations, social systems are also affected. Workers who cannot work productively create adverse conditions in the workplace and may place an economic burden on the rest of society.[74] Children who do not learn to care for themselves require extra efforts from families, which strains the family system.[44,47] Older persons who lose the capacity to perform tasks of daily living independently may require socially expensive supports and/or living arrangements.[35] In short, occupational dysfunction results in lost potential for persons to contribute to the social order and in increased costs to society to support occupationally dysfunctional members.

This theme is likely to take on increasing importance as health care systems in various countries are concerned with containing health care costs and optimizing outcomes. The intrinsic worth of occupational therapy derives from the fact that occupational dysfunction has a high social cost. To the extent that occupational therapy services are able to prevent, reverse, or lessen occupational dysfunction, their worth to society is enhanced.

Summary. This section identified and discussed core constructs (Table 4–2) of the emerging paradigm that pertain to occupational dysfunction, which occurs when persons are prevented from or limited in doing those occupations they want and/or need to do. These constructs not only identify the nature and consequences of occupational dysfunction, but also delineate the generic nature of the human problems that occupational therapy services address.

Occupation and the Dynamics of Therapy

The third thematic area of the core constructs relates to occupational therapy's vision of how the field addresses the occupational dysfunctions of its patients and clients. These constructs concern the means and the goals of

Table 4–2. **Core Constructs Related to Occupational Dysfunction**

The Personal Impact of Occupational Dysfunction	• When persons are denied access to or have restrictions in their occupations, they experience a reduction in quality of life. • Occupational dysfunction disrupts the life story.
Consequences of Occupational Dysfunction	• When disease, trauma, or other factors disrupt or prevent participation in occupation, the lack of occupational performance may lead to further deterioration. • Maladaptive patterns of occupational performance also may be a factor in the etiology of some problems.
Disruption of Performance Components	Disruption of motor, cognitive, emotional, and other performance components may affect the ability to perform occupations.
Multidimensional Nature of Occupational Dysfunction	Occupational dysfunctions are multidimensional problems resulting from the interplay of biological, psychological, and ecological factors.
The Social Cost of Occupational Dysfunction	When individuals cannot adequately perform their occupations, social systems are also affected.

therapy. Together they define the fundamental nature of services offered by occupational therapy. Four constructs define these dynamics of therapy:

1. Participation in occupation as the core of therapy
2. Occupation as the level of intervention
3. Meaning in therapy
4. Occupation as the goal or outcome of therapy

We will examine each of these constructs in the following sections.

Participation in Occupation as the Core of Therapy. Reilly[82] identified as the essential premise of occupational therapy that "man through the use of his hands as they are energized by mind and will, can influence the state of his own health." This statement acknowledges that when humans engage in occupations using their physical and mental powers they can affect their biological and psychological status. It also calls attention to the fact that the use of occupation to improve health status is the basic dynamic of occupational therapy. The philosophical basis of occupational therapy adopted by the American Occupational Therapy Association[84] in 1979 articulates this premise further when it notes: "The common core of occupational therapy is active participation of the patient/client in occupation for purposes of improving performance."

Therapists employ the therapeutic agency of occupation though four primary pathways (Fig. 4–1). First, therapists provide direct opportunities to perform occupations that have been designed with specific therapeutic goals in mind. This occurs when a therapist provides an occupational form

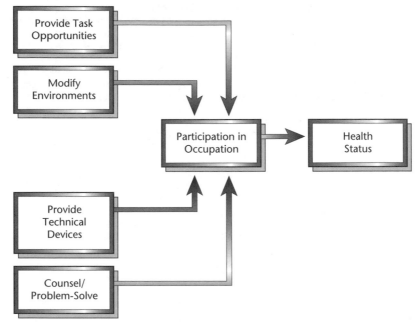

Figure 4–1. Pathways to employ occupation as therapy.

in which a patient or client is invited to participate. The occupational form can be simple sensory motor play, craft, work tasks, group projects, or any of an infinite variety of occupational forms selected for their anticipated therapeutic value.

Second, therapists enable people to engage in occupations by modifying the occupational forms a person does and the environment in which the person performs.[28,56] Therapists can modify occupational forms through strategies such as simplifying steps, providing special sensory or memory cues, or reducing expectations for outcomes. Environmental modifications include such things as removing architectural and structural barriers. Alteration of the human context to reduce complexity or stress in task performance is another form of environmental modification. Modification of the social environment has long been a part of occupational therapy, but the new emphasis on home health care, family involvement, industrial intervention, and school setting practice is making environmental modification an increasingly important aspect of intervention.

Third, occupational therapists provide the use of various technical devices that extend limited capacity or compensate for lost capacity. This technology ranges from simple adaptive equipment that has been modified to accommodate motor limitations, to complex, computer-based equipment that is used for communication and environmental control. As technology has improved, the potential to use it to create a better match between persons of limited capacities and the occupations they wish to perform has greatly increased.

Fourth, therapists may enable persons to engage in occupations through counseling and problem solving. The therapeutic goal is to facilitate the *client or patient's* ability to participate in occupations. Because the effects of occupation pervade the person's life in a way that extends well beyond the therapeutic session, therapy can have far-reaching effects. This is especially true when therapy influences how persons engage in occupation outside of therapy.

To summarize, therapists may employ the therapeutic agency of occupation to influence the health of the individual in a variety of ways. Participation in occupation is both the dynamic and the defining characteristic of occupational therapy.

Occupation as the Level of Intervention. As the field has changed from the prior mechanistic model to the emerging paradigm of practice, substantial debate has centered on the appropriate methodology of practice. The crux of this debate can be characterized as whether occupational therapy should "treat at the micro level of performance components and subskills . . . or at the macro level of actual performance of relevant occupations."[107] Another way of characterizing the debate, according to Trombly,[100] is the bottom-up versus the top-down approach.

The mechanistic paradigm focused occupational therapy's attention downward to the underlying occupational performance components. It assumed that improvement in these components would yield corresponding improvement in occupational performance. The new view recognizes two important flaws with this approach.

First, when underlying performance components cannot be fully restored, the adaptation to permanent disability requires something different: a reorganization of the whole. This reorganization can only be attended to at the level of the occupations that make up the parts of the person's everyday life and the level of the whole occupational life and its meanings for the persons. The bottom-up approach is insufficient for the adaptation that most persons with disabilities must make in their lives.

Second, performance is naturally organized from the top down. As we have already noted, people move their bodies, process sensory information, and think in context. Thus, performance is dependent not only on underlying components but also on the goal of the occupation and the context.[56,102] For example, new understandings of the nervous system argue that people do not move their bodies according to some inner instructions or motor schema. Rather, performance is nested in the intentions of the person (which are profoundly influenced by the occupational form the person is pursuing) and in the physical context.

Performance is occupationally embedded. When therapy seeks to restore, alter, or reorganize performance, it must employ methods that are occupationally embedded, that proceed from the occupational whole. As Wood[107] argued, "a wide variance in performance abilities in real-life occupations cannot be explained by the status of, or by improvements in, performance components at the micro level of occupational functioning." Rather they are due to the alignment of these components within the occupational context.

This construct is calling attention to the need to reinvent the methods of therapy that became stripped of their occupational context in the mechanistic paradigm era. It calls attention to the occupations that are employed in therapy so that their organizing effects may be carefully selected to invite and direct the organization of performance.

Therapy and Meaning. According to Yerxa,[110] "engagement in occupation encompasses not only the observable performance of individuals, but also their subjective reactions to the activity and objects with which they are occupied." Therefore, the patient or client must find meaning in the actions that constitute therapy. This meaning ordinarily derives from the patient's experiential background, the current impact of the dysfunction on the patient's experience, and the significance of the therapeutic activity negotiated between the therapist and the patient.

Meanings vary tremendously. A child with sensory motor problems may find meaning in therapy simply by experiencing fun in activities that would ordinarily be threatening. In an occupation, a person with spinal cord injury may find what kind of life is still possible, despite limitations in physical capacities. The person with severe cognitive dysfunction may find the meaning of increased control, security, and coherence.

Respect for individual relevance of activities is important in therapy. This means taking the time and effort to discover the meaning that each performance has for a person in the context of his or her disability and other life experiences.[51,52] In the end, the meaning that is experienced in the therapeutic process determines the impact of the activity on the individual. Negotiating meaning in therapy requires mutual cooperation between the therapist and the patient or client.[110]

Just as the concept of narrative has augmented the construct of meaning in occupation, it has also contributed to an understanding of how meaning operates in therapy. Helfrich, Kielhofner, and Mattingly[40] argue that therapy is an event that enters into and becomes part of the life story of the patient. The meaning that therapy has for the patient is related to its relevance and impact upon the patient's life story. Clark[25] argues that therapy involves occupational story-making, in which the therapist helps the patient to reinvent his or her life story, finding, as it were, new possibilities for continuing what has happened in one's life. Hence, new life meaning is discovered and enacted in the course of therapy.

Summary. The broad assumption that occupation can be employed as a therapeutic means defines the basic dynamic of occupational therapy. Table 4–3 lists the constructs that define the use of occupation as a therapeutic tool. These themes define conditions under which occupation has a therapeutic effect and the type of impact it can have.

Focal Viewpoint

The focal viewpoint is the field's way of making sense of that with which it is concerned. Through the focal viewpoint, occupational therapy frames the phenomena that are within its domain of interest. In the previous chapter, we saw that, during the first occupational therapy paradigm, the focal viewpoint embraced a holistic picture of the interdependence of mind, body, and environment. We also saw how this focal viewpoint was replaced during the second paradigm with a reductionistic focus on underlying musculoskeletal, neurological, and intrapsychic mechanisms.

The focal viewpoint is, once again, undergoing rapid transformation. In the 1980s occupational therapists began to re-emphasize a holistic per-

*Table 4–3. **Occupation and the Dynamics of Therapy***

Participation in Occupation as Core of Therapy	• When humans engage in occupations using their physical and mental powers, they can affect their biological and psychological status.
	• Use of occupation to improve health status is the basic dynamic of occupational therapy.
	• Therapists may employ the therapeutic agency of occupation through four primary pathways:
	  1. Provide opportunities to perform occupations
	  2. Enable people to engage in occupations by modifying environments and tasks
	  3. Provide the use of technical devices that extend limited capacity or compensate for lost capacity
	  4. Enable persons to engage in occupations through counseling and problem solving

Occupation as the Level of Intervention	When therapy seeks to restore, alter, or reorganize performance, it must employ methods that are occupationally embedded.
Therapy and Meaning	• The patient or client must find meaning in the actions that constitute the therapy. • Respect for individual relevance of activities is important in therapy. • Therapy is an event that enters into and becomes part of the life story of the patient. • Therapy involves occupational story making in which the therapist helps the patient to reinvent his or her life story. • New life meaning is discovered and enacted in the course of therapy.

spective. Much of this viewpoint was influenced by systems theory, which emerged in the life sciences, but quickly became a grand or metatheory with applications across a range of disciplines and applied fields such as occupational therapy.

Early systems theorists criticized reductionism, arguing that it failed to recognize how human beings functioned as wholes and that they were intimately tied to their environments.[6,7,11,17,59] Systems theory also emphasized that living systems evolved and changed, demonstrating a kind of complexity that could not be grasped from the mechanistic metaphors of reductionism. Recognizing that these criticisms of reductionism were also relevant to occupational therapy's mechanistic paradigm, many occupational therapy writers began to incorporate systems concepts as new ways to think about the phenomena with which they were concerned.*

Within the last decade, a new set of concepts referred to as *dynamical systems theory* began to be introduced into occupational therapy. While building upon the original aims of systems theory, dynamical systems theory has brought forward concepts and arguments that replace earlier formulations.†

As was the case with earlier systems theory, the concepts of dynamical systems are being applied in a variety of fields.[80] Dynamical systems theory is, in the words of Vallacher and Nowak,[104] "a broad metatheory from which to generate topic-specific principles and a set of paradigmatic guidelines . . .". In occupational therapy, different authors and researchers concerned with a range of phenomena have already begun to apply dynamical systems concepts to the particular problems in which they are interested (e.g., movement, cognition, and motivation).

---

*Since systems theory has been changing rapidly, occupational therapy writings may reflect different "generations" or branches of systems thought. Thus occupational therapy writings from a few years ago may employ concepts and arguments that have been replaced in systems theory with newer ones.

†One example of how recent dynamical systems theory has replaced earlier systems concepts is the concept of hierarchy.[11] Systems theory originally emphasized that nature was organized into a hierarchy of levels of phenomena in which lower levels were integrated into higher more complex levels. It emphasized that the higher level represented an emergent complexity and order that could not be attributed entirely to the underlying parts of which it was composed. Hierarchies were proposed as fixed orders having fairly invariant relationships between levels (e.g., higher levels governing lower levels, lower levels constraining higher levels).

Hierarchy was proposed as part of the grand architecture of nature, and systems literature emphasized the hierarchical structure of many different types of systems, including, for example, the brain. Current systems thinking recognizes that hierarchical arrangements can be found in the brain and in other parts of nature, but it emphasizes that these are "functional hierarchies" realized as part of a dynamic process, and not rigid structures. Moreover, the older concept of hierarchy left unanswered the question of how the new emergent order at each new level of complexity came about. Dynamical systems theory has introduced a set of concepts that do a much better job of explaining emergent, self-organizing complexity. Thus, while dynamical systems theory recognizes and addresses many of the same problems as earlier systems theory, it often "reframes" some of the problems and offers new concepts that give more detailed descriptions and explanations.

Since dynamical systems concepts address many, if not all, the problems originally posed by older systems ideas in a more complete and contemporary fashion, it is reasonable to expect that the concepts and perspectives of dynamical systems theory will fundamentally shape occupational therapy's focal viewpoint. It is also important that many features of dynamical systems theory strongly resonate with other aspects of occupational therapy's contemporary paradigm.

The Systems Approach to Understanding Organized Complexity

When a carpenter builds a house, a child stacks blocks, a cook prepares a meal, or a professor delivers a lecture, many different kinds of phenomena are involved. All performers have goals *in mind*, which they pursue employing their bodies (e.g., *musculoskeletal and nervous systems*), following methods and experiencing meanings derived from their *sociocultural contexts*. Hence, as Mosey[69] notes, occupational therapy spans the spectrum of biological, psychological, and social phenomena. Moreover, as Yerxa[113] points out, this range of phenomena challenges occupational therapy to adopt ways of knowing that can grasp this complexity. The importance of earlier and current systems concepts is that they provide a way of understanding the organized complexity of occupation.

To consider how systems theory approaches the problem of organized complexity, let us begin with two simple observations. When an individual performs a simple motor activity such as reaching out to grasp a door knob, he or she never does it in the same way, that is, never uses exactly the same movements or contracts exactly the same muscles. Similarly, when a person greets a neighbor, he or she never uses exactly the same words with exactly the same inflection of tone. While the goal of such tasks may not vary, the details of how the neuromuscular and mental performance components fulfill the goals is highly variable and highly sensitive, both to the context of performance and to the state of the person (e.g., level of fatigue or mood) at the time of the performance.[101]

Importantly, when persons perform, they are definitely not following a specific preset pattern. Nonetheless, this is precisely how reductionism explained behavior. Reductionist strategies such as those employed during the mechanistic paradigm assumed that grasping a doorknob or greeting someone could be explained by recourse to underlying musculoskeletal structures, nervous system instructions, cognitive scripts, and personality traits that were present before and merely evoked during the performance. Reductionism viewed the human being as analogous to a machine with all the instructions and causal connections for functioning "built-in." Consequently, reductionism led us to believe that once all the parts of a system were catalogued and understood, we could explain behavior from the bottom up. In retrospect, we can see that this was a mistaken approach.

Systems concepts take up where reductionism has let off in helping occupational therapy understand how persons engage in their occupational behavior. Reductionistic strategies have given us an important view of the complex structures involved in the biopsychosocial phenomena with which occupational therapy is concerned. For example, we now have detailed information about the structure of the musculoskeletal and nervous systems and about some of the stable patterns that underlie such phenomena as cognition and motivation. While reductionism revealed how the potential for grasping and greeting exists in the make-up of the musculoskeletal, neurological, and mental systems, it did not explain how these systems actually manage to do a "grasp" or a "greeting."*

Self-Organizing Processes. Dynamical systems theory asserts that human behavior is *self-organizing*.[49,104]

Hence, the act of grasping an object cannot be fully explained by recourse to the musculoskeletal and nervous systems because grasping is an emergent, self-organizing process. Specifically, this means that behavior only gets put together when the performance is happening. This forces us to look to the process itself to understand what is going on rather than looking "behind the scenes" as reductionism did.

Dynamical systems' explanation of self-organization involved a number of key concepts. The first of these is *degrees of freedom*.[32,49] Simply stated, degrees of freedom refers to the number of possibilities that are built into existing structures or patterns of the human being. Consider the musculoskeletal system; it is composed of approximately 100 joints. Each of these joints allows motions such as flexion, extension, and rotation. These motions can be combined simultaneously and sequentially and at varying velocities, thus creating an enormous number of possibilities for movement. The brain contains approximately a hundred billion neurons.[49] Each neuron has connections with hundreds to thousands of other neurons, making possible more patterns of neuronal firing than the imagination can grasp. Consider further the vast number of ideas, feelings, associations, and memories of which the human psyche is capable. Human beings, by virtue of the degrees of freedom in their musculoskeletal, neurological, and mental structures, represent the potential for an incomprehensive number of possibilities for behavior. Add to this that much of behavior takes place in a

---

*Another way of contrasting the mechanistic approach with the systems approach is that the former placed a high degree of emphasis on understanding the architecture underlying occupational behavior. Hence, occupational therapists sought to understand the *structures* that influenced how people chose, did, and reacted to their occupations. The current emphasis of dynamical systems is on *process*. It is concerned with how behavior unfolds in time and recurs over time.

sociocultural context in which other actors embody the same degrees of freedom. And how all the persons involved can combine their behaviors further multiplies the number of possibilities. We now begin to have a picture of the degrees of freedom available for completing everyday occupational behaviors.

Yet, each instance of occupational behavior (doing a chore, talking with a friend, driving to work in traffic, reading a book, sweeping the floor, hammering a nail, dancing with a partner, writing a report) harnesses a very small subset of those potentials into a unique organized pattern. Thus, while degrees of freedom in the biological and psychological make-up and in the sociocultural context of the person are legion, the actual patterns of motion, neuronal firings, mental imagery, and social interaction that converge in occupational performance are relatively constrained. These elements come together in an organized pattern. As we noted earlier, reductionism tried to explain this organized pattern by recourse to the underlying components; but the underlying components only give rise to possibilities: Something else is involved when a subset of those possibilities are utilized in the behavior.

Soft Assembly and Synergies. Dynamical systems theory observes that states of order, including organized behavior, arise spontaneously in complex systems without any central agent or underlying causal mechanism. Many parts "cooperate together," achieving some higher, emergent order.[37]

The concept of emergent order is widely demonstrated in the physical sciences. An everyday example is the formation of a whirlpool when water drains out of a sink or tub. The molecules of water provide the necessary degrees of freedom; that is, water molecules are appropriately "sticky" and "slippery" to give water its liquid properties. However, the formation of a whirlpool is not simply determined by the molecular structure of water. Rather, it occurs as a dynamic process. Millions of water molecules cooperate together to form the highly organized pattern of the whirlpool without any prior chemical or physical instructions. The whirlpool occurs under a set of dynamic conditions (i.e., the flow of water pulled by gravity and constrained by the physical context of the sink with its drain opening).

A necessary condition of the emergence of all organized patterns is a flow of energy or information.[49] An analogous flow occurs in humans when, for instance, the body is metabolizing nutrients, body parts are moving in space, or information is coursing through the brain. Ongoing action and experience are, then, to the organization of grasping or greeting what the flow of water is to the organization of a whirlpool.

According to dynamical systems theory, behavior is organized by being put together or assembled when the process of the behavior is happening. This process of self-organization is referred to as *soft assembly*.[95,103] For soft assembly in human behavior to occur, the relevant musculoskeletal, neurological, and mental components must be coupled with the task being performed and with the environment. Just as the whirlpool does not emerge unless there is a dynamic flow occurring in a particular kind of constrained environment, particular human behaviors only occur when the biological and psychological components are involved in dynamic action within certain task and contextual constraints. In the case of grasping an object with the musculoskeletal apparatus of the upper extremity, the nervous system, the intention* to grasp the object, gravity, and the location, size, and shape of the object are all involved.

It is not necessary that complete instructions for performance are stored beforehand in the brain since, as Kelso[49] argues, the behavior emerges "in a self-organized fashion, without any agent-like entity ordering the elements, telling them where to go." Rather, as Fogel and Thelen[32] point out, the way in which all the elements cooperate together "is not rigidly fixed beforehand, but is strictly a function of the status of the organism in a particular task context."

During any performance, the degrees of freedom are "not controlled directly but are constrained to relate among themselves."[49] This constrained relationship among elements is referred to as a *synergy*, which is a functional unit that assembles for the purposes of and during a particular kind of performance.[49,95] Here is an example of such a synergy that you can readily demonstrate to yourself. Place two objects in front of yourself—one closer and the other a bit farther away. Now, reach out to grasp the two objects (one in each hand) starting with both hands simultaneously. Notice what happens. If you look carefully, you will see that the two reaches are coordinated together as a single functional synergy, that is, both hands terminate at their target objects at the same time. To accomplish this, the hand reaching for the more distant object travels at a higher speed than the other hand reaching for the nearer object.[49] So long as you begin both movements at the same time, you will notice that what "feels most natural" is to move your two arms in such a way that the two different movements are functionally linked. This coupling of the two movements together (a synergy in dynamical systems terms) does not exist outside the actual process of performance. Like other synergies, it emerges

---

*One might object that an intention is needed to precede and direct the action. Then it might be argued that the intention represents the instructions that precede and direct the behavior. However, intention itself is conceptualized as arising dynamically out of its own set of relevant conditions. Moreover, the intention to move does not need to proceed or even exist outside the purposeful act of movement itself. It can be implicit in the behavior as when one unthinkingly reaches for the doorknob while anticipating what is on the other side of the door. In fact, what is most remarkable about the influence of intention on action is that it need not be directly focused on the action itself. For example, Trombly[102] discusses an experiment in which persons were to grasp a coin with the intention either to toss it or to place it in a slot. It turns out that the act of grasping the coin was organized differently when the intention was to put it in a slot versus to toss it.

during the performance of a specific task and disappears once the performance is over.

The synergy itself emerges out of the confluence of these elements: the musculoskeletal and nervous system performance components, the physical distances of the two objects, and the task. The latter elements, namely, the specific thing that is being performed and the physical conditions under which it is being performed, are as important to the emergence of the synergy as are the performance components. No single aspect dictates or instructs the behavior. It occurs as an emergent property when all those elements are brought together in a dynamic process.

A second feature of synergies is worth noting. They are not rigid, fixed structures. If you really concentrate on it, you can vary the act of reaching for two objects so that it breaks out of this synergy, so to speak. For example, you can force one hand to get where it's going before the other, but you will have to concentrate and, perhaps, move more slowly, and the behavior will not feel as smooth or natural. It is not inaccurate to say that we feel ourselves attracted toward doing the activity in a particular way.

Dynamic Attractors and Parameters. While each instance of behavior is unique, the overall pattern of a behavioral synergy has similar characteristics. Thus, when a person goes about any particular task, the way in which elements are recruited together (in the case of the previous example, movements of the two arms) tends to take on a particular configuration or pattern. The tendency for this configuration or pattern to occur is termed a dynamic attractor.[95] As Thelen and Ulrich explain, the attractor exists "strictly as a result of the cooperativeness of the participating elements in a particular context."[95] While the dynamic attractor is a preferred way for the system to behave (or the way it is statistically most likely to behave), it is not fixed or obligatory.[37,49,95] As in the example above, one can, with effort, disturb the synergy that results from the dynamic attractor.

The stability of an attractor state is linked to its ability to dissipate the information or energy that threatens to destabilize it. So, for example, when persons hold certain attitudes, they will tend to dissipate information that threatens to disrupt that attitude. A person who believes he or she is not competent will dismiss a certain amount of feedback to the contrary, as all experienced therapists are aware.* The way in which dynamic attractors dissipate information actually serves to reinforce the relative strength of the attractor.

Phase Shifts and Control Parameters. While dynamic attractors have a probability of arising when conditions are right, they are also sensitive to

---

*Different dynamic attractors account for the disparate reactions that different people may have to the same situation. For example, a person for whom confidence is a dynamic attractor will tend to interpret a personal mistake as an exception to his or her competence, while someone else whose attractor state is insecurity will interpret it as more evidence of his or her incompetence.

the characteristics of those elements or variables that are interacting together as part of the synergy. These characteristics of variables that are part of the synergy are referred to as *parameters*.[49] So, for example, in the act of reaching out to grasp an object, some of the relevant parameters are the distance and size of the object, strength in the upper extremity, and the amount of bodily fatigue or energy.

In addition, one does not, for example, reach and grasp objects from some intentional and behavioral vacuum, but rather one does it as part of a history of unfolding action.[49] Hence, all behavior represents a transition from one organized state to another. Understanding behavior requires that we pay attention to how one pattern of behavior transforms or shifts into another dynamic pattern. A dynamic attractor exists when the values or characteristics of all the contributing elements are within certain parameters. When one of the parameters exceeds a critical value, it can result in dissolution of the synergy or it can result in a whole new, qualitatively different pattern.[49,95] For example, when we attempt to persuade a hesitant friend or loved one to join us in some activity, we hold an expectation of success as we talk on and on about how much fun it will be. As we continue unsuccessfully to persuade the second person, confidence decreases. Once our confidence wanes to a certain level, what follows might be the dissolution of the behavior (i.e., we just give up on convincing the other person). On the other hand, a new pattern may emerge as when we switch to a different emotional and tactical strategy (e.g., the angry response "you never want do anything I want to do").

As the preceding example illustrates, a system will tend to "resist or dampen perturbations up to a point, beyond which there is a rapid collapse of the attractor."[104] While we may maintain a behavioral strategy to a point as our confidence in its efficacy wanes, when we reach a critical threshold, our behavior will qualitatively change. In this way, dynamic attractors react like the proverbial camel's back, broken by the addition of a single straw.

Transformations from one dynamic pattern of behavior to another are referred to as *phase shifts*, and the parameter whose change in value triggered the phase shift is referred to as the *control parameter*.[95,104] The control parameter does not prescribe or contain a code for the new pattern of organized behavior that emerges; it simply creates new dynamics within which the relevant variables will cooperate together to assemble to new behavior.[49]

Locomotion provides a useful example of how phase shifts from one dynamic attractor to another operate. The dynamic attractor for locomotion in the sufficiently mature human is walking with an alternation of stepping and weight bearing by the lower extremities. Relevant variables include the available joints and musculature of the lower extremity, a stepping reflex, gravitational forces, the walking surface, and the task (or intention) of getting from here to there.

If one of the parameters changes sufficiently, the overall organization of locomotion will qualitatively change. One need only watch footage of

Neil Armstrong walking on the moon to see that, when one parameter is altered (e.g., strength of gravitational pull), gait also takes on different qualitative characteristics. Of course, one need not go to the moon to see a phase shift in ambulation. For example, observe a parent teaching his or her child to ride a bicycle. The task of staying alongside a child who is speeding up can shift someone's ambulation from walking to running. In this case, the phase shift from walking to running is triggered by the change in the control parameter, speed.

Such phase shifts occur across domains of behavior; motivation is another good example. The motivation for an occupation is often engendered by the excitement posed by the challenge, that is, the relationship between one's abilities and the demands of the activity. However, as one engages in the activity, skill increases and the challenge decreases, and one tires of the activity. Hence, a qualitative shift in organization of motivation, that is, from enjoying an activity to being bored by it, can be precipitated by a change in skill. Conversely, if the gap is widened too much (as in a loss of skill due to a physical impairment, or a change of context in which the occupation is performed), enjoyment may be transformed to anxiety or anger.

Large qualitative shifts can result when a control parameter changes by a small amount if the change crosses a critical threshold. On the other hand, no change in behavior may result from even greater amounts of change in parameters that are within the range of values for which a dynamic attractor still holds.[49,95] Moreover, when behavioral synergies change following a change in some system variable, the former is not necessarily proportional to or even in the same direction as the latter. For example, increasing one's empathy for another sometimes results in the other's withdrawing. Such seemingly paradoxical aspects of human behavior can be explained as dynamic attractors. This lack of correspondence between changes in parameter values and behavioral synergies is referred to as *nonlinearity*.[95] The property of nonlinearity accounts for the difficulty of predicting much of human behavior.

Viewing Occupation Through a Systems Perspective

In the stream of everyday occupational life, behavioral strategies emerge, dissolve, and transform. Systems concepts argue that underlying this ongoing flow of behavior is not a preprogrammed set of instructions and structures but rather the effect of dynamic attractors.* Relevant per-

---

*As Haken[37] and Vallacher and Nowak[104] have observed, it is likely that biological and psychological systems are not entirely governed by dynamical principles. We are most likely to find dynamic processes at work when there is a significant flow of energy in the system. Indeed, it may be a feature of some aspects of occupational dysfunction that the flow of energy or information is insufficient to maintain dynamic patterns that are important to adaptive functioning. In such cases, the system may collapse back toward a much more mechanistic state.

sonal, environmental, and task variables coalesce to form the dynamic conditions out of which our emotions, thoughts, and actions take shape. Systems theory offers a picture in which we see occupational behavior patterns emerging and transforming across time.

Another part of the system's picture is the coordination of patterns across levels. To consider how this works, let us return to the example of ambulation. The ambulating human is a biopsychological system (i.e., a system involving the musculoskeletal, neurological, and mental or intentional elements) engaged in a particular task (walking). Now consider the situation of two persons going for a walk together. The new system is a biopsychosocial system in which two separate musculoskeletal, neurological, and mental systems must be coupled together.

The synergy that exists in the musculoskeletal and neurological systems of each of the two walkers are nested within the social system. Moreover, the emergent social pattern between the two walkers adds new dimensionality to environmental conditions, influencing the organized pattern of each walker. The occupational task of going for a walk together requires both persons to move forward at the same speed. Unless the two persons naturally walk at exactly the same pace, one or both persons must adjust their stride. But, because the overarching system is now a social system, new variables come into play. For example, the pace of walking that emerges (a dynamic attractor) includes the relative dominance of the personalities of the walking partners.[4] This kind of influence across levels (e.g., biological, psychological, and social) is a feature of complex systems.[49]

Systems theory provides occupational therapy with a picture of organized complexity in which the human being must be viewed as a biopsychosocial entity, with performance components that are recruited into behavioral synergies in the context of actual performance in a task and environmental context. The picture also includes levels of phenomena in which synergies are nested within larger synergies. Finally, the view underscores the importance of considering behavior in time, and of understanding how behavior shifts from one pattern to another.

The Importance of Occupation in the Systems Perspective

System theory's explanation of how behavior is organized arose outside occupational therapy. However, the concepts strongly support the long-standing idea that having a specific occupation to perform recruits and organizes behavior. Dynamical systems theory underscores the idea that the task (or in contemporary occupational therapy terminology, the occupational form) is essential to any dynamic attractor. Without the occupations that specify what it is that the human being is accomplishing, musculoskeletal, neurological, and mental components do not get coupled together into organized patterns.

Let us return for just a moment to the greeting card I introduced in Chapter 1. The man who painted the postcard was judged by the psychiatrist to be unable to concentrate. Assuming that the psychiatrist was a trained observer who accurately saw the patient having extreme difficulty concentrating, why was the patient able to paint a watercolor that obviously required substantial concentration? The answer lies in the fact that concentration is not something that a person has or doesn't have. Concentration does not exist as a feature of the brain or mental structures that precede and instruct behavior. Rather, concentration is a dynamic pattern of behavior that happens when the neurological and mental systems coordinate in the midst of doing an occupation. The organized behavior that we refer to as concentration is a quality of this emergent order. There is a kind of sorcery in occupations that recruits organized behavior that apparently was absent before. We now recognize such behavioral patterns as emergent properties.

This is an important lesson. Occupational therapy's previous paradigm attributed performance to underlying mechanisms or performance components. We now understand that, while these underlying components (e.g., neuromuscular) are necessary to performance, they are not enough to produce the kind of competent action needed for everyday life. What completes the picture is the occupation that the person is doing.

The Impact of Dynamical Systems Concepts in Occupational Therapy

It should be clear that the systems concepts offer a viewpoint on the phenomena with which occupational therapy is concerned that is distinctly different from the previous mechanistic perspective. This viewpoint will influence how occupational therapists think about and investigate what they do. In the end it will also influence how they go about therapy.

As Newston[72] notes, dynamical systems theory has an important "heuristic and metaphorical" value; that is, the theory provides a means of beginning to map onto reality some possible explanations for behavior processes that previously could not be fully explained. For example, qualitative changes in motor behavior and dramatic reversals of motivation that could not be accounted for in linear models are more fully explained from a dynamical systems perspective.[56] Systems concepts also provide a useful heuristic framework of clinical reasoning. When, for example, a behavioral process undergoes a transformation from one state to another, therapists can ask if the transformation represents a phase shift resulting from some critical change in some parameter value. By giving the field alternative ways to frame situations, it opens clinical reasoning up to new ways to examine and understand patient behavior.

Systems concepts have also triggered new methods of investigation in occupational therapy. For example, occupational therapy researchers have begun to study how dynamic synergies emerge in the context of performing occupations.[48,64,108]

Finally, systems theory offers this new way of understanding the therapeutic process. It goes something like the following. The effects of therapy are not limited to simple linear changes in underlying performance components (e.g., strengthening muscles or increasing confidence). Rather, therapeutic change involves complex reorganization. Performance components, occupational forms, and environmental conditions are part of the multiple factors that may be realigned, altered, and coordinated into a new order. Occupational therapy, by providing individuals with opportunities to achieve new patterns of behavior within the context of occupational forms, empowers them to reshape and reorganize themselves and their lives into adaptive patterns.

Focal Viewpoint: Summary

In this section I provided an overview of the focal viewpoint. I have argued that the current focal viewpoint of occupational therapy is strongly determined by systems theory. This section examined some of the main arguments and concepts from systems theory and their impact on occupational therapy thinking. Table 4–4 summarizes these themes.

Integrative Values

Values play a strong role in shaping the collective vision of occupational therapy.[33,45] Moreover, the practice of occupational therapy requires decision making that must be guided by values.[88] Therefore, the integrative values of the paradigm define the goals toward which the profession and the practitioner should strive. Values identify what occupational therapy should be in order to understand and serve the needs of human beings.

Dialogue over values in occupational therapy has been intense and international in the last two decades. To some degree, the international dialogue has arisen out of concern that the values of occupational therapy expressed a biased, Western point of view. As therapists representing diverse cultures have joined the dialogue, there has been an increasingly thoughtful and critical discourse concerning what values should guide occupational therapy. This dialogue is certainly not finished. Nor should it be. Values require constant attention and scrutiny.

Occupational therapy shares many values with other professions and scholarly disciplines. However, it also possesses a value orientation that reflects the unique ongoing dialogue within the field. Not all the values expressed here are confined to occupational therapists, but the configura-

Table 4–4. Systems Thought and the Focal Viewpoint

The Systems Approach to Understanding Organized Complexity	• Occupation spans a complex spectrum of biological, psychological, and social phenomena. • Systems concepts provide a way of understanding the organized complexity of occupation.
Self-Organizing Processes	Human behavior is self-organizing: • Degrees of freedom refers to the possibilities built into structures or the patterns of the human being. • Occupational behavior harnesses a very small subset of those potentials into a unique organized pattern.
Soft Assembly and Synergies	Organized behavior arises spontaneously in complex systems without any central agent or underlying causal mechanism: • Many parts "cooperate together" to achieve an emergent order. • A necessary condition is a flow of energy or information. • Behavior is organized by soft assembly, i.e., being put together or assembled when the process of the behavior is happening. • Elements cooperate together in a synergy as a function of the organism in a particular task context.
Dynamic Attractors and Parameters	• A dynamic attractor is a preferred (i.e., statistically probable) way for the system to behave. • The stability of a dynamic attractor is linked to its ability to dissipate information or energy that threatens to destabilize it.
Phase Shifts and Control Parameters	Dynamic attractors are sensitive to the characteristics (i.e., parameters) of those elements or variables that are interacting together as part of the synergy: • A dynamic attractor exists when the values or characteristics of all the contributing elements are within certain parameters. • When one parameter exceeds a critical value it can result in dissolution of the synergy or in a qualitatively different pattern. • Transformation from one dynamic pattern of behavior to another is referred to as a phase shift. • The parameter whose change in value triggered the phase shift is referred to as the control parameter. • The lack of correspondence between changes in parameter values and behavioral synergies is referred to as nonlinearity.
Viewing Occupation through a Systems Perspective	Systems theory provides occupational therapy with the following picture of organized complexity in the human being: • A biopsychosocial being with performance components that are recruited into behavioral synergies in the context of actual performance in a task and an environmental context. • Levels of phenomena in which synergies are nested within larger synergies. • Behavior occurring in time with shifts from one pattern to another.

Table 4–4. Systems Thought and the Focal Viewpoint (Continued)

Importance of Occupation in the Systems Perspective	Systems theory underscores that the task (or in contemporary occupational therapy terminology, the occupational form) is essential to any dynamic attractor.
The Impact of Dynamical Systems Concepts in Occupational Therapy	Systems theory: • Has an important "heuristic and metaphorical functions" for mapping onto reality possible explanations for behavior. • Provides a useful heuristic framework for clinical reasoning. • Has triggered new methods of investigation in occupational therapy. • Offers a new picture of the therapeutic process: 　○ Effects of therapy are not limited to simple linear changes in underlying performance components. 　○ Therapeutic change involves complex reorganization. 　○ Therapy provides opportunities to achieve new patterns of behavior within the context of occupational forms.

tion of these values together, as well as the emphases that are placed on certain value themes, reflect a unique occupational therapy perspective.

My aim is to highlight those values that have the most influence on the field, emphasizing those themes that are unique to occupational therapy. Moreover, each value reflects a theme with several related subthemes. The way in which I have catalogued these values represents an interpretation of the literature and will not necessarily correspond with how others have categorized values.

Client-Centered Practice

Under the leadership of occupational therapists from Canada, the theme of client-centered practice has been articulated. This theme asserts that the client must be the focal point of the therapeutic process.

The client-centered theme begins with the assertion of each person's essential humanity and worth. It is recognized that, while dignity is a birthright,[42] the worth of the individual is enhanced when persons actualize potential and enhance their own competence.[1,73] Moreover, the entire process of therapy and the relationship between clients and therapists must be guided by a profound respect for and understanding of the client's perspectives, desires, and needs.

Client-centered practice is most critical in the therapist-client relationship; it involves:

an involvement on the therapist's part which creates expectations; it is goal-directed toward the client's self-understanding and self-responsibility. In this process, the occupational therapist is a mirror or a sounding board helping the client develop awareness of emotions, perceptions of self and of reality; a model for identification; and a source of gratification in providing the client with the experience of a positive relationship, of being understood and cared for.[73]

Underlying the therapist's use of self should be an attitude of altruism that reflects "unselfish concern for the welfare of others."[1]* And this means that the therapist may alternately take on different roles, including those of a technician with particular knowledge, a collaborating partner, or a friend who genuinely cares about the client.[77]

Client-centered practice requires an attitude of empathy toward the circumstances of the patient. Empathy involves:

> (a) an expression of *being there*, (b) a turning of the soul, (c) a recognition of likeness and uniqueness, (d) an entry into the other's experience, (e) a connection with the other's feelings, (f) a power to recover from that connection, and (g) a personal enrichment that derives from these actions.[79]

This empathy is carried out uniquely in occupational therapy through a form of *doing with* the patient, reaching for both the hands and heart of the patient in the midst of the patient's performing occupations.[79]

Occupation

During the mechanistic era many occupational therapists experienced embarrassment over their involvement with everyday occupations. As Reilly[82] notes, "The wide and gaping chasm which exists between the complexity of illness and the commonplaceness of our treatment tools is, and always will be, both the pride and anguish of our profession." Over the past two decades, however, there has been a return of respect and value for occupation. Occupational therapy seems to have rediscovered the centrality of occupation to human life and well-being.

The field increasingly embraces the view that occupations have intrinsic value for human life and that persons need to participate in occupations.[8,33] As Yerxa notes,[111] occupational therapy holds as critically important "participation . . . in the stream of life." Johnson[45] echoes this theme that occupations connect people to life:

---

*It should be noted that the concept of altruism has been challenged as being "centered in occupational therapists, rather than the practice of occupational therapy."[42] Moreover, it is suggested that this value can "connote a power relationship of *doing unto* and *doing for* the recipient of the altruistic act.[42] Such a connotation is in opposition to the idea of doing with the client in therapy. This criticism is certainly worth considering. However, it seems that the idea of altruism is still an important reminder that the therapeutic process is one in which the therapist is emotionally and intellectually involved and that, in the midst of such involvement, the therapist should not lose sight of the fact that therapy exists for the benefit of the client. Personal satisfaction and gain from the process must be weighed as secondary.

> We value [patients'] desire to integrate themselves into life to the extent possible for them—and we seek to help them enter the mainstream of life: to shop in markets, to attend movies, to listen to the music of great symphonies; to see and feel the beauty of ballet, to work, to play, to watch, to feel.

The value of occupation in developing the human potential is also an important theme. It is asserted that participation in occupation

> plays a major role in developing and exercising self-direction, initiative, interdependence, and relatedness to the world. Activities verify the individual's ability to adapt, and they establish a satisfying balance between autonomy and societal membership.[1]

The centrality of occupation to a "good life" and the charge of occupational therapy to promote and support occupation in persons' lives is a resonant theme in the field today. Bing[9] stated the imperative a decade ago in these words:

> The grand tasks of occupational therapy are to attend to the multiple, complex, interrelated, and critical human activities of not just living, but living well.

Value of the Patient's/Client's Perspective

Occupational therapy holds that it is important to know and respect the unique perspective of the patient or client.[41,56,68] Therapists see the client's experiences and desires as the background against which judgments about adaptivity and the need for change should be made.[31,45,78,111] As McColl[68] argues, the client knows

> what it feels like to experience a balance or imbalance in occupational areas, and at some level, he or she knows what needs to be done to recalibrate the difference"

Such a way of looking is non-normative; it extols the right of individuals to define and pursue their own problems and needs. This value includes the recognition that disability is a personal matter, experienced uniquely by each person. According to this value, the experiential world of the patient or client should be the focal point of the therapeutic process.[52] This means a commitment to the patient's right to make choices and exercise decisions.[45]

An increasingly important theme has been that culture constitutes the subjective perspective of the patient or client. Culture determines persons' views of occupational life and of disease and disability.[60] Moreover, it influences persons' ways of thinking, feeling, communicating, and, ultimately, of participating in therapy.[41,60] Therefore, therapy should affirm and validate the client's cultural beliefs and perspectives.[41] This requires that occupational therapists must avoid imposing values derived from their own professional perspectives that may clash with those of the client.*

Active Engagement and Empowerment

Occupational therapists see the individual as the locus of the dynamics that will determine health outcomes. Occupational therapy requires the active, and meaning-driven participation of the patients who, through the quality of their participation, determine the value and effectiveness of the therapy.[107]

This value requires a collaborative relationship in which the patient is considered an equal participant in the health care process.[111] This also means that therapists must reject hierarchical models in which the therapist is considered the "expert" with a degree of authority over the patient.[41] The client (and sometimes the client's family) also have natural expertise concerning what the experience of disability means and what goals make sense within the cultural and social context. This native expertise that comes from life experience requires that the therapist share power with the client in the therapeutic process.[99]

Related to this theme is the idea that therapy should empower clients. Therapists should work alongside clients, and participate and share with them.[41] As Lyons describes it, therapy should help clients be "active participants in their own lives, and in the life of the community."[62]

---

*Hocking[41] provides several examples of such potential clashes. She notes, for example, that the traditional occupational therapy values of independence and self-determination may conflict with cultural values of clients that emphasize interdependence. As a result of growing awareness of what it means to respect the patient's perspective, occupational therapists are having to re-examine and replace some older values. In the previous edition of this book I included independence and self-determination as part of the occupational therapy values. For reasons that should be obvious, I have not included these values here. In some discussions of occupational therapy and, certainly, in some therapists' practice, independence and self-determination are still important values. As I have examined different arguments, it seems that the following is a useful perspective: When persons embrace independence and self-determination as a value, or when they clearly come from a cultural perspective that embraces such values, occupational therapy can provide assistance to enable patients or clients toward these goals. When patients or clients express interdependence or a desire to be taken care of by family members as part of a cultural perspective, this viewpoint must be respected. Occupational therapy may be useful in helping the clients and their families achieve patterns of behavior that, on the one hand respect traditional cultural view, but on the other hand allow for learning how to cope with the burden of disability, employing resources that may not be available within the cultural perspective. A practical example is an elderly disabled person who considers it a sign of honor and respect that family members care for him. Such a perspective may result in the person acquiring secondary disability as a result of inactivity and placing a heavy burden on other members of the family. While the cultural perspective must be respected, therapists might help all concerned explore ways that honor and respect can be maintained while the elderly person takes somewhat more responsibility for his own care. Such negotiations are never easy and sometimes not successful, since cultural values are strongly held and deeply emotional. As the example demonstrates, values do not tend to line up neatly for application, and often therapists must work within a context of competing or clashing values.

Balancing Art and Science

The mechanistic paradigm ushered into occupational therapy a concern for scientific soundness. Over the past quarter century in particular, occupational therapy has matured significantly in its scholarly work. The importance of research in discovering and testing the concepts of the field has been underscored.[1,2,75]

At the same time there remains a recognition that science must be balanced with art.[9,51,107] Much of the art of occupational therapy is linked to the media of the field. Cultural practices, craft, celebration, art, music, everyday intimate acts of self-care, and work are among the types of occupations into which therapists invite patients. Bringing persons into the presence of those practices that constitute the fabric of everyday life requires a special care. Bateson[5] once characterized the practice of occupational therapy through the metaphor of sacramental transformation, that is, an inner change wrought by participation in an outward act. He went on to remind therapists that the inner transformation of the patient would depend to a large extent on the therapists' reverence for the activities into which patients were led. Both the therapist and the patient must experience the activity as having significance.

Managing the intersection of scientific understanding and judgment with artful practice is challenging work. It requires occupational therapists to balance different ways of knowing and thinking in action.[67] It means "evolving a blend of competence and caring."[77]

Integrative Values: Summary

Dialogue in occupational therapy about values is ongoing. Major themes in occupational therapy (Table 4–5) affirm the value of occupation and emphasize a client-centered practice and respect for the subjective perspectives of clients and patients. These themes also affirm that therapy is a process of active engagement and empowerment that must be guided by a balance of art and science.

Table 4–5. **Integrative Values**

Client-Centered Practice	Asserts each person's essential humanity and worth:
	• Dignity is a birthright.
	• The worth of the individual is enhanced when persons actualize potential and enhance their own competence.
	• The relationship between client and therapists must be guided by:
	  ○ Profound respect for and understanding of client's perspectives, desires, and needs
	  ○ Altruism reflecting concern for the welfare of the others
	  ○ Empathy toward the circumstances of the patient carried out through a form of doing with the patient

Table 4–5. **Integrative Values** *(Continued)*

Occupation	• Occupations have intrinsic value for human life.
	• Persons need to participate in occupations.
	• Occupation develops human potential:
	  ○ Exercises self-direction, initiative, interdependence, and relatedness
	  ○ Verifies the ability to adapt
	  ○ Establishes a satisfying balance between autonomy and societal membership

Value of the Patient's/ Client's Perspective	• Respect the unique perspective of the patient or client:
	  ○ It is the right of individuals to define their own problems and pursue their own needs.
	  ○ The experiential world of the patient is the focal point of therapy.
	• Culture:
	  ○ Determines persons' views of occupational life, and of disease and disability
	  ○ Influences persons ways of thinking, feeling, communicating, and participating in therapy
	• Therapy should affirm and validate the client's cultural beliefs and perspectives.

Active Engagement and Empowerment	• Therapy requires:
	  ○ The active and meaning-driven participation of the patient
	  ○ A collaborative relationship in which the patient is considered an equal participant
	• Therapy should empower clients to be active participants in their own lives and in the community.

Balancing Art and Science	• Science must be balanced with art.
	• Managing scientific understanding with artful practice requires:
	  ○ Balancing different ways of knowing and thinking in action
	  ○ The blending of competence and caring

Conclusion

For a profession to be coherent, members must share a common culture and a vision of their work.* This common culture and vision is the

---

*It is also important to remember that the field's paradigm is contained in three voices. One voice is that of practice; therapists exemplify the paradigm in the collective ways they carry our practice. A second voice is the oral tradition of the field—what therapists say to each other in formal and informal conversations about practice. A third voice is that found in the literature. In any profession, literature is a powerful force, since it formally codifies and serves to disseminate the concepts, viewpoint, and values of the profession. The emerging paradigm is maintained and elaborated through all three voices; that is, it is found in the literature of the field, in how therapists talk about practice, and in the identity and practice of individual therapists. Paradigms first become evident in the literature. Indeed, changes in how the paradigm is reflected in writing may precede changes in practice. In this chapter, I rely mainly on the literature of the field to exemplify the paradigm.

field's paradigm. The paradigm expresses core constructs, a focal viewpoint, and values that reflect and contribute to a collective definition of the field's nature and scope. Nevertheless, a paradigm does not imply perfect consensus or uniformity throughout the field. Even within a period of paradigm stability, there will be debates and disagreements.[16] There is, however, a shared field of discourse.

This chapter described the emerging paradigm of occupational therapy. I discussed core constructs that elucidate the occupational nature of humans, problems of occupational dysfunction, and occupation as a health determinant. I identified as the focal viewpoint a systems perspective on the biopsychosocial phenomena with which the field is concerned. Finally, I discussed value themes that provide a sense of what the field considers important.

These elements of the paradigm provide a broad backdrop against which detailed explanatory and prescriptive concepts for practice can be articulated in the field's conceptual practice models. The paradigm both reflects and guides the development of these models, which I will discuss in the following chapters.

Tornebohm[97,98] points out that paradigms are often transparent. By this he means that, although persons employ paradigms in their professional work, they are not necessarily aware of them. One of my goals in this chapter is to make the occupational therapy paradigm more apparent. This goal is based on Tornebohm's[97,98] assertion that members of a field should be able to express, criticize, and develop the paradigm of the field. Thus, I have sought to interpret and synthesize themes that are dispersed throughout the field. It would be naive to assume that all members of the occupational therapy profession share all of the views that I have proposed as constituting the emerging paradigm. Nevertheless, I argue that many of the themes in this chapter reflect and shape the reality that members of the profession see when they go about their work. Moreover, I argue that the emerging identity of occupational therapy will be closely linked to the kinds of themes discussed herein.

References

1. American Occupational Therapy Association: Core values and attitudes of occupational therapy practice. Am J Occup Ther 47:1085–1086, 1993.
2. American Occupational Therapy Association: Position Paper: Occupation. Am J Occup Ther 49:1015–1017, 1995.
3. Banus, BS, et al: The Developmental Therapist. Slack, Thorofare, NJ, 1979.
4. Baron, RM, Amazeen, PG, and Beek, PJ: Local and global dynamics of social relations In Vallacher, RR, and Nowak, A. (eds): Dynamical Systems in Social Psychology. Academic Press, New York, 1994.
5. Bateson, G: Communication in occupational therapy. Am J Occup Ther 10:188, 1956.
6. von Bertalanffy, L: General systems theory: A new approach to unity of science. Hum Biol 23:347, 1951.
7. von Bertalanffy, L: Chance or law. In Koestler, A, and Smythies, JR (eds): Beyond Reductionism. Beacon Press, Boston, 1968.

8. Bing, RK: Professional nationalism. Am J Occup Ther 37:301, 1983.
9. Bing, RK, The subject is health: Not of facts, but of values. Am J Occup Ther 40:667–671, 1986.
10. Black, MM: The occupational career. Am J Occup Ther 30:225, 1976.
11. Boulding, K: General systems theory: The skeleton of science. In Buckley, W (ed): Modern Systems Research for the Behavioral Scientist. Aldine, Chicago, 1968.
12. Bruce, MA, and Borg, B: Frames of Reference in Psychosocial Occupational Therapy. Slack, Thorofare, NJ, 1987, p 193.
13. Bruner, J: The organization of early skilled action. Child Development 44:1, 1973.
14. Bruner, J: Acts of Meaning. Harvard University Press, Cambridge, 1990.
15. Burke, JP: Defining occupation: Importing and organizing interdisciplinary knowledge. In Kielhofner, G (ed): Health through Occupation: Theory and Practice in Occupational Therapy. FA Davis, Philadelphia, 1983, p 136.
16. Burrell, G, and Morgan, G: Sociological Paradigms and Organizational Analysis: Elements of the Sociology of Corporate Life. Heinemann, London, 1979.
17. Capra, F: The turning point: A new vision of reality. Futurist 16:19, 1982.
18. Cassell, EJ: The nature of suffering and the goals of medicine. N Engl J Med 306:639, 1982.
19. Chapple, E: Rehabilitation: Dynamic of Change. Center for Research in Education, Cornell University, Ithaca, NY, 1970.
20. Christiansen, C: Toward a resolution of crisis: Research requisites in occupational therapy. Occupational Therapy Journal of Research 1:115, 1981.
21. Christiansen, C: Occupational therapy: Intervention for life performance. In Christiansen, C, and Baum, C (eds): Occupational Therapy: Overcoming Human Performance Deficits. Slack, Thorofare, NJ, 1991.
22. Christiansen, C: Ways of Living: Self Care Strategies for Special Needs. American Occupational Therapy Association, Rockville, MD, 1994.
23. Christiansen, C: Three perspectives on balance in occupation. In Clark, F, and Zemke, R (eds): Occupation Science. FA Davis, Philadelphia, 1996.
24. Clark, FA, et al: Occupation science: Academic innovation in the service of occupational therapy's future. Am J Occup Ther 45:300, 1990.
25. Clark, FA: Occupation embedded in a real life: Interweaving occupational science and occupational therapy. Am J Occup Ther 47:1067–1077, 1993.
26. Clark, PN: Human development through occupation: Theoretical frameworks in contemporary occupational therapy practices, Part 1. Am J Occup Ther 33:505, 1979.
27. DeCharms, R: Personal Causation. Academic Press, New York, 1968.
28. Dunn, W, Brown, C, and McGuigan, A: The ecology of human performance: A framework for considering the effect of context. Am J Occup Ther 48:595–607, 1994.
29. Englehardt, T: Defining occupational therapy: The meaning of therapy and the virtues of occupation. Am J Occup Ther 31:666–672, 1977.
30. Fidler, G, and Fidler, J: Doing and becoming: Purposeful action and self-actualization. Am J Occup Ther 32:305, 1978.
31. Florey, L: Intrinsic motivation: The dynamics of occupational therapy theory. Am J Occup Ther 23:319, 1969.
32. Fogel, A, and Thelen, E: Development of early expressive and communicative action: Reinterpreting the evidence from a dynamic systems perspective. Developmental Psychology 23:747–761, 1987.
33. Fondiller, ED, Rosage, L, and Neuhas, B: Values influencing clinical reasoning in occupational therapy: An exploratory study. Occupational Therapy Journal of Research 10:41, 1990.
34. Gilfoyle, EM: Eleanor Clarke Slagle Lecture: Leadership: Transformation of a profession. Am J Occup Ther 38:575, 1984.
35. Gilfoyle, EM: Nationally speaking—partnerships for the future. Am J Occup Ther 42:485, 1988.
36. Groves, EJ, and Rider, BA: A comparison of treatment approaches used after carpal tunnel release surgery. Am J Occup Ther 43:398, 1989.
37. Haken, H: Synergetics: An approach to self-organization. In Yates, FE (ed): Self-Organizing Systems: The Emergence of Order. Plenum Press, New York, 1987.

38. Harvey-Krefting, L: The concept of work in occupational therapy, Am J Occup Ther 39:301, 1985.
39. Heard, C: Occupational role acquisition: A perspective on the chronically disabled. Am J Occup Ther 31:243, 1977.
40. Helfrich, C, Kielhofner, G, and Mattingly, C: Volition as narrative: Understanding motivation in chronic illness. Am J Occup Ther 48:311–317, 1994.
41. Hocking, C: The art of being therapeutic: Cultural safety. Paper presented at the Australian Association of Occupational Therapists' 18th Federal and Inaugural Pacific Rim Conference, Hobart, Australia, 1995.
42. Hocking, C, Whiteford, G, and Henare, D: What constitutes core values in occupational therapy practice? (Letter to the editor) Am J Occup Ther 49:175–176, 1995.
43. Huizinga, J: Homo Ludens. Beacon Press, Boston, 1955.
44. Jacobs, P, and McDermott, S: Family caregiver costs of chronically ill and handicapped children: Method and literature review. Pub Health Rep 104:158, 1989.
45. Johnson, J: Old values—new directions: Competence, adaptation, integration. Am J Occup Ther 35:597, 1981.
46. Johnsson, H, Borell, L, and Kielhofner, G: Anticipating retirement: The formation of attitudes and expectations concerning an occupational transition. Am J Occup Ther (in press).
47. Kaiser, AP, and Hemmeter, ML: Value-based approaches to family intervention. Early Childhood Special Education 8:72, Winter, 1989.
48. Kamm, K, Thelen, E, and Jensen, J: A dynamical systems approach to motor development. Physical Therapy 70:763–772, 1990.
49. Kelso, JAS: Dynamic Patterns: The Self Organization of Brain and Behavior. MIT Press, Cambridge, 1995.
50. Kielhofner, G: Temporal Adaptation: A conceptual framework for occupational therapy. Am J Occup Ther 31:235–242, 1977.
51. Kielhofner, G (ed): Health Through Occupation: Theory and Practice in Occupational Therapy. FA Davis, Philadelphia, 1983.
52. Kielhofner, G, and Miyake, S: Rose-colored lenses for clinical practice: From a deficit to a competing model. In Kielhofner, G (ed): Health through Occupation: Theory and Practice in Occupational Therapy. FA Davis, Philadelphia, 1983.
53. Kielhofner, G, et al: A comparison of play behavior in nonhospitalized and hospitalized children. Am J Occup Ther 37:305, 1983.
54. Kielhofner, G: Occupation. In Hopkins, H, and Smith, H (eds): Willard and Spackman's Occupational Therapy, ed 7. Lippincott, Philadelphia, 1989.
55. Kielhofner, G: Functional assessment: Toward a dialectical view of person-environment relations. Am J Occup Ther 47:248–251, 1993.
56. Kielhofner, G: A model of human occupation; Theory and application, ed 2. Williams & Wilkins, Baltimore, 1995.
57. Kielhofner, G, Borell, L, Burke, J, Helfrich, C, and Nygard, L: Volition subsystem. In Kielhofner, G (ed): A Model of Human Occupation; Theory and Application, ed 2. Williams & Wilkins, Baltimore, 1995.
58. King, LJ: Toward a science of adaptive responses. Am J Occup Ther 32:429, 1978.
59. Koestler, A, and Smithies, JR (eds): Beyond Reductionism. Beacon Press, Boston, 1969.
60. Krefting, LH, and Krefting, DV: Cultural influences on performance. In Christiansen, C, Baum, C (eds): Occupational Therapy: Overcoming Human Performance Deficits. Slack, Thorofare, NJ, 1991.
61. Llorens, L: Facilitating growth and development. Am J Occup Ther 24:93, 1970.
62. Lyons, M: Enabling or disabling? Students attitudes toward persons with disabilities. Am J Occup Ther 45:311–316, 1991.
63. Mallinson, T, Kielhofner, G, and Mattingly, C: Like being stuck in flypaper. Am J Occup Ther (in press).
64. Mathiowetz, V: Informational support and functional motor performance. Paper presented at the American Occupational Therapy Association National Conference, Boston, 1994.
65. Matsutsuyu, J: Occupational behavior—a perspective on work and play. Am J Occup Ther 25:291, 1971.

66. Mattingly, C: The narrative nature of clinical reasoning. Am J Occup Ther 45:998–1005, 1991.
67. Mattingly, C, and Flemming, M: Clinical Reasoning: Forms of Inquiry in a Therapeutic Practice. FA Davis, Philadelphia, 1994.
68. McColl, MA, Law, M, and Stewart, D: Theoretical Basis of Occupational Therapy. Slack, Thorofare, NJ, 1993.
69. Mosey, AC: An alternative: The biopsychosocial model. Am J Occup Ther 28:137, 1974.
70. Mosey, AC: Psychosocial Components of Occupational Therapy. Raven Press, New York, 1986.
71. Nelson, D: Occupation: Form and performance. Am J Occup Ther 42:633, 1988.
72. Newston, D: The perception and coupling of behavior waves. In Vallacher, RR, and Nowak, A (eds): Dynamical Systems in Social Psychology. Academic Press, New York, 1994.
73. Occupational Therapy: Guidelines for Client-Centered Practice. Canadian Association of Occupational Therapists, Toronto, 1991.
74. Ogden-Niemeyer, L, and Jacobs, K: Work Hardening: State of the Art. Slack, Thorofare, NJ, 1989.
75. Ottenbacher, KJ: Research: Its importance to clinical practice in occupational therapy. Am J Occup Ther 41:213–215, 1987.
76. Parent, LH: Effects of a low-stimulus environment on behavior. Am J Occup Ther 32:19, 1978.
77. Peloquin, SM: The patient-therapist relationship in occupational therapy: Understanding visions and images. Am J Occup Ther 44:13–21, 1990.
78. Peloquin, SM: The depersonalization of patients: A profile gleaned form narratives. Am J Occup Ther 47:830–837, 1993.
79. Peloquin, SM: The fullness of empathy: Reflections and illustrations. Am J Occup Ther 49:24–31, 1995.
80. Prigogine, I, and Stengers, I: Order Out of Chaos. Bantam Books, New York, 1984.
81. Polatajko, HJ: Dreams, dilemmas, and decisions for occupational therapy practice in a new millennium: A Canadian perspective. Am J Occup Ther 48:590–594, 1994.
82. Reilly, M: Occupational therapy can be one of the great ideas of 20th century medicine. Am J Occup Ther 16:1, 1962.
83. Reilly, M: Play as Exploratory Learning. Sage, Beverly Hills, CA, 1974.
84. Resolution # 532-79: Occupation as the common core of occupational therapy. Representative Assembly Minutes, Detroit, MI. Am J Occup Ther 33.785, 1979.
85. Robinson, A: Play: The arena for acquisition of rules for competent behavior. Am J Occup Ther 31:248, 1977.
86. Rogers, J: Order and disorder in occupational therapy and in medicine. Am J Occup Ther 36:29, 1982.
87. Rogers, J: The study of human occupation. In Kielhofner, G (ed): Health through Occupation: Theory and Practice in Occupational Therapy. FA Davis, Philadelphia, 1983.
88. Rogers, J: Clinical reasoning: The ethics of science and art. Am J Occup Ther 37:601, 1983.
89. Schkade, JK, and Schultz, S: Occupational adaptation: Toward a holistic approach for contemporary practice, Part 1. Am J Occup Ther 46:829–837, 1992.
90. Shannon, P: The work-play model: A basis for occupational therapy programming. Am J Occup Ther 24:215, 1970.
91. Shannon, PD: Project to identify the philosophy of occupational therapy. Unpublished report, American Occupational Therapy Association, Rockville, MD, 1983.
92. Sharott, GW: Occupational therapy's role in the client's creation and affirmation of meaning. In Kielhofner, G (ed): Health through Occupation: Theory and Practice in Occupational Therapy. FA Davis, Philadelphia, 1983.
93. Smith, MB: Competence and adaptation: A perspective on therapeutic ends and means. Am J Occup Ther 28:11, 1974.
94. Spencer, JC: The physical environment and performance. In Christiansen, C, and Baum, C (eds): Occupational Therapy: Overcoming Performance Deficits. Slack, Thorofare, NJ, 1991.
95. Thelen, E, and Ulrich, BD: Hidden skills: A dynamic systems analysis of treadmill stepping during the first year. Monographs of the Society for Research in Child Development 565 (1, Serial No. 223), 1991.

96. Toglia, JP: A dynamic interaction approach to cognitive rehabilitation. In Katz, N (ed): Cognitive Rehabilitation: Models for Intervention in Occupational Therapy. Andover Medical Publishers, Boston, 1992.
97. Tornebohm, H: Reflections on practice-oriented research. Unpublished paper, University of Goteborg, Goteborg, October 10, 1985.
98. Tornebohm, H: Caring, knowing and paradigms. Unpublished paper, University of Goteborg, Goteborg, December 10, 1986.
99. Townsend, E: Muriel Driver Lecture. Occupational Therapy's social vision. Canadian Journal of Occupational Therapy 60:174–184, 1993.
100. Trombly, CA: Occupational Therapy for Physical Dysfunctions, ed. 3. Williams & Wilkins, Baltimore, 1989.
101. Trombly, CA: Anticipating the future: Assessment of occupational function. Am J Occup Ther 47:253–257, 1993.
102. Trombly, CA: Occupation: Purposefulness and meaningfulness as therapeutic mechanisms. Am J Occup Ther 49:960–972, 1995.
103. Turvey, MT: Coordination. American Psychologist 45:938–953, 1990.
104. Vallacher, RR, and Nowak, A: The chaos in social psychology. In Vallacher, RR, and Nowak, A (eds): Dynamical Systems in Social Psychology. Academic Press, New York, 1994.
105. Vandenberg, B, and Kielhofner, G: Play in evolution, culture, and individual adaptation: Implications for therapy. Am J Occup Ther 36:20, 1982.
106. Wiemer, R: Traditional and nontraditional practice arenas. In Occupational Therapy: 2001. American Occupational Therapy Association, Rockville, MD, 1979, p 43.
107. Wood, W: Weaving the warp and weft of occupational therapy: An art and science for all times. Am J Occup Ther 49:44–52, 1995.
108. Wu, C-Y, Trombly, C, Lin, K-C: The relationship between occupational form and occupational performance: A kinematic perspective. Am J Occup Ther 48:679–687, 1994.
109. Yerxa, EJ: Authentic occupational therapy. Am J Occup Ther 21:1, 1967.
110. Yerxa, EJ: Occupational therapy's role in creating a future climate of caring. Am J Occup Ther 34:529, 1980.
111. Yerxa, EJ: Audacious values: The energy source of occupational therapy practice. In Kielhofner, G (ed): Health Through Occupation: Theory and Practice in Occupational Therapy. FA Davis, Philadelphia, 1983, p 152.
112. Yerxa, EJ, et al: An introduction to occupation science: A foundation for occupational therapy in the 21st century. Occup Ther Health Care 6:1, 1989.
113. Yerxa, EJ: Seeking a relevant, ethical and realistic way of knowing for occupational therapy. Am J Occup Ther 45:199–204, 1991.

CHAPTER 5

CONCEPTUAL PRACTICE MODELS

I n Chapters 3 and 4 we explored the historical and current development of occupational therapy's paradigm. Through the values, viewpoint, and constructs it offers, the paradigm paints a picture of the field in a broad stroke. While the paradigm serves the essential purposes of providing an identity and outlook for occupational therapy, it can only say the most general things about practice. Conceptual practice models address the specifics.

The emerging paradigm reflects the fact that practice is biopsychosocial. This means that therapists encounter a wide range of phenomena for which they require understanding and guidelines for action. The diversity of these many phenomena compels the field toward more than a single theoretical and practical system. Quite expectedly, occupational therapy has many models of practice that address different phenomena within the biological, psychological, and social spectrum.

The practice of occupational therapy creates a particular set of demands for knowledge. Ordinary practice challenges therapists with the following kinds of questions: How does one understand the sense of hopelessness in a patient who has lost physical capacities necessary to his accustomed way of life? And, more, how does one help this patient overcome the inertia of this helplessness? How does one comprehend the nature of the pain, the limited mobility, and the reduced strength of a person with arthritis? Relatedly, how does one minimize the consequences of these physical impairments for the person experiencing them? What underlies the problems that a child with cerebral palsy has in moving her body? What might enable this child to achieve more control over her movements?

These types of questions demand answers of a different kind from the more philosophical discourse of the field's paradigm. They demand particular knowledge that can be applied to solving real problems faced by patients and clients. Conceptual practice models are developed to address these types of questions.

In this and several following chapters, I will examine the nature of conceptual practice models and the current state of model development in occupational therapy. This chapter explores in more detail what a conceptual model of practice is and why knowledge development in occupational therapy has taken on the shape of conceptual practice models.

Why Conceptual Practice Models Exist

My thesis about conceptual models of practice has emerged from consideration of others' ideas about organizing knowledge for practice, from examination of how developed bodies of knowledge in the field were organized, and from my own efforts to create a conceptual model of practice—the model of human occupation. I believe that models, as defined in this book, occur more or less naturally in the field because they reflect the practical needs and considerations of occupational therapy.

Various terms such as practice theory, conceptual framework, and frame of reference have also been used to describe applied bodies of knowledge in occupational therapy. My definition of a conceptual model of practice most closely parallels what Mosey[2,3] identified as a frame of reference, with one very important difference. She argues that frames of reference organize existing theory (usually nonoccupational therapy theory from outside the discipline) for use in practice. I emphasize, instead, that conceptual practice models articulate unique occupational therapy theory. The intersection of these viewpoints is probably as good a place as any to begin illustrating what I mean by a conceptual practice model.

Occupational therapists can solve practical problems because they have an understanding of the nature of those problems, how they have arisen, and what factors they involve. Therapists confronted with patient problems have puzzled about their nature and about what can be done to resolve them. The riddles of practice have naturally sent some therapists off to create explanations of these problems. It must be remembered that the paradigm of the field helps to frame problems in a way that is unique to the field. Because of this kind of "problem setting," therapists have inevitably sought to develop explanations of problems in unique ways. Hence, therapists engage in the development of unique occupational therapy theory.

Since the theory development has taken place in response to practical problems, it must connect back to the resolution of those problems.

Consequently, occupational therapists have developed their theories as explanations for application. This has meant that the theoretical arguments they make take on a particular form (i.e., talking about how aspects of human occupation ordinarily work, how things go wrong, and how they can be corrected). This kind of theory for application is peculiar to practice fields. For example, scholars in fields such as sociology or anatomy feel no onus to organize their theoretical arguments in this way. A social scientist can spend his or her entire career happily seeking a better understanding of some aspect of social life. This is not how those engaged in theory development in occupational therapy see their work. Their theories should talk about problem identification and problem solution.

It is not enough, however, to direct one's theorizing toward making sense of practical problems and their resolution. I remember vividly how, after the first four articles on the model of human occupation were published in 1980, requests seemed to come from every corner of practice for more practical tools to apply the model. Some therapists wanted to know what kinds of assessments should be used with this model. Others wanted specific examples and guidelines for applying the theory with a particular population or in a specific setting. Consequently, those of us working on the model realized that we needed to create new assessment tools for applying concepts. We also realized that we needed to develop clear links between the concepts we were developing and the everyday work of therapists. No doubt, others developing theory for practice felt this same need to direct their work to practical concerns.

Another influence on the development of conceptual practice models is the expectation of empirical verification. With the mechanistic paradigm came a maturation of occupational therapy's concern for research to validate the concepts used in practice. Consequently, as therapists develop theory to explain patient problems and their resolution, they also must use research to scrutinize and refine their theory.

Hence, conceptual practice models get organized as they do because of natural forces and expectations in the field. Occupational therapists seeking to make sense of the puzzles of practice end up doing so in ways that resemble what I am calling a conceptual model of practice.

The Nature and Purpose of Conceptual Practice Models

A conceptual practice model involves, above all, a dynamic process of knowledge development; that is, a model is never a finished product. Rather, a model is a way of thinking about and doing practice that is constantly being refined and improved. Models do get articulated in articles,

and books, and this can make them seem like a static set of facts and procedures. Nevertheless, nothing could be further from what constitutes a useful
model of practice.

Since each model involves an ongoing process of development, it is
most useful to begin by considering what models seek to accomplish.
Conceptual practice models aim to create explanations of some phenomena
of practical concern in the field, while providing a rationale and methods for
therapeutic interventions. Thus, a model has the dual purpose of explaining
a group of phenomena and guiding practice related to those phenomena. It
is the combined concern for both theoretical explanation and practical action
that make conceptual models of practice unique in their organization.

Components and Dynamic Processes of Models

As I argued in Chapter 2, a well-developed model has the following
characteristics:

- Each model is built on an interdisciplinary base of knowledge.
- Each model addresses a particular group of phenomena, making theoretical arguments concerning order (i.e., organization and function); disorder (i.e., dysfunction); and the processes of therapeutic
  intervention (i.e., planned change and/or preservation).
- Because models are used in practice, they also accumulate technology (i.e., procedures and materials) for therapeutic application.
- Models are subjected to research that provides evidence concerning
  their theoretical arguments and therapeutic efficacy.

These components of a model exist in a dynamic flow of information, as
illustrated in Figure 5–1. The interdisciplinary base provides information to
support the theoretical arguments; the theoretical arguments provide the
rationale for and guide the development of clinical application; feedback
from clinical application and research provides information for further theory
development; basic research tests the theoretical arguments; and applied
research tests application of the theory in practice. Finally, models not only
draw from but contribute theory and research to other disciplines and to
other models in the field. This ongoing process of developing a model is influenced by and influences the field's paradigm. In the following sections we will
examine the characteristics of conceptual practice models in more detail.

Interdisciplinary Base

Models of practice in occupational therapy are influenced by and borrow interdisciplinary concepts. Those who develop models select theoreti-

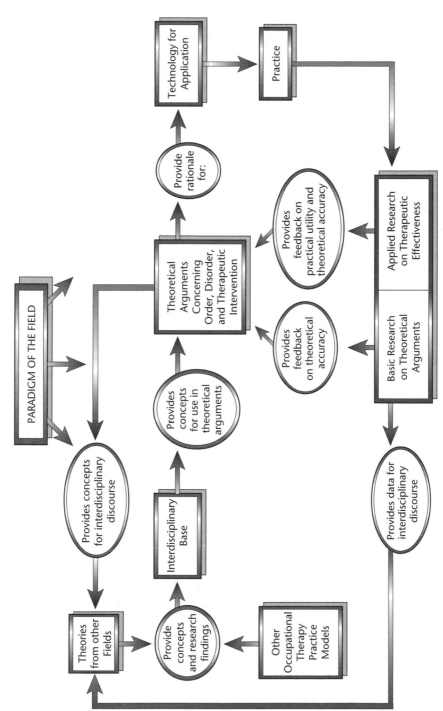

Figure 5–1. Components and process of a conceptual model of practice.

cal concepts from both outside and inside the field that are relevant to the phenomena they are trying to explain. For example, therapists who have contributed to the development of concepts for understanding problems of perception following brain injury have familiarized themselves with inter-disciplinary knowledge about perception and its relationship to brain func-tion. Their views and the theoretical arguments they have made are influenced by arguments in this interdisciplinary literature and they have directly imported concepts from this literature. This use of concepts from other disciplines is not unique to occupational therapy. Because of the nature of knowledge development and the inevitable overlap between vari-ous fields, the theoretical structures in both academic disciplines and applied fields are strongly influenced by developing knowledge in other dis-ciplines. This is especially true today, since disciplinary boundaries are not nearly as rigid as they have been in the past.

Theoretical Arguments

Conceptual models of practice do not merely borrow interdisciplinary knowledge; they reinterpret, reorganize, and add to interdisciplinary con-cepts, creating new theoretical arguments. This is where the influence of the field's paradigm is important. The core constructs, focal viewpoint, and val-ues of the paradigm provide a kind of intellectual framework within which occupational therapists go about their theorizing. The perspective provided by the field's paradigm influences both what knowledge is selected and how it is used in models.

For example, the paradigm constructs that identify occupation as the focus for therapy influence those developing models related to sensory pro-cessing and perception to link their concepts to occupational performance, and to create explanations of how engaging in occupations might amelio-rate problems of sensory processing and perception. Moreover, they are likely to frame their arguments using systems concepts from the focal view-point of the paradigm. This happens not because the paradigm is ensconced somewhere as a set of rules for theory developers to follow. Rather, the par-adigm exists as a discourse, that is, as a set of ideas, concepts, and arguments that are being discussed in the literature, in conferences, and other contexts. As those who develop theory read, listen to presentations, and enter into discussions, they become part of that discourse and are influenced by it in their own work. Not everyone is influenced in the same way, but the para-digmatic discourse leaves its imprint on models of practice. Those working on the models of practice are also likely to enter into the paradigmatic dis-course, so that the influence between models and the paradigm is mutual.

Order, Disorder, and Intervention. The paradigm defines occupational therapy as concerned with occupational functioning, occupational dysfunction, and the use of occupation as therapy. Conceptual practice models address specific phenomena (e.g., perception, motivation, movement, cognition). The way in which models address these phenomena also reflects the aforementioned paradigmatic concerns. Theoretical arguments in conceptual practice models are concerned with:

- The interrelationship between phenomena addressed in the model and performance in daily occupations
- The impact of disorder in the phenomena addressed in the model on occupation
- The ways in which occupations can be used as therapy to counteract disorder in the phenomena addressed by the model

Hence theoretical arguments in each model of practice can be readily recognized as addressing order, disorder, and therapeutic intervention. Moreover, they do so in reference to the paradigmatic focus on occupation. Importantly, by relating the theoretical arguments to the paradigm's assumptions, views, and values, the occupational therapist who is creating a conceptual model of practice develops theory that reflects the unique scholarly perspective of occupational therapy.

Let us see how this is so. One occupational therapy model explains the biomechanics of movement, movement problems that occur when the musculoskeletal system is impaired, and how to accomplish musculoskeletal system changes to preserve movement for participation in occupations. Another model explains the motivation for occupation, the ways that motivation can be disrupted by disability, and how to maintain or change motivation.

While motivation and biomechanics are concepts borrowed from other disciplines, they are discussed specifically in terms of their relationship to performance in everyday occupations; that is, these models seek to explain how motivation and movement, respectively, operate to influence occupational behavior. Some interdisciplinary concepts related to motivation and of biomechanics are selected and emphasized while others are not. This happens because therapists are seeking specifically to explain how movement and motivation operate in relationship to occupation.

The models concerned with such phenomena as movement or motivation will seek to explain disorders of movement or motion as they affect and are affected by occupation. Finally, the models will be concerned with explaining how participation in occupations can be maximized in the face of problems of movement or motivation, as well as how occupation can be used to positively influence dysfunctional movement or motivation.

Conceptualizations of order, disorder, and intervention are part of an interrelated whole. For example, the biomechanical model (see Chapter 6) postulates that movement against resistance is required to maintain muscle strength; the model also holds that the absence of such movement leads to muscle atrophy—a form of dysfunction. The model of human occupation (see Chapter 10) holds that individuals need to experience success to maintain a belief in their abilities. Further, the model associates lack of success with a lack of confidence in abilities. Thus, identification of how things go wrong is constructed from a conceptualization of what happens when things go right.

Each model's conceptualization of dysfunction poses a problem or puzzle that must be solved in practice. By "framing" or naming the problem, the model determines the nature of the solutions that can be used in practice. For example, the biomechanical model may frame the dysfunction as the inability to do a work task, reflecting inadequate strength. Because of the way the problem is framed, therapy will be aimed at improving strength or compensating for inadequate strength. The model of human occupation may define one dysfunction as the inability of a worker to return to the job because of the fear of failing at the work tasks. The problem is framed as a problem of belief in one's own efficacy. Thus, therapy must affect this belief.

Theoretical arguments related to intervention typically address both preservation and change in therapy. *Preservation* is the process whereby order is maintained in the phenomena of concern. Theoretical arguments concerning preservation guide therapy aimed at health maintenance, prevention of further dysfunction, or maximal retention of function in the course of progressive diseases. *Change* is the process of altering or minimizing disorder and achieving new states of organization. So, for example, the biomechanical model explains how strength can be improved following injury and how tasks can be appropriately modified when weakness will be an ongoing problem. The model of human occupation explains how the sense of efficacy can be increased and how the environment can be structured to be less threatening to a person who lacks a sense of efficacy. Thus, the model's theoretical arguments usually address both change-oriented remedial approaches (change) and compensatory approaches aimed at adjusting to limitations.

Technology for Application

Those who use models in practice require supporting technology to apply the models. The technology of models includes procedures, equipment, materials for assessment and intervention, and exemplars that illustrate application of the theory in practice.

Assessment. Application of a model in practice always requires a way to gather and analyze data about the phenomena addressed. This process is generally referred to as assessment. In assessment, data is gathered about the concepts of a model. For example, a key concept of the biomechanical model is strength; consequently, methods of gathering data about strength have been developed. These methods include standardized procedures such as using the dynamometer (a mechanical device to measure grip strength). There are also more naturalistic methods such as observing strength in a work task to determine work fitness.

Therapists analyze and interpret the data they collect in the context of the theoretical arguments. For example, the biomechanical model postulates that strength depends on movement against resistance. If assessment reveals subnormal strength along with the observation that a person has become inactive over a period of time, the therapist concludes that inactivity has contributed to observed weakness. In this way the theoretical arguments provide a context within which the therapists can make sense of and draw conclusions about the information gathered.

Intervention. Application of a model in practice yields intervention procedures or strategies. Procedures are generally represented as guidelines or principles. They may concern such things as how to motivate patients or clients in the midst of performing an occupation or how to adapt activities so that someone with limited movement can perform them. Sometimes procedures include methods for physically handling or interacting with patients or clients.

That models may have specified procedures should not be taken to suggest that procedures can be substituted for theory in practice. Therapists must understand theoretical arguments to make good decisions about selecting among procedures in practice. Moreover, procedures can only be specified at a level of abstraction, so the therapist must match what is specified more generally by the model with the particulars of a given patient or client. If theory is understood well, then effective use of procedures and strategies will follow.

Models are not only prescriptive (i.e., giving specific guidelines for intervention), but also suggestive, providing opportunities for creative new applications. Further, models always require a degree of interpretation in their applications because of the inevitable gap between abstract concepts and real life. The therapist must translate between the general construct and the particular instance.

Another way that application of a model may be illustrated is through exemplars, which illustrate how a model can be applied. The most common exemplars are case examples and program examples. Textbooks and articles that discuss application of models typically include cases to show how the model's concepts are used in practice. One value of cases is that they illustrate the process of translating the general concepts to particular situations. Cases can also be effective ways to show how models can be used to develop creative applications.

Writers frequently illustrate the utility of a conceptual model of practice by discussing how it was used to design and implement a program of service. Programs refer to packages of services offered in a specific context and/or to a particular population. Such articles or chapters generally discuss how the model conceptualizes the problems that the population typically experiences and how the model guides selection of assessments. They also include a discussion of how the model is translated into services or strategies used in the program.

Empirical Support

Research allows therapists to ascertain how well the theoretical arguments of a model explain reality. This type of investigation is often referred to as basic research. Another form of investigation, applied research, studies application of the model in practice. Applied research *can* be used to scrutinize theory, but its main objective is to assess technical results. Such results include whether assessments based on the model provide dependable information and whether procedures based on the model improve the function and well-being of patients or clients.

As empirical evidence mounts, theoretical models can be altered to correct or elaborate existing theoretical arguments. This process ultimately strengthens the explanatory power of the theoretical arguments. Empirical evidence that a model has practical utility is, of course, quite important in the context of modern health care systems that are demanding demonstrations of positive outcomes from service.

Development of Models of Practice

Each conceptual practice model has its own unique course of development. A model may begin as a collection of techniques or ideas in practice to which a comprehensive and coherent theory is added. This is an inductive approach; it begins with practical observations, born out of clinical trial and error, that lead to articulation of the theory. The deductive approach begins with theory that addresses known problems in therapy; clinical applications are worked out in response to the theoretical arguments. Most models are developed by a combination of both approaches, although one approach or another may be dominant at different points in the model's development.

To gain acceptance and remain in use, a model of practice must have certain characteristics. First, the model has to be formally articulated. Model developers must publish articles and/or books on the model. Sometimes, however, model articulation begins with manuals, workshops, and other forms of organizing and sharing knowledge.

Another important characteristic is the model's appeal to practitioners. A model is appealing when it is simple enough to be understood, yet complex enough to offer some fresh, intriguing insight. A model should "ring true." That is, the model should make sense in terms of both personal and professional experience.

Models are made more credible when they have been subjected to research. Generally, research not only serves to test and refine the theoretical arguments, but it supports the development of technology for application. An example is the use of research to develop assessment tools.

Finally, the model must be serviceable. Unless the ideas can be applied in some very concrete ways, they are not useful in a practice discipline. The technology for application is what allows therapists to apply a model.

Models, of course, vary in how well each of these elements is developed. Some models have well-articulated theoretical arguments, but are weak in application. Other models have appealing methods for application although their theoretical arguments and research base are not as well developed. While models may be adopted and survive for a while because of strength in one area, it is unlikely that such models can endure unless all elements are developed.

Models in Perspective

Conceptual practice models are the sources of major theory building in occupational therapy. Moreover, they guide the research and clinical application efforts of the field. The availability and use of conceptual practice models will determine to a large extent the competence of occupational therapists.

I emphasized in this chapter that models are dynamic and changing. This means not only that models will change over time, but also that new models may emerge in the field and that some models may eventually fade out of use.

Current Models in Occupational Therapy

One of the most perplexing challenges I faced in writing this book was to decide how to characterize the current conceptual practice models in occupational therapy. In some cases identifying a model of practice was relatively easy since its authors had organized their work in much the way I have used to describe a model in this chapter. In other cases, it appeared that work in progress was becoming a conceptual practice model. Yet in other cases, it appeared that a set of ideas and their application in practice was waning in the field.

My desire was to describe conceptual models of practice that were either mature or rapidly maturing and were currently in use. I used the structures and dynamic processes that I have characterized as underlying models to determine which models met the criteria of being mature or maturing models; that is, I asked whether approaches had articulated theoretical arguments about order, disorder, and therapeutic intervention, whether they had accumulated a technology for application, and whether they had at least a beginning research base. Based on these criteria I identified eight models of practice that are presented in the next eight chapters. They are:

- The Biomechanical Model
- The Cognitive Disabilities Model
- The Cognitive-Perceptual Model
- The Group Work Model
- The Model of Human Occupation
- The Motor Control Model
- The Sensory Integration Model
- The Spatiotemporal Adaptation Model

Admittedly, the models I selected met these criteria unevenly. In some cases, I selected models primarily on the weight of one or more of these criteria and because of significant potential for future development.

One could ask whether the biomechanical, motor control, and cognitive-perceptual approaches are really models, since it is not clear that unique occupational therapy theory is being articulated in them. I have incorporated them because their technology is in wide use by therapists and because they appear to have strong potential to develop theoretical arguments unique to the field.

The spatiotemporal adaptation model lacks its own well-developed technology for application. However, the authors have made substantial theoretical arguments that are closely tied to the unique concerns of occupational therapy. The group work model is fundamentally different from other models. This model focuses on the group, rather than the individual human being, as the unit of concern. Other models are all concerned with properties of the individual. Although this model has made some theoretical arguments, provided some technology for application, and begun to generate research, it is at an early stage of development. It can be argued that this model is concerned with one of the media of occupational therapy, that is, the therapeutic use of groups. I have included this model because I believe that a theoretical model that deals specifically with sociocultural phenomena must and will emerge. Also, the increasing need of therapists to deal with groups (not only therapeutic groups, but also natural groups such as families, coworkers, schoolmates) calls for a model focused on occupational groups. Although the group work model focuses on therapeutic groups, it could be extended to address naturally occurring occupational groups.

Something must also be said about approaches that were excluded from this text. Early in the formulation of the first edition of this book I expected to include a chapter on a developmental model of practice. The prevalence of development as a theme in occupational therapy suggested that a developmental model was present or in the making. My examination of the literature suggested that there was no single developmental model meeting the criteria set out (i.e., articulation of occupational therapy theory, technology for application, and research). On the other hand, developmental themes were present throughout models of practice. Thus, it seemed that development is more appropriately seen as a paradigmatic theme present in many models, rather than as a model per se.

Object relations is another perspective I considered for inclusion. The themes that make up object relations theory come from a wide range of sources (most related to the psychoanalytic tradition). The themes stress intrapersonal and interpersonal elements of motivation and behavior. These themes have been present throughout much of occupational therapy's history (see Chapter 3). Mosey[2] first proposed object relations as a frame of reference, noting that it pertained to the "process wherein the individual becomes attached to or invests in objects—people and things— which satisfy his need." In a more recent discussion, she revised this frame of reference, referring to it as analytic. According to Mosey, the analytic frame of reference is concerned with an individual's reconciliation of universal issues, including reality, trust, intimacy, adequacy, dependence/independence, sexuality, aggression, and loss. Bruce and Borg[1] present the object relations frame of reference in their occupational therapy mental health text. In this discussion, which is the most complete presentation of the potential use of object relations in occupational therapy, they discuss technology for application, including assessments and treatment guidelines. As they note, this approach is highly subjective and lacks a research base. It is not included in this text because I believe that object relations theory is best considered related knowledge; that is, it is helpful to the therapist in understanding elements of the patient's motivation that affect occupation and in understanding the therapeutic relationship, but it does not define the occupational therapy process. The emphasis that object relations places on unconscious and intrapersonal themes contrasts with the emphasis of occupational therapy on everyday performance. In this sense, the mainstream concerns of object relations diverges from the concerns of occupational therapy. This exclusion does not rule out a possible reinterpretation of object relations themes in the future to bring them more squarely within the concerns of occupational therapy.

Mosey[3] has presented another frame of reference, which she terms role acquisition. This approach embodies many themes related to the emerging paradigm as I have described it. It includes some theoretical arguments, suggested assessment approaches, and clinical strategies. No unique technology for application has been developed, and no research on this approach has been reported. Moreover, Mosey proposes it as a frame of reference; this concept, as we have seen, differs in some important ways from the concept of a conceptual practice model. For these reasons it is not included here as a model, although it may be that this approach will be developed into a model of practice in the future.

In conclusion, I have chosen in this volume to treat a collection of models that appear to best characterize the state of the art and future potentials. History will be the true judge of the wisdom of my selections and prognostications.

References

1. Bruce, MA, and Borg, B: Frames of References in Psychosocial Occupational Therapy. Slack, Thorofare, NJ, 1987.
2. Mosey, AC: Three Frames of Reference for Mental Health. Slack, Thorofare, NJ, 1970, p 37.
3. Mosey, AC: Psychosocial Components of Occupational Therapy. Raven Press, New York, 1986.

CHAPTER 6

THE BIOMECHANICAL MODEL

The biomechanical model has been present in some form throughout occupational therapy history. The basic concern of biomechanics is the musculoskeletal capacities that underlie functional motion in everyday occupational performance. The model seeks to explain how the body is designed for and used to accomplish motion. At one time this approach was called kinetic occupational therapy, a term that emphasized the goal of restoring abilities for motion.[11]

Although much of the conceptual and empirical knowledge for this model comes from basic science, the practical applications have been accumulating throughout the profession's history. Many of the approaches and devices used in the model of practice today are based on decades of development.

The biomechanical model is applied to persons who experience limitations in moving freely, with adequate strength, and in a sustained fashion. These limitations result from problems with the musculoskeletal system, peripheral nervous system, integumentary system, or cardiopulmonary system. Problems of coordinated movement due to central nervous system dysfunction are more typically addressed through the motor control model or the sensory integrative model. Even in those cases, however, some biomechanical concerns, such as maintaining normal joint movement, are usually addressed.

Interdisciplinary Base

The biomechanical approach is based on principles of kinetics and kinematics. These disciplines concern the nature of movement and the forces acting on the human body as it moves. The field of anatomy, particularly as it concerns the musculoskeletal system, is also basic to this model. Finally, physiology as it concerns bone, connective tissue, and muscle is part of the theoretical base of the model. This knowledge is applied to such factors as tissue elasticity, tissue healing, muscle strengthening, and the energy cost of activities. In addition, knowledge of how the cardiopulmonary system supports functioning of the musculoskeletal system is incorporated into this model.

Theoretical Arguments

Motion underlies all performance in occupations. Whether for manipulation of objects, gesturing in communication, or body orientation to receive information, all purposeful behavior in daily occupations is built on the ability of persons to move their bodies.[14] The theoretical arguments of the biomechanical model concern this ability to move while performing occupations.

Order

The biomechanical model addresses the capacity for functional motion (i.e., the movement required to perform one's occupations). The capacity for motion has three components. The first is the potential for motion at the joints, or *joint range of motion*. The second is *strength*, or the ability of muscles to produce tension to maintain postural control and move body parts. The third is *endurance*, which is the ability to sustain effort (i.e., intensity or rate) over the time required to do a particular task.

Joint Range of Motion. Understanding of the available motion at each joint comes from knowledge of the structure and function of the joint. "Each joint is potentially able to move in certain directions and to certain limits of motion due to its structure and the integrity of surrounding tissues."[20] The connective tissue, muscle, and skin that surround joints have elasticity, which is the ability to stretch and to return to the original shape and size after movement. The degree of elasticity of these tissues affects the degree of possible movement.

Active range of motion refers to the range of movement that a person can produce using his or her own strength. Passive range of motion refers to the range of movement through which a joint can be externally manipulated.

Strength. Stability and motion are produced when skeletal muscles act on the joints of the body. Muscles cross one or more joints and exert force to control or produce movements allowed by the structure of the joints. Thus, tension produced in the muscles is necessary to stabilize or move joints.

The strength or ability of a muscle to produce tension is a function of the number and size of fibers in the muscle. The size, or diameter, of muscle fibers increases when the muscle is used to produce tension. Thus, the use to which a muscle is put in the course of everyday activities affects its strength.

In daily life, normal movement is not limited to the action of a single muscle across a single joint. Performance depends on the simultaneous action of muscles across many joints. This produces the stability and movement required for a task. Moreover, groups of muscles work together to produce each movement.[12,20]

Endurance. The ability to sustain muscle activity (i.e., endurance) is a function of muscle physiology. The variables involved are the work being done and the supply of oxygen and energy materials from the cardiopulmonary system. Thus, endurance is a somewhat more complex phenomena than strength and motion, since it not only depends on the musculoskeletal system but also entails the function of other body systems.

Dynamics of Movement Capacity. Several factors are considered in understanding movement. The potential for movement (joint range of motion) is a function of the anatomy of joints and soft tissues around joints. The production of movement is a function of muscle placement on the musculoskeletal system, of the coordinated work of muscles, and of the strength of individual muscles. Endurance is a function of both muscle physiology and the ability of the body systems to transport needed material to muscle tissue and to remove waste material.

Early understanding of how muscles produced movement was based primarily on the anatomical study of their position with respect to the skeletal system (i.e., where the muscles attached to bones and how they crossed joints). Such observations of anatomical organization led to the belief that specific movements and muscles were used to perform a given task.[22]

As more sophisticated methods have become available to study the process of movement, the understanding of how movement is used to accomplish occupations has changed. The actual movements produced during occupational performance can be described in terms of kinematics. For example, movement can be characterized by the actual movement path or displacement of a body part and the velocity (i.e., speed) and acceleration (i.e., rate of change in speed). Kinematics are an important part of the understanding of how the body actually accomplishes purposeful movements. For example, it is now understood that different persons will use different combinations of movement to achieve the same purposeful task and that the same person will use different combinations of movements to perform the same task at different times.[22] Dynamical systems ideas have recently been applied to the kinematic study of movements in tasks. As discussed in Chapter 4, variability in component movements and muscles for task performance across time and persons is expected, given the emergent nature of organized movement.

Self-Maintenance of the Musculoskeletal System. One of the most important observations of this model is that the capacity for movement (i.e., strength, range of motion, and endurance) is correlated with occupational performance; that is, muscle strength increases and decreases according to how much muscles are stressed in the course of everyday occupations. Similarly, the structure of bones is also positively affected by how much weight bearing they do, and joint mobility is affected by the nature of ongoing joint movement. Finally, the capacity for endurance waxes and wanes over time with changes in activity level.

Disorder

Dysfunction exists when a restriction of joint motion, strength, and/or endurance interferes with everyday occupational functioning.[20] Thus, the central concern of the model is a limitation of sustained stability or movement that produces an incapacity to perform occupations. A variety of diseases or traumas may lead to movement problems.

Joint range of motion may be limited because of joint damage, edema of tissues around the joint, pain, skin tightness, muscle spasticity (excess muscle tone producing tightness), or muscle and tendon shortening (due to immobilization). Examples of conditions that affect joint mobility are arthritis, trauma to the joint or surrounding connective tissue, and burns that limit the elasticity of skin over the joint.

Muscle weakness (reduced tension-producing capacity) can occur as a result of disuse or because of disease affecting muscle physiology. Loss of muscle strength may be due to diseases and trauma of the lower motor neurons (e.g., polio or amyotrophic lateral sclerosis), the spinal cord, or peripheral nerves, all of which may result in deinnervation of muscles. If muscles lose their innervation, they may completely atrophy and be incapable of producing tension. Muscle diseases such as muscular dystrophy directly affect muscle tissue. Finally, extended disuse or immobilization can result in weakness that impairs everyday performance.[12,20]

Like strength, endurance can be reduced with any extended confinement or limitation of activity. Other factors, including pathology of the cardiovascular or respiratory systems and muscular diseases, can also reduce endurance.

Therapeutic Intervention

Interventions based on the biomechanical model focus on the intersection of motion and occupational performance. These interventions can be divided into three approaches. The first approach seeks to prevent deformity and maintain existing capacity for motion. The second, restoration, aims at improving diminished capacity for motion. The third is compensation for limited motion. In all three approaches, the overriding criterion for intervention is to minimize any gap between persons' existing capacity for movement and the functional requirements of their ordinary occupational tasks.

Maintenance and Prevention. Reasonable use is necessary to maintain function of the musculoskeletal system. The biomechanical model extends this principle to argue that muscles still able to produce contractions and move joints should be used to maintain the capacity for functional motion. When the person is not able to control stability or movement, joint range should be maintained passively (i.e., by externally manipulating joints through their range of motion). Joint positioning, including the use of splints that maintain joints in proper positions, is also used to prevent joint deformity. The exception to this practice occurs when immobility of a joint is functionally advantageous for an individual.

Research has shown, and more and more people are aware, that many biomechanical problems are caused by how persons perform tasks in their daily occupations. Examples are back injury due to use of poor body mechanics while lifting and damage to soft tissues due to repetitive motions performed in work.[20] This awareness has fueled interest in efforts to prevent occurrence or recurrence of such problems, especially in the workplace. Occupational therapists can teach proper body mechanics or recommend work task or work site modifications to avoid such problems.

Restoration. Restoration aims at increasing available motion, strength, and endurance. Principles of restoration are based on the understanding of normal biomechanical functioning. This model asserts that because movement in tasks maintains normal range, strength, and endurance, movement can be used to restore or improve these as well. Therapists design programs in which joint movements and muscle tension produced are gradually increased. These increases in demand result in increases in capacity, until a desired level of functioning is reached. Goals for movement, strength, and endurance are determined according to the residual potential and the occupations the person needs to perform. For a person with quadriplegia, a goal may be to achieve the necessary motion, strength, and endurance for independence in self-care. For a person recovering from coronary bypass surgery, the goal may be to achieve the capacity to work 8 hours a day throughout a normal work week.

Compensation. Many people experience extended, permanent, or progressively greater limitations in their capacity for movement. Compensatory treatment aims to offset these limitations.[20] Compensation involves the use of devices that are attached to the body or that are used to mediate between the body and objects that need to be manipulated. Compensation may also involve modifying or replacing the objects used to perform routine tasks; the approach can also include modifications in the physical environment. Finally, compensation may involve altering procedures for accomplishing tasks, including the use of other persons as assistants in accomplishing these tasks.

Technology for Application

An extensive technology has been developed to support the application of this model. Information about the technology exists in a wide variety of published sources, including those that focus on particular kinds of musculoskeletal disorders.

Assessment

Range of motion is usually measured with a goniometer calibrated to the degrees of movement about an axis. If the patient is not capable of moving a joint voluntarily, the therapist passively moves it to evaluate available range. Range of motion is measured in degrees of movement about the axis of a joint.

Strength is normally tested as "maximum tension produced under voluntary effort."[20] The strength assessment most often used is manual muscle testing, in which the therapist (alone or using some instrument) tests the ability of the person to produce resistance and/or movement under standardized circumstances. In addition to examining strength of individual muscles and muscle groups, the evaluator may assess the pattern of muscle strength and weakness.

Endurance is usually measured by determining the duration or the number of repetitions before fatigue occurs. Several kinds of apparatus are available for muscle strength and endurance testing. These can produce very sophisticated analyses of muscle action.

Intervention

Methods of intervention for biomechanical dysfunction are clearly delineated. The method must match not only the targeted limitations of motion, strength, and endurance but also their underlying causes because the latter may determine what is the most appropriate intervention. For example, if limited range of motion is due to tightness, stretching may be used; if it is due to edema, compression may be used to reduce the edema. Active and passive range of motion and appropriate positioning may be used to prevent deformities. Special splints and other devices may also be used for these purposes.

Strength is developed by increasing the stress on a muscle through:

1. The amount of resistance offered to the movement
2. The duration of resistance required
3. The rate (speed of movement) of an exercise session
4. Frequency of sessions

Different types of exercise regimens are available. Current approaches (such as work hardening) emphasize strengthening by performing tasks required in the person's occupation.[11]

Therapists using this model may be involved in the prescription, design, fabrication, and checkouts of orthoses (special devices attached to the body to substitute for lost function) and in training patients in their use. Orthoses can be used to support, immobilize, or position the joint to enhance function. The orthosis can be used to correct for deformities or to increase function; it may be temporary or permanent. Orthotic splints either use existing movements to achieve functional motion or rely on sources of power external to the body.

Role of Occupation in Maintenance, Prevention, and Restoration

The traditional view in occupational therapy was that occupations provided natural and motivating circumstances for maintaining musculoskeletal functioning. This belief was based on the argument that involvement in meaningful occupations employed attention, thereby encouraging greater effort, diminishing fatigue, and diverting attention from pain or fear of movement. Additionally, therapists argued that occupations provided a form of conditioning that more nearly replicated the normal demands for movement in everyday life. Reflecting this perspective, Trombly[20] argues for the following approach to selecting activities used as therapeutic media. The selected activity must be interesting to the patient and must intrinsically demand the correct motion. This means that the performance of the activity as it is set up for the patient must involve the desired motion, without unreasonable contrivance or necessity for the patient to concentrate on the movement itself rather than the goal of the activity.

This implies that the therapist requires knowledge of the kind of functional movements that an activity will require from the participant. As noted earlier, it was assumed in the past that a therapist could determine what discrete movements would be required by doing a biomechanical activity analysis. Now it is recognized that, while it may be possible to determine the overall type of movement required to compete a specific activity, it is not possible to predict the exact pattern of muscle action and joint motion with which a person will accomplish a given task. As Trombly notes:

> The next time the person does the same thing, his or her muscles may be more warmed up, or there may be a slight difference in placement of task object in relation to the active limb, so a new coordinative structure evolves. That is, different muscles may be recruited, or the same muscles used before may be more or less active in order to accomplish the movement goal in the most efficient way. The motor goal is constant or invariant and requires a constant or invariant response, but this response can be fulfilled by a varying set of muscular contractions.[22]

Perhaps for this reason, research shows that therapists lack significant agreement about the biomechanical demands of activities.[22]

It appears that biomechanical analysis of activities will be understood somewhat differently in the future. First of all, therapists will pay more attention to the functional purpose of a task, since purpose does appear to exert an organizing influence on movement.[22] This means that when therapists analyze activities, they will need to think about the requisite movement in more functional terms, such as grasping, lifting, climbing, carrying, and so on. These are the kinds of functional movements that may remain stable within occupations, while the underlying combinations of muscle action and joint motion that accomplish the functional movements may vary considerably.

While in the future the process of analyzing an activity will be viewed differently, it will remain an important element of this model since therapists need to modify occupational activities in order to achieve therapeutic goals. Activity may be modified so as to reduce or alter task demands and thereby prevent musculoskeletal problems. Therapists may also adapt activity to better match permanently reduced musculoskeletal capacity. Finally, activity may be progressively modified to intensify task demands that will increase musculoskeletal capacity.

Therapists have several ways to modify an activity, including:

- Positioning the task
- Adding weights or other devices that provide assistance or resistance to movements performed in the activity
- Modifying tools to reduce or increase demands
- Changing materials or size of objects used
- Changing the method of accomplishing the task

In doing activity adaptation, Trombly[20] cautions that the therapist should not contrive the activity so much that it becomes meaningless. In all cases of using adapted activities it is important that the client be involved in occupational performance that has some meaning and relevance.

Compensatory Technology*

Compensatory technology is used for patients who will live with a disability either temporarily or permanently. Underlying this technology is the principle that when persons do not have the biomechanical capacity to perform daily living, leisure, and work tasks in ordinary ways, special equipment and modified procedures can compensate. They are used to close the gap between the person's capacities and the task demands. As Trombly notes, the desired goal of the treatment is for the person to be able to use his or her remaining capacities (and by using maintain them), while exercising the highest level of possible independence in occupational performance.

Evaluation includes assessment of actual performance in activities of daily living (e.g., toileting, bathing, feeding, grooming, dressing, mobility, and communication), leisure, work, and community living. When assessment is completed and the person's inability to perform necessary tasks is identified, the therapist determines the biomechanical limitations and assets. With this information, the therapist can recommend and train persons in the use of special equipment, modified procedures, or altered environments that make it possible for the person to perform the task. A wide range of adaptive equipment (commercially available or fabricated in therapy) is used to assist persons in performing every aspect of their daily occupations. The technology of adaptive equipment exists to interface between musculoskeletal capacities and environment and task demands. Some technology is quite simple, involving modification of ordinary tools and implements of life to make them easier to grasp and manipulate. Some technology involves modification of the environment (i.e., adding ramps and grab bars) to make it easier for a persons with limited biomechanical capacity to get around. There also exists more sophisticated technology for both restoration and compensation. This includes a wide range of equipment such as motorized wheelchairs, special communication devices, environmental controls, and modified workstations.

In collaboration with the client, the occupational therapist identifies the most appropriate device and/or modified procedure to use in occupational tasks. The therapist also provides instruction and practice in how to make use of compensatory devices and procedures. This can include instructing persons in how to organize their tasks and time to make the best use of existing capacity to accomplish their occupational tasks.

---

*Trombly[20] describes what she calls the rehabilitation approach as an alternative or complement to the biomechanical approach. However, the purpose of this technology is to support compensation for biomechanical limitations. These rehabilitation techniques do not have an independent theoretical base. Rather, the biomechanical model provides the rationale for the various rehabilitation strategies and equipment. Therefore, I am including what she calls rehabilitation techniques as a compensatory technology of the biomechanical model.

The occupational therapy setting is often used for persons to try out adapted equipment and procedures. Also, as therapists increasingly provide services in homes, schools, and workplaces, they can work even more specifically in the natural setting in which the task is to be performed. Therapists may assist individuals in planning changes in their homes (if this is financially feasible) and in learning to access specialized transportation and community facilities.

Work Hardening

Work hardening is an individualized biomechanical approach to treatment aimed at returning an individual to work—usually to a specific job. One of the main methods used in work hardening is physical reconditioning, the use of simulated and real work activities along with exercise to improve the person's ability to perform specific work tasks.

Work hardening programs employ a range of equipment including exercise and aerobic conditioning equipment, work capacity evaluation devices (which simulate the required movements of work tasks), work samples and workstations that simulate real jobs, and individualized simulations that reproduce a specific job requirement.[4,13]

Research

Research related to the interdisciplinary theoretical base of the biomechanical model is substantial. This research is producing new understanding of muscle physiology, the effects of exercise, and the dynamic role of muscles and muscle groups in movement.[4] As this body of knowledge grows, it influences the occupational therapy biomechanical model.

The proper area of occupational therapy research related to the biomechanical model will need further clarification, but some promising directions are emerging. One area of study is the relationship between musculoskeletal functioning and success in occupations.[16] For example, one study examined the ability of measures of physical capacities to predict injured workers' return to work.[7] Another study examined the potential for persons with muscular dystrophy to participate in specific occupational tasks.[15] A third study examined the relationship of wrist muscle tone to self-care abilities.[17]

Other studies are beginning to examine the actual muscle action and kinematics patterns used in different task conditions.[5,8,9,18,19,26] Such research helps to clarify how the movement is produced and used in occupational performance.

In one promising area of inquiry, studies examine how the purpose or meaning of activities affects compliance, effort, fatigue, and improvement in movement capacity. Studies have demonstrated the advantages of a dance program over normal range-of-motion exercises.[12,23,24] A study of elderly women supported the conclusion that adding imagery to movement is more effective than rote exercise in eliciting frequency and duration of movement.[13] A study of normal women demonstrated that perceived exertion was less in a task with purpose than in a purposeless task in which the same effort was exerted.[7] A new dimension to the biomechanical model appears to be emerging from this line of research, that is, the incorporation of the themes of experience and motivation into the understanding of human movement. Nelson and Peterson,[10] for example, differentiate between two motives that are intrinsic to movement:

1. Pleasure in the sensory experience of moving and exerting effort
2. The purpose added when movement is used to accomplish a goal

They argue that activities that add purpose to movement may enhance the quality of exercise, both by increasing the goal orientation of the client and by providing environmental support that guides the client's attention and motor planning.

As Trombly[21] notes, research on this model in occupational therapy is still very preliminary, and much more investigation will need to be done to clarify relationships between musculoskeletal and occupational functioning and to "establish the effects on occupational function of therapy applied according to the model."

Discussion

The use of biomechanical knowledge is not unique to occupational therapy. For example, physical therapy also applies biomechanics. What makes the biomechanical model a unique model of practice in occupational therapy is the way biomechanical principles are applied to understanding occupational performance. Additionally, occupational therapy is unique in the use of occupations to influence changes in range, strength, and endurance. Increasingly, the health care system is demanding functional outcomes from intervention (e.g., whether the person will return to work or remain living at home). This trend encourages the use of occupations that present clients with real-life demands.

The use of physical agents (e.g., heat or electrical stimulation), passive manipulation (e.g., massage or joint mobilization), and pure exercise has been controversial in occupational therapy. Physical agents, passive manipulation, and pure exercise are used extensively in physical therapy and, in fact, characterize much of how that profession applies biomechanics. Nonetheless, occupational therapists do also use these methods.

While the debates over occupational therapists' use of physical agents, exercise, and passive techniques have been heated, it seems that there are two legitimate sides to the argument. First of all, there is concern that occupational therapists applying biomechanical knowledge can become overly reliant, if not exclusively focused on, the nonoccupational aspects of musculoskeletal function.[25] Such practice brings into question whether occupational therapy is being practiced as it should be,[6] that is, in accordance with how the field's paradigm identifies practice. On the other hand, it is argued that there is a legitimate place for nonoccupational techniques that may be used as an adjunct or prelude to occupational therapy's unique focus on occupational functioning.[1] Current thinking (and official policy in the United States) suggests that use of these methods is "adjunctive" and has a legitimate purpose when they are necessary to develop or support the ability to engage in occupations.[2,3] The focus on occupation is, thus, affirmed while the use of adjunctive methods is recognized.

Given the centrality of movement problems to occupational therapy patients and clients, and the long history of this approach in occupational therapy practice, there is no doubt that the model will continue to be a vital part of occupational therapy science and practice. Further development is needed to increase its coherence and to articulate its position as a unique occupational therapy model of practice.

It is useful to consider that the biomechanical model was first developed as an occupational therapy approach under the previous paradigm and necessarily reflected the focus of that paradigm on inner mechanisms (i.e., musculoskeletal). As the field's paradigm has shifted to a focus on occupation, this model has had to be and is still being redefined.

TERMS OF THE MODEL

active range of motion	Degree of self-initiated movement possible at the joint.
biomechanical activity analysis	Examination of the endurance, range of motion, and muscle strength needed for the completion of an activity.
body mechanics	Position and movements of the body during the performance of occupations.
compensatory treatment	Therapy involving adaptations to deal with existing limitations.
elasticity	The capability of tissue to stretch and to return to its original shape and size.
endurance	The ability to sustain effort over the time required to do a particular task.
functional motion	Movement required for daily occupations.
joint range of motion	The potential for motion at the joints.
kinematics	The study of how the body moves in terms of the movement path, velocity, and acceleration.
manual muscle testing	Examination of an individual's muscle strength by asking the client to produce movement against manual resistance.
muscle strength	The ability of muscles to produce tension to maintain postural control and move body parts.
orthosis (pl., orthoses)	Device used to correct joint misalignment or to substitute for lost function.
passive range of motion	Amount of movement at the joint when it is moved by means other than the individual.
physical reconditioning	The process of returning the body to a state of fitness.
tendon	Connective tissue that connects a muscle to the bone.
work hardening	Program applying biomechanical principles by using simulations of the physical requirements of a work situation to recondition persons for work.

SUMMARY

The Biomechanical Model

FOCUS

- Musculoskeletal capacities that underlie functional motion in everyday occupational performance
- How the body is designed and used to accomplish motion for occupational performance
- Applied to persons who experience limitations in moving freely, with adequate strength, and/or in a sustained fashion

INTERDISCIPLINARY BASE

- Kinetic and kinematic principles concerning the nature of movement and the forces acting on the human body as it moves
- Anatomy of the musculoskeletal system
- Physiology of bone, connective tissue, muscle and cardiopulmonary function

THEORETICAL ARGUMENTS
Order

- Capacity for functional motion is based on:
  - The potential for motion at the joints (joint range of motion)
  - Muscle strength (ability of muscles to produce tension to maintain postural control and move body parts)
  - Endurance (ability to sustain effort [i.e., intensity or rate] over the time required to do a particular task)
- Joint range of motion depends on the structure and function of the joint and the integrity of surrounding connective tissue, muscle, and skin.
- Muscles cross one or more joints and exert force to control or produce movements allowed by the structure of the joints.
- Performance depends on the simultaneous action of muscles across many joints producing the stability and movement required for a task.
- The ability to sustain muscle activity (i.e., endurance) is a function of muscle physiology in relationship to the work being done and the supply of oxygen and energy materials from the cardiopulmonary system.
- The movements produced during occupational performance are as much a function of the dynamic circumstances of performance as they are of the structure of the musculoskeletal system.
- The capacity for movement (i.e., strength, range of motion, and endurance) both affects and is affected by one's occupational performance.

Disorder

- Dysfunction exists when a restriction of joint motion, strength, and/or endurance interferes with everyday occupations.
- Joint range of motion may be limited by joint damage, edema, pain, skin tightness, muscle spasticity (excess muscle tone producing tightness), or muscle and tendon shortening (due to immobilization).
- Muscle weakness can occur as a result of:
  - Disuse
  - Disease affecting muscle physiology (e.g., muscular dystrophy)
  - Diseases and trauma of the lower motor neurons (e.g., polio), the spinal cord, or peripheral nerves that result in deinnervation of muscles
  - Endurance can be reduced by:
  - Extended confinement or limitation of activity
  - Pathology of the cardiovascular or respiratory systems and muscular diseases

Therapeutic Intervention

- Interventions focus on the intersection of motion and occupational performance and can be divided into three approaches:
  1. Prevention of deformity and maintenance of existing capacity for motion
  2. Restoration by improving diminished capacity for motion
  3. Compensation for limited motion
- Intervention aims to minimize any gap between existing capacity for movement and the functional requirements of ordinary occupational tasks.

TECHNOLOGY FOR APPLICATION

- Range of motion is usually measured with a goniometer calibrated to the degrees of movement about an axis.
- Strength is normally tested through manual muscle testing, in which the therapist (alone or using some instrument) tests the ability of the person to produce resistance and/or movement under standardized circumstances.
- Endurance is usually measured by determining the duration or the number of repetitions before fatigue occurs.
- Methods of intervention match not only the targeted limitations of motion, strength, and endurance, but also their underlying causes, because the latter may determine what is the most appropriate intervention.
- Strength is developed by increasing the stress on a muscle through the:
  - Amount of resistance offered to the movement
  - Duration of resistance required

- ○ Rate (speed of movement) of an exercise session
- ○ Frequency of sessions
- Current approaches (such as work hardening) emphasize strengthening by performing tasks required by the person's occupation.
- Prescription, design, fabrication, checkout, and training in the use of orthoses to support, immobilize, or position the joint can prevent/correct deformities and/or enhance function.
- Occupations:
  - ○ Provide natural and motivating circumstances for maintaining musculoskeletal functioning
  - ○ Employ attention, thereby encouraging greater effort, diminishing fatigue, and diverting attention from pain or fear of movement
  - ○ Provide conditioning that more nearly replicates the normal demands for movement in everyday life
- Attention to the functional purpose of a task is important since purpose appears to exert an organizing influence on movement.
- Activity may be modified to:
  - ○ Reduce or alter task demands and prevent musculoskeletal problems
  - ○ Match permanently reduced musculoskeletal capacity
  - ○ Intensity task demands that will increase musculoskeletal capacity
- Ways to modify an activity include:
  - ○ Positioning the task
  - ○ Adding weights or other devices that provide assistance or resistance to movements performed in the activity
  - ○ Modifying tools to reduce or increase demands
  - ○ Changing materials or size of objects used
  - ○ Changing the method of accomplishing the task
- When using adapted activities, it is important that the client be involved in occupational performance that has some meaning and relevance.
- When persons do not have the biomechanical capacity to perform daily living, leisure, and work tasks in ordinary ways, special equipment and modified procedures can compensate (i.e., close the gap between the person's capacities and the task demands).

RESEARCH

- Areas of study:
  - ○ The relationship between musculoskeletal functioning and success in occupations
  - ○ Muscle action and kinematics patterns used in different task conditions
  - ○ How the purpose or meaning of activities affects compliance, effort, fatigue, and improvement in movement capacity

References

1. Ahlschwede, K: Views on physical agent modalities and specialization within occupational therapy: A rebuttal. Am J Occup Ther 46:650–652, 1992.
2. American Occupational Therapy Association. Use of adjunctive modalities in occupational therapy. Am J Occup Ther 46:1075–1081, 1992.
3. American Occupational Therapy Association Position Paper: Physical Agent Modalities. Am J Occup Ther 46:1090–1091, 1992.
4. Basmajian, JV, and Wolf, SL: Therapeutic Exercise, ed 5. Williams & Wilkins, Baltimore, 1990.
5. Follows, A: Electromyographical analysis of the extrinsic muscles of the long finger during pinch activities. Occupational Therapy Journal of Research 7:163, 1987.
6. Heater, SL: Specialization or uniformity within the profession? Am J Occup Ther 46:172–173, 1992.
7. Kircher, MA: Motivation as a factor of perceived exertion in purposeful versus nonpurposeful activity. Am J Occup Ther 38:165, 1984.
8. Mathiowetz, VG: Informational support and functional motor performance. Unpublished doctoral dissertation, University of Minnesota, 1991.
9. McGrain, P, and Hague, MA: An electromyographic study of the middle deltoid and middle trapezius muscles during warping. Occupational Therapy Journal of Research 7:225, 1987.
10. Nelson, DL, and Peterson, CQ: Enhancing therapeutic exercise through purposeful activity: A theoretical analysis. Topics in Geriatric Rehabilitation 4:12, 1989.
11. Ogden-Niemeyer, L, and Jacobs, K: Work Hardening: State of the Art. Slack, Thorofare, NJ, 1989.
12. Pedretti, LW, and Zoltan, B: Occupational Therapy Practice Skills for Physical Dysfunction. CV Mosby, St. Louis, 1996.
13. Riccio, CM, Nelson, DL, and Bush, MA: Adding purpose to the repetitive exercise of elderly women. Am J Occup Ther 44:714, 1990.
14. Robert, S, and Falkenburg, S: Biomechanics: Problem Solving for Functional Activity. CV Mosby, St. Louis, 1992.
15. Schkade, JK, Feilbelman, A, and Cook, JD: Occupational potential in a population with Duchenne Muscular Dystrophy. Occupational Therapy Journal of Research 7:289, 1987.
16. Smith, SL, Cunningham, S, and Weinberg, R: Predicting reemployment of the physically disabled worker. Occupational Therapy Journal of Research 3:178, 1983.
17. Spaulding, SJ, et al.: Wrist muscle tone and self-care skill in persons with hemiparesis. Am J Occup Ther 44:11, 1989.
18. Trombly, CA, and Cole, JM: Electromyographic study of four hand muscles during selected activities. Am J Occup Ther 33:440–449, 1979.
19. Trombly, CA, and Quintana, LE: Activity analysis: Electromyographic and electrogoniometric verification. Occupational Therapy Journal of Research 3:178, 1983.
20. Trombly, CA: Occupation Therapy for Physical Dysfunction, ed 3. Williams & Wilkins, Baltimore, 1989, p 184, p 231, p 290.
21. Trombly, CA: Occupational Therapy for Physical Dysfuction, ed 4. Williams & Wilkins, Baltimore 1995.
22. Trombly, CA: Occupation: Purposefulness and meaningfulness as therapeutic mechanisms. 1995 Eleanor Clarke Slagle Lecture. Am J Occup Ther 49:960–972, 1995
23. Van Deusen, J, and Marlowe, D: A comparison of the ROM dance, home exercise/rest program with traditional routines. Occupational Therapy Journal of Research 7:349, 1987.
24. Van Deusen, J, and Marlowe, D: The efficacy of the ROM Dance Program for adults with rheumatoid arthritis. Am J Occup Ther 41:90, 1987.
25. West, WL, and Wiemer, RB: Should the Representative Assembly have voted as it did, when it did, on occupational therapists' use of physical modalities? Am J Occup Ther 45:1143–1147, 1991
26. Wu, C-Y, Trombly, CA, and Lin, K-C: The relationship between occupational form and occupational performance: A kinematic perspective. Am J Occup Ther 48:679–687, 1994.

CHAPTER 7

THE COGNITIVE DISABILITIES MODEL

The cognitive disabilities model originated as an approach to persons with mental illness, and it is now applied to other groups of patients in whom cognitive limitations are observed (e.g., those with traumatic brain injury and dementia). A cognitive disability refers to an "incapacity to process information necessary to do ordinary activities safely."[7]

As the title of the model implies, the approach to functional limitations is based on concern for underlying cognitive capacity. This model began with a primary interest in describing the kinds of limitations persons exhibited for processing information in task performance. The central arguments of this model are that cognitive ability exists in a single hierarchical continuum, and that cognitive disability is determined by "a medical condition [that] restricts the way the brain operates."[7]

This model focuses on residual limitations imposed by health problems and emphasizes evaluation of patients' functional limitations.[8] The model seeks to achieve an accurate description of cognitive impairment from which therapists can determine appropriate intervention goals and advise others about the potential of patients to be safe and to learn. There is a strong emphasis on issuing cautions and warnings about patients' restricted capacity and on achieving necessary supervision, environmental modification, and/or legal restriction of patients to prevent "hazardous situations."[8]

The model describes the cognitive abilities and limitations in terms of cognitive levels graded hierarchically from normal to profoundly impaired function. Use of these cognitive levels to describe the degree of functional limitation and to guide the therapist's decision making about patient care is the core feature of how this model is applied.

Interdisciplinary Base

The cognitive disabilities model is derived from several sources. It began with attempts by Allen[3] to classify the performance difficulties of patients using concepts from Piaget's work on cognition, particularly his description of the sensorimotor period of development. Allen originally expected that cognitive capacities could be redeveloped in persons who had lost them, but she later abandoned this idea.

This model originally claimed to be based on the concepts of neuroscience. However, minimal reference is made to current neurological concepts. Moreover, the model draws different conclusions about the possibility of improving functioning than other occupational therapy approaches based on neuroscience. The latter emphasize neuroplasticity and the potential for bringing about change through therapy. The cognitive disabilities model recommends against a focus on changing the individual through therapy. Allen[3] points out that she avoided theories that assumed learning or normal memory because she presumes that these capacities are permanently impaired in persons with chronic psychiatric disease and other persons with brain damage.

The cognitive disabilities model is influenced by the medical view that functional limitations are directly mediated by neurological damage and change according to the natural history of the disease and/or with medical interventions that directly alter the brain. More recent work[7,8] seeks to establish a unique focus apart from the medical model. While the medical model stresses the disease process and its eradication and/or control, the cognitive disabilities model focuses on the consequences of the disease (i.e., cognitive limitations that result from diseases). In developing this focus, Allen has used the World Health Organization's[12] system for classifying impairment, disabilities, and handicaps. This classification system is not disease-based; instead, it focuses on incapacitation resulting from diseases.

The model also stresses occupational therapy's concentration on adjustment to residual limitations as differentiating occupational therapy from medicine, which is concerned with producing biological change.* According to this model, occupational therapy should acknowledge and focus on the measurement and management of permanent residual limitations rather than their alteration.

---

*Some would take issue with the assertion that biological change is the exclusive domain of medicine. Certainly many of the models discussed in this book assert that participation in occupation can influence biological changes (e.g., muscle fiber size and synaptic connections) that are also manifest as functional changes (e.g., strength, sensory and perceptual abilities).

Theoretical Arguments

Although the model assumes that brain function and dysfunction are the bases of cognitive processes and disorders, the model does not seek to explain the brain–behavior relationship or how specific brain disorders impair the quality of cognition underlying action. Rather, the emphasis of the model is on how impairment of cognition affects performance of daily living tasks.[7,8]

Voluntary motor action was originally specified as the focus for this model. The model defined voluntary motor action as "a behavior response to a sensory cue guided by the mind."[2] Allen concentrated on voluntary motor behaviors that occur in routine tasks, arguing that these are usually the most important to patients and most valued by others in the patient's environment. More recently, communication abilities also have been incorporated into the model. Communication abilities are viewed as being a function of cognitive level; therefore, this model anticipates restrictions in communication when cognition is impaired.

Order

The model defines normal function in terms of the relationship of brain, cognition, and task behavior. According to the model, the brain determines cognition, which in turn guides behavior (voluntary motor actions). As noted previously, the explanatory focus is not on the brain–cognition relationship but on the role of cognition in determining task performance. The model has concentrated on two features of cognition: (1) the cognitive dimensions of task performance and (2) the continuum of cognitive functioning (i.e., the levels of cognitive functioning).

Cognitive Dimensions of Task Performance. Although she does not define cognition per se, Allen identifies cognition with the response to sensory cues by forming purposes and processing information to guide motor activity.[2] This view of cognition is further explicated in the identification of the following dimensions of task performance: attention, behavior, purpose, experience, process, and time. *Attention* is selective responsiveness to sensory cues. *Behavior* refers to the motor actions exhibited in task performance. *Purpose* connotes the person's intended objective, which guides the motor response to a sensory cue. *Experience* is what a person goes through when he or she is involved in a task. *Process* refers to the course of action that is followed to achieve a purpose, and *time* refers to the duration over which a person sustains sensorimotor associations as manifest in ongoing voluntary motor responses to sensory cues. These dimensions were originally used as a basis for describing qualities of task performance across the cognitive levels.

Cognitive Levels. As noted earlier, the model proposes a hierarchical continuum of function and dysfunction. This continuum is divided into six cognitive levels.* While detailed criteria for each level has been developed, the following is an overview of how the levels describe function and dysfunction:[7]

> **Level 0: Coma.** Coma is a prolonged state of unconsciousness with a lack of specific response to stimuli.
> **Level 1: Automatic Actions.** Automatic actions are a response to a stimulus initiated by someone else and are invariable reactions to the stimulus.
> **Level 2: Postural Actions.** Postural actions are self-initiated, gross body movements that overcome the effects of gravity and move the whole body in space.
> **Level 3: Manual Actions.** Manual actions are those using the hands, and occasionally other parts of the body, to manipulate material objects.
> **Level 4: Goal-Directed Actions.** Goal-directed actions sequence the self through a series of steps to match a concrete sample or a known standard of how the finished product should appear.
> **Level 5: Exploratory Actions.** Exploratory actions are discoveries of how changes in neuromuscular control can produce different effects on material objects.
> **Level 6: Planned Actions.** Planned actions estimate the effect of actions on material objects, but the objects do not have to be present for the estimate to occur. The significance of the effects of a sequence of steps permits anticipation of secondary effects.

These levels have been a part of the cognitive disabilities model from its beginning although some revision of the definitions of levels has occurred. More recently intermediate levels have been identified. For example, level 1 has been subdivided into 1.0 withdrawing, 1.2 responding, 1.4 locating stimuli, 1.6 rolling in bed, and 1.8 raising body part. Allen[7] notes that the addition of these intermediate levels allows a finer discrimination of cognitive function/limitation.

Disorder

The cognitive disabilities model originally defined dysfunction as "a restriction in voluntary motor action originating in the physical or chemical structures of the brain and producing observable limitations in routine task behavior."[2] As the more recent definition given at the beginning of this

---

*Although technically there are seven levels when coma is included as a level, the literature consistently refers to six cognitive levels, so that convention is followed here.

chapter suggests, the current emphasis is in information processing for safe performance of ordinary activities.

The model still assumes that brain abnormality underlies a deficit in mental processes or cognition that, in turn, restricts functional capacity. The model does not attempt to explain the nature or etiology of various brain disorders that lead to cognitive disabilities. Rather, the medical model is recommended as the source of explanations of diseases. Medical explanations of the underlying causes of the disability are recommended as important background information for occupational therapy.[8] The medical model also provides information about prognoses, such as the expected length of current symptoms and prospects for improvement of the person's condition.

The unique view of dysfunction this model achieves is a description of the restrictions in task performance that occur in association with disease. Thus the cognitive levels, which describe the extent of cognitive disability and the degree of functional limitation, are the core of the model's view of dysfunction.

Therapeutic Intervention

This model makes two important assertions about change. The first is that occupational therapy does not change the cognitive level of patients who have cognitive limitations resulting from brain pathology. Changes in cognitive level are considered either part of the natural course of the disease process or due to the effects of medication. More recently, Allen has stated that occupational therapy may be associated with changes in cognitive level, but she does not claim a causative link.[8] She argues that other factors, such as natural healing and psychotropic drugs, have more effects than therapy on brain pathology and, therefore, on cognitive changes.

The second assertion is that brain disorders place restrictions on learning; persons at or below level 4 are considered to have severe restrictions in learning new behaviors. Specifically, it is argued that patients at or below level 4 do not generalize[7] and that "Novelty is ignored at Levels One through Four, making it impossible to teach new skills."[1]

Given these two assertions, the approach to intervention emphasizes monitoring changes in cognitive level and adapting intervention to fit the level at which the patient is functioning. Once a patient's cognitive level of function is determined to be stable or deteriorating (as in progressive dementias), then the interventions focus on training, environmental modification, providing information and guidelines to caregivers, and other strategies designed to accommodate and manage the patient's functional limitations/capacities.

The following are offered as guidelines for intervention once a patient's level of function is determined. Patients should be offered the opportunity to process information at a higher level for a brief period but should not be forced to sustain function that produces discomfort, frustration, or confusion. Patients can struggle with higher function if they desire but should not be pushed. This approach argues that it is not useful for persons to work toward function requiring a cognitive level higher than that of which they are judged capable.

Phases of Treatment. This model divides treatment into four phases of illness (acute, postacute, rehabilitation, and long-term), each having its own implications for treatment. During the acute phase, therapists' use of this model consists of evaluating the patient's cognitive level. In the postacute phase, patients can engage in activities suited to their cognitive level, the therapist continues to monitor any changes in cognitive level and makes recommendations for how much assistance will be needed upon discharge. Allen[7] argues that when patients are in the rehabilitation phase, little or no change in cognitive level is expected. Therefore the emphasis is on improving patient performance by providing adaptive equipment, modifying the environment, and teaching caregivers to provide assistance. At this stage, activity analysis allows therapists to provide activities of an appropriate level to the patient. Moreover, activities beyond the patient's level of ability can be avoided or done with appropriate modification/supervision. Long-term care refers to the "provision of a community-based activity program for people who are functioning at cognitive levels 3 and 4."[7]

Allen[7] notes that successful outcomes during the rehabilitation and long-term care phases depends on psychological and social factors. Because the cognitive disabilities model does not provide guidelines for how to evaluate or influence these factors, the assumption must be that other models are necessary to guide the occupational therapist's decision making about these factors.

Environmental Compensation. The main approach to treatment is *environmental compensation* for the patient's limitations in functional capacity. This approach differs from medical treatment in that it emphasizes making adjustments to the residual effects of disease rather than addressing the disease process itself.[8] According to the model, occupational therapy services are not presumed to affect the cognitive level of patients, so cognitive improvement is not a goal or outcome of occupational therapy. Rather, the occupational therapist documents the level of cognitive dysfunction and provides a task environment in which a patient can function. Such "environmental compensations offset the defects in the structure of function of the organism through the modification of a task."[1] Giving patients tasks that they can do, even with their cognitive limitations, enables them to be more functional. A further goal of therapy is to enable patients to comprehend and accept their permanent limitations. This is accomplished by providing concrete feedback to the patient on task performance. The occupational therapist uses the model to assess the patient's functional level to determine when the patient is ready for discharge and in what type of environment the patient can function on discharge. The goal is to identify the least restrictive environment in which a person with cognitive disabilities can function safely.[4,8] The therapist's role also includes providing caregivers with realistic information about disabled persons' limits and about necessary supports to allow the disabled person to function.

Although it is acknowledged that patients functioning at levels 5 and 6 may exhibit some deficits and are capable of learning, this model does not provide guidelines for programming aimed at allowing these persons to capitalize on their learning capacity. Although Allen does not say so, one may presume that such concerns are the domain of other models.

Technology for Application

The cognitive disabilities model provides detailed, specific procedures for patient assessment, task analysis, and task selection in treatment.

Assessment

Detailed assessments of functional level have been developed for use with the cognitive disabilities model; they include the Routine Task Inventory, the Allen Cognitive Level Test, and the Cognitive Performance Test.

The Routine Task Inventory (RTI) is administered by interviewing the patient or by observing the patient's performance. Because the reliability of this assessment for patients at levels 1 through 4 is considered questionable, the RTI may be administered by interviewing a caregiver.[8,10] When observation is used, it is recommended that more than a single activity be observed since a single performance may give a biased reading of the patient's level. The RTI consists of 32 routine activities, such as grooming, dressing, bathing, shopping, doing laundry, as well as more general behavior items such as following instructions, cooperating, and supervising. Each task is described according to each of the six cognitive levels of performance. Matching the patient's reported or observed performance to the descriptions under each task enables the therapist to determine the patient's level of cognitive functioning.

The Allen Cognitive Level (ACL) test uses performance in a single activity to provide a quick estimate of the patient's cognitive level.[9] Leather lacing is the activity; the cognitive level is determined by the complexity of leather-lacing stitch that the patient can imitate. Allen has standardized the method of presenting the task and scoring patient performance. The ACL has three versions. The first version (ACL-O) is designed to measure persons whose cognitive level ranges from 2 to 6. "Lack of sensitivity and other flaws"[9] led to the development of the two other versions. The ACL-E has a more detailed score sheet and a modified administration procedure (i.e., the therapist twists the leather lacing to see if the patient can correct it). The ACL-PS modifies the presentation of the leather lacing task to see if the patient can do it by looking or requires verbal instructions or demonstration. Further revision of the ACL has resulted in yet another version, the ACL-90; this version is commercially available and it is the version of the ACL that is typically used.

The Cognitive Performance Test is composed of six activities of daily living tasks: Dress, Shop, Toast, Telephone, Wash, and Travel.[9] Each task employs standardized equipment and administration. For example, the Dress task consists of asking a patient to choose the appropriate attire for a cold rainy day. The patient chooses among a man and a woman's heavy-weight raincoat, a man and a woman's robe, a man's straw hat, a man's rain hat, a woman's plastic rain scarf, a woman's sheer scarf, and an umbrella. The patient's choice and behavior in putting on appropriate clothes is used to determine the cognitive level at which a patient is functioning.

Besides these more structured assessments, therapists make informal observations of task performance to monitor patients' cognitive level. Guidelines are provided for identifying the patient's cognitive level. Further, the use of tasks with known levels of complexity can be used to gauge the patient's functional level. That is, the therapist analyzes the task to determine its cognitive demands and then observes whether the person can perform it.

Use of Evaluation Data

The central theme in this model is evaluation of cognitive disability. An emphasis is also made on how evaluation data are to be used. Depending on the phase of the patient's illness and/or treatment, the data may be used to evaluate the course of the disease or effects of medication, or to make determinations of the appropriateness of rehabilitation, discharge, supervision, and environmental accommodations. Evaluation is also used to make recommendations for appropriate placement of the patient.

Allen and Earhardt[8] emphasize that careful evaluation of a patient's cognitive limitations has important implications for what a patient can be considered capable of doing safely, what legal restrictions may be placed on a person, and the kinds of environmental safeguards and support that are necessary to manage a person in the community. They link the idea of cognitive disability closely to the legal definitions of competence and the associated idea of ordinary care. *Ordinary care* is a legal term that refers to reasonable effort and judgment according to prevailing cultural norms. They indicate that cognitive level 6 corresponds to what is legally defined as competence. Allen[7] underscores the role of the occupational therapist in issuing warnings about patients' cognitive limitations. She indicates that "[w]hen necessary, therapists should take steps to initiate legal action (such as removing a driver's license or obtaining a legal guardian) (p 14)."

Task Analysis

This model emphasizes the importance of *task analysis*.[2,5,6] The current text on this model includes a number of performance actions (e.g., sanding, glueing, cutting) and activities (e.g., grooming, dressing) that are analyzed according to the cognitive levels.[8] Analysis of the complexity of tasks underlies the entire assessment approach. Moreover, selection and adaptation of tasks for patient performance is central to this model's treatment approach. Task analysis begins with determining the normal procedure for performing a task. Then the therapist identifies the relative complexity of steps in the task. It is argued that task analysis can be applied to any activity. Therefore, the patient's cognitive level (functional ability) can be matched to any task, and it can be determined whether the patient has the capacity to perform the task, given its complexity. Then, if necessary, the task can be adapted by changing or eliminating a troublesome step or adjusting the complexity of the task. For example, Allen[1] notes the differences in complexity of pattern a patient can create:

> At Level Three we see a disorganized use of one color, at Level Four the person can follow a checkerboard pattern, at Level Five the person follows a simple pattern and those people at Level Six create a unique pattern.

The final goal of all task analysis is to identify steps in the process that the patient cannot do. Tasks can then be adapted to avoid procedures that patients are unable to perform, while allowing them to use remaining abilities. As Allen[1] notes, the therapist uses "elements of the physical environment as substitutes for deficient patterns of thought that would normally be used to guide behavior." Figure 7–1 illustrates the relationship of patients' task behavior, task analysis, and adjustment of task demands. According to this figure, task behavior is a function of the patient (including the patient's cognitive limitations) and the task demand. The model argues that, since the patient's cognitive level cannot be changed, the therapist must analyze the task and adjust the task demand to accommodate the cognitive limitation of the patient. This concept (whether applied in selecting tasks for use in therapy or in creating a functional environment for living) is central to how this model is applied.

A more recent feature of this model's approach to task analysis is the provision of guidelines for training in specific tasks that take into consideration different levels of cognitive impairment. Guidelines are provided for

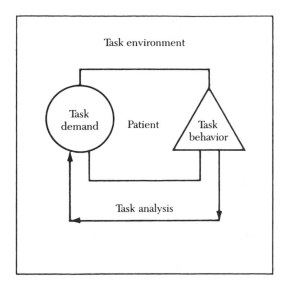

Figure 7–1. The therapist's awareness of the task environment.

determining what a person of a given cognitive level can do within given types of tasks, along with information about how that person can be trained to do the task.

Treatment Applications

Application of the model is straightforward and requires very little adaptation for different settings. The model uses a very specific approach to identifying cognitive levels, to analyzing tasks of which persons are capable at those levels, and to providing such tasks as therapy. Descriptions of applications of the model in the literature address a range of persons deemed to have cognitive limitations. These include, for example, papers illustrating use of the model with persons with dementia,[14] persons with mental illness,[15] and persons recovering from cerebrovascular accidents (CVAs) and traumatic brain injury.[6]

Allen believes that purposeful activity is the treatment method of occupational therapy. She discusses the importance of focusing on routine tasks in the patient's life. Allen[3] writes that activity provides persons with the opportunity to use remaining capacities, thereby achieving meaningful involvement and a rightful place in community life. This treatment model strongly emphasizes the use of crafts during the acute phase of illness. According to the model, psychiatric patients prefer crafts because they are easily adapted to the patient's functional level and provide tangible evidence of functional capacity.[2,7]

Research

The cognitive disabilities model is relatively new. Consequently, limited research on this model exists. Most studies focus on determining the reliability and validity of the ACL and RTI. Two studies found good agreement between raters using the ACL.[2,8] Other studies have demonstrated evidence of an association between the ACL and measures of mental status and psychiatric symptomatology.[2,16]

One study demonstrated an association between ACL scores and functional performance in patients with dementia.[16] Another study found that a group of psychiatric adolescents were functioning at lower cognitive levels than a nonpsychiatric group.[13] This evidence supports the thesis that persons with psychiatric problems may experience limitation of cognitive abilities.

Two studies have examined the ability of cognitive level to predict community functioning. One study examined whether cognitive level at discharge would predict schizophrenic patients' social adjustment in the community. The relationship was negligible. Cognitive level was a poorer predictor of community adjustment than demographic variables, such as age, sex, work history, record of hospitalization, and marital history.[13] A more recent study asked whether cognitive level could predict future community adaptation of young persons with serious mental illness.[11] This investigation found that cognitive level is inversely related to community adaptation (i.e., persons at lower cognitive levels were more adaptive and persons at higher levels were less adaptive), although the association was slight. These two studies alone do not provide definitive findings; however, they do raise questions about whether cognitive levels are accurate and useful for predicting community adjustment. These are especially important questions to answer since one of the primary uses of cognitive levels is to make decisions about the person's ability for and needs in community functioning.

Discussion

The cognitive disabilities model seeks to objectively describe limitations in functional performance. The model's view of the nature of cognitive dysfunction is concise and provides specific methods of assessment and intervention. The model provides specific means for assessing patient capacity and matching that capacity to task demands.

The cognitive disabilities model proposes a nontraditional view of the role of participation in activities and its relationship to functional capacity. The issue of whether patients improve and/or maintain capacity from participation in occupation is an important one that will need further scrutiny.

Allen argues that occupational therapists have overstated the effect of activity in producing change as reflected in treatment goals of increasing, or enhancing patient capacity.[2] She further argues that alternative explanations for improvement, such as the natural course of healing and the effects of other treatments, such as medication, have not been sufficiently ruled out. Moreover, she asserts that occupational therapy has failed to recognize the permanent deficits of patients with cognitive disabilities, reasoning that, "To deny mental deficits has led to false hope about our ability to resolve them."[1]

Caution about possibly overstated claims for the impact of activity is useful. Further, it is a useful argument that failure to recognize real limitations in persons' capacities may result in blaming them (i.e., attributing lack of performance on motivational factors) and in failing to provide them with necessary supports for functioning. On the other hand, denying that therapy can affect cognitive level and subsequent function is inconsistent with other views of the potential for changing or maintaining capacity in persons with brain injury or disease. While it is important to acknowledge any permanent limitations of capacity, the therapist must be careful not to limit unwittingly the patient's opportunities to learn or to develop functional performance. Significant change in a person's functional capacity may take time and concentrated efforts. Therefore, it is possible to conclude that change cannot be affected by therapy when, instead, the current health care delivery system does not provide enough resources to bring about change. Moreover, the emphasis on patients' limitations could be used by those who control health policy to justify not expending time and resources to support patients to regain function.

The claim that learning does not occur within a wide range of functioning (levels 1 through 4) is not yet substantiated. Because of the seriousness of this claim, it is critical to demonstrate through research whether permanent deficits exist in the learning capacities of persons with cognitive impairment. One pilot study suggested that, while learning differed in groups with different cognitive levels, all patients learned to master some new skills.[13] This single study cannot rule out Allen's hypothesis that learning does not occur, but it indicates the importance of research to assess it. Moreover, it will be important to distinguish between those situations in which participation in occupation can produce an improvement and those in which significant improvement in discrete areas of function is not possible or likely.

Allen points out that disease can be a powerful explanation for much of the dysfunction therapists observe in patients with mental disorders.[2] Equally plausible is that the lack of opportunity to use or develop capacities is a source of functional limitation.

Since this model grew out of practice in psychiatric settings, it should also be noted that it represents a departure from traditional psychosocial models, which emphasize motivational and emotional factors in functioning. This model has not been concerned directly with motivation, although Allen acknowledges humans have a "need to engage in desirable activities."[2] Moreover, she notes that persons suffer when left with nothing to do, and she argues that persons with disabilities should have access to activities that reflect their interests and desires.[1] Her main concern is the distress that occurs when persons do not have access to task performance. In recent work, Allen has recognized motivation as a possible factor influencing quality of performance.[8] This concern addresses the problem of how to achieve an accurate assessment of ability that is free of motivational factors. Allen's lack of emphasis on motivational factors is based on her view that differences in individual performance are more directly linked to actual functional limitations (i.e., the cognitive limitations) than to problems in motivation. No research, however, has demonstrated the relative importance of functional limitations and motivational factors.

Finally, the proposal that cognition can be reduced to a single hierarchical continuum differs from other occupational therapy approaches (see Chap. 8, e.g.), which argue that cognition is multidimensional. Such approaches suggest that an individualized picture of cognitive strengths and weaknesses is necessary and that a simple categorization of a person's cognitive capacity fails to recognize individual variability in cognitive styles and deficits.

Thus, while the cognitive disabilities model offers a concise formulation of cognitive factors that affect occupational performance, this precision may be achieved at the expense of oversimplification. Finding the right balance between an adequate conceptualization of the phenomena of concern and having straightforward ideas for application is always difficult. No doubt, this issue will continue to challenge occupational therapists in the future, both with regard to this and other conceptual practice models.

TERMS OF THE MODEL

attention	Selected responsiveness to sensory cues.
behavior	The motor actions exhibited in task performance.
cognitive capacity	The potential for mental processing.
cognitive dimensions of task performance	The observable aspects of mental activity, including behavior, process, time, experience, and attention.
cognitive disability	Incapacity to process information necessary to do ordinary activities safely.
cognitive levels	System of classification based on the complexity of sensorimotor associations demonstrated during performance of a task.
cognitive limitations	Deficits in mental processing that can be observed during task performance.
environmental compensation	Changing the task to accommodate cognitive deficits.
experience	What one goes through when involved in a task.
ordinary care	Reasonable effort and judgment according to prevailing cultural norms; this concept is the point of reference for legally determining neglect.
process	The course of action that is followed to achieve a purpose.
purpose	The intended objective that guides the motor response to a sensory cue.
symbolic cues	Information conveyed by symbols (e.g., diagrams, written directions).
task analysis	Determination of the cognitive demands of an activity.
time	The duration over which a person sustains sensorimotor associations as shown by ongoing voluntary motor responses to sensory cues.
voluntary motor action	A behavioral response to a sensory cue that is guided by the mind.

SUMMARY

The Cognitive Disabilities Model

FOCUS

- Originally an approach to persons with mental illness, it is now applied to other groups of patients in whom cognitive limitations are observed (e.g., those with traumatic brain injury and dementia).
- Focuses on residual limitations and emphasizes:
  - Evaluation of patients' functional limitations
  - Issuing cautions and warnings about patients' restricted capacity
  - Achieving necessary supervision
  - Environmental modification
  - Legal restriction of patients to prevent hazards
- Cognitive levels (graded from normal to profoundly impaired function) are used to describe the degree of functional limitation.

INTERDISCIPLINARY BASE

- Piaget's work on cognition, particularly his description of the sensori-motor period of development
- Neuroscience (however, the model rejects neuroplasticity and the potential for bringing about change through therapy in persons with chronic psychiatric disease and brain damage)
- Emphasis on medical view that functional limitations result from neurological damage and change according to the natural history of the disease and/or with medical interventions that directly alter the brain
- World Health Organization classification of impairment, disabilities, and handicaps, which focuses on incapacitation resulting from diseases

THEORETICAL ARGUMENTS

Order

- Normal function is based on the relationship of brain, cognition, and task behavior:
  - Brain determines cognition.
  - Cognition guides behavior (voluntary motor actions).
- Concentrates on two features of cognition:
  - The cognitive dimensions of task performance
  - The continuum of cognitive functioning (i.e., the levels of cognitive functioning)
- Cognitive dimensions of task performance (originally used as a basis for describing performance across the cognitive levels):
  - Attention (selective responsiveness to sensory cues)
  - Behavior (motor actions exhibited in task performance)
  - Purpose (person's intended objective)

- ○ Experience (what a person goes through when involved in a task)
- ○ Process (course of action followed to achieve a purpose)
- ○ Time (duration over which a person sustains sensorimotor associations)
- Hierarchical continuum of function and dysfunction is divided into six cognitive levels:
  - ○ Coma (prolonged state of unconsciousness without response to stimuli—not counted as a cognitive level since cognition is absent)
  - ○ Automatic actions (response to stimulus initiated by someone else; invariable reactions to the stimulus)
  - ○ Postural actions (self-initiated, gross body movements that move the whole body in space)
  - ○ Manual actions (using hands, and occasionally other body parts, to manipulate objects)
  - ○ Goal-directed actions (series of steps that match a sample or standard of a finished product)
  - ○ Exploratory actions (discovers how changes in neuromuscular control produce different effects on objects).
  - ○ Planned actions (estimates effect of actions on objects that are present; anticipates secondary effects)

Disorder

- Brain abnormality underlies a deficit in cognition, producing restrictions in task performance.
- Cognitive levels describe the extent of cognitive disability and the degree of functional limitation.

Therapeutic Intervention

- Assertions about change:
  - ○ Occupational therapy does not change the cognitive level of patients who have cognitive limitations resulting from brain pathology. (Changes reflect the natural course of disease or effects of medication.)
  - ○ Brain disorders place restrictions on learning. (Persons at or below level 4 have severe restrictions with regard to learning new behaviors.)
- Approach to intervention emphasizes:
  - ○ Measuring and monitoring changes in cognitive level
  - ○ Adapting intervention to fit the level at which the patient is functioning
- While therapy can offer opportunity to process information at a higher level for a brief periods, patients should not be pushed to struggle with higher function.
- Treatment divided into four phases:
  - ○ Acute (therapists evaluate patient's cognitive level)
  - ○ Postacute (patients can engage in activities; therapist monitors cognitive level and recommends how much assistance will be needed at discharge)

- ○ Rehabilitation (improves patient performance by providing adaptive equipment, modifying the environment, and teaching caregivers to provide assistance; provides activities at an appropriate level to the patient, avoiding/supervising activities beyond the patient's level of ability)
- ○ Long-term care (providing community-based activity program for people at cognitive levels 3 and 4)
- • Main approach to treatment is environmental compensation—i.e., making adjustments to the residual effects of disease rather than addressing the disease process itself.
- • Since occupational therapy services are not presumed to affect the cognitive level of patients, cognitive improvement is not a goal or outcome of occupational therapy.
- • Goals are:
  - ○ Giving patients tasks that they can do
  - ○ Enabling patients to comprehend and accept permanent limitations
  - ○ Identifying the least restrictive environment in which a person can function safely
  - ○ Providing caregivers with information about disabled persons' limits and necessary supports to function

TECHNOLOGY FOR CLINICAL APPLICATION

- • Detailed, specific procedures are given for patient assessment, task analysis, and therapeutic task selection.
- • Four formal assessments of functional level have been developed:
  - ○ Routine Task Inventory (administered by interviewing the patient or caregiver, or by observing patient's performance; consists of 32 routine tasks, each described according to the six cognitive levels)
  - ○ Allen Cognitive Level Test (performance in leather lacing is used to determine cognitive level)
  - ○ Cognitive Performance Test (composed of six daily living tasks, it employs standardized equipment and administration
- • Informal observations of task performance and use of tasks with known levels of complexity are also used to gauge the patient's functional level.
- • Evaluation of cognitive limitations is considered important to determine:
  - ○ What a patient can be considered capable of doing safely
  - ○ What legal restrictions may be placed on a person
- • Task analysis is central to treatment and includes:
- • Determining the normal procedure for performing a task
  - ○ Identifying the relative complexity of steps in the task
  - ○ Identifying steps in the process that the patient cannot do
  - ○ Adapting tasks to avoid procedures that patients are unable to perform

RESEARCH

- Model is relatively new, and limited research exists.
- Studies focus on:
  - Determining the reliability and validity of assessments
  - Demonstrating associations between cognitive level and measures of mental status and psychiatric symptomatology
- Two studies raise questions about the utility of cognitive level for predicting community adaptation.

References

1. Allen, CK: Independence through activity: The practice of occupational therapy (psychiatry). Am J Occup Ther 36:731, 1982.
2. Allen, CK: Occupational Therapy for Psychiatric Diseases: Measurement and Management of Cognitive Disabilities. Little Brown, Boston, 1985, pp xiii, 6, 31, 22, 573.
3. Allen, CK: Cognitive disabilities: Measuring the social consequences of mental disorders. J Clin Psychiatry 48:185, 1987.
4. Allen, CK: Occupational therapy: Functional assessment of the severity of mental disorders. Hosp Community Psychiatry 39:140, 1988.
5. Earhart, CA, and Allen, CA: Cognitive Disabilities: Expanded Activity Analysis. Los Angeles County/University of Southern California Medical Center, Los Angeles, 1988.
6. Allen, CK: Treatment plans in cognitive rehabilitation. Occupational Therapy Practice 1:1, 1989.
7. Allen, CK: Cognitive disabilities. In Katz, N (ed) Cognitive Rehabilitation: Models for Intervention in Occupational Therapy. Andover Medical, Boston, 1992, pp 4–6.
8. Allen, CK, and Earhart, CA: Occupational Therapy Treatment Goals for the Physically and Cognitively Disabled. American Occupational Therapy Association, Rockville, MD, 1992.
9. Allen, CK, Kehrberg, K, and Burns, T: Evaluation instruments. In Allen, CK, Earhart, CA, and Blue, T (eds): Occupational Therapy Treatment Goals for the Physically and Cognitively Disabled. American Occupational Therapy Association, Rockville, MD, 1992.
10. Heimann, NE, Allen, CK, and Yerxa, EJ: The routine task inventory: A tool for describing the functional behavior of the cognitively disabled. Occupational Therapy Practice 1:67, 1990.
11. Henry, A, Tohen, M, Coster, W, and Tickle-Degnen, L: Predicting Psychosocial Functioning and Symptomatic Recovery of Adolescents and Young Adults Following a First Psychotic Episode. Paper presented at the Joint Annual Conference of the American Occupational Therapy Association and the Canadian Association of Occupational Therapists, Boston, 1994.
12. International Classification of Impairments, Disabilities, and Handicaps: World Health Organization, Geneva, 1980.
13. Katz, N, Josman, N, and Steinmetz, N. Relationship between cognitive disability theory and the model of human occupation in the assessment of psychiatric and nonpsychiatric adolescents. Occupational Therapy in Mental Health 8:31, 1988.
14. Levy, LL: Psychosocial intervention and dementia, Part II: The cognitive disability perspective. Occupational Therapy in Mental Health 7:13, 1988.
15. Weissenberg, R, and Giladi, N: Home Economics Day: A program for disturbed adolescents to promote acquisition of habits and skills. Occupational Therapy in Mental Health 9:89, 1989.
16. Wilson, DS, et al: Cognitive disability and routine task behaviors in a community-based population with senile dementia. Occupational Therapy Practice 1:58, 1990.

CHAPTER 8

THE COGNITIVE-PERCEPTUAL MODEL

Persons with damage to the central nervous system (CNS) may experience a variety of perceptual and cognitive deficits. Approaches to remediating perceptual and cognitive problems* are widely represented in occupational therapy practice.[17,19] Moreover, cognitive-perceptual literature and practice have grown dramatically in the last decade. Nonetheless, instead of a single, widely accepted formulation, there are a number of related conceptual schemes for understanding and remediating cognitive and perceptual problems. These schemes overlap to an extent, and the trend in the literature appears to be toward an increasingly consistent view of cognitive-perceptual problems and their remediation. Recent efforts by a few authors to synthesize cognitive-perceptual themes and therapeutic approaches suggest that a cognitive-perceptual model of practice is being articulated and applied.

In this chapter I will highlight the main concepts and applications that characterize this emerging conceptual practice model. My aim is to present convergent themes, concepts, and practices. Because the model is still being shaped, authors' use of terminology varies, including how the model or approach is labeled. In particular, it should be noted that the term *cognitive-perceptual*, which I am using to label this model, refers to what some have

---

*The sensory integration and motor control treatment models (discussed in later chapters) have some overlapping concepts and methods with the cognitive-perceptual model.[20] However, they differ in that both the sensory integration and the motor control models are primarily concerned with motor behavior, while the cognitive-perceptual model is more concerned with behavioral strategies. In addition the sensory integration model was developed to address problems of sensory processing unrelated to frank brain damage, whereas the cognitive-perceptual model is mainly applied to persons who have brain damage.

145

called cognitive/perceptual retraining or cognitive rehabilitation. This chapter integrates the work of several authors; I have used the terminology of particular authors when discussing their concepts.

The cognitive-perceptual model is built upon an understanding of the brain's information processing ability and its impairment in cases of brain injury. The model is concerned with how impaired cognitive and perceptual processes restrict occupational performance. One of the notable trends in the formulation of this model is toward an understanding of how cognitive and perceptual strategies and deficits are manifest in the midst of performing occupations.

Definitions of Perception and Cognition

Quintana[28] defines *perception* as the "integration of sensory impressions into psychologically meaningful information." Abreu and Toglia[3] present perception as a dynamic process involving "sensory detection, sensory analysis, hypothesis formation, and a decision response." *Cognition* is defined by Quintana[28] as the "ability of the brain to process, store, retrieve, and manipulate information." Abreu and Toglia[3] note that cognition involves the abilities to "attend to, organize, and assimilate information." Cognition is identified as a process of using hindsight, foresight, and insight in determining a course of action.[3,28] Thus, attention, memory, initiation, planning, reflection, and adaptive problem solving are processes generally recognized as part of cognition. Noting that cognition is a global concept, Katz[16] incorporates the following range of processes within cognition:

> attention, orientation, perception, praxis, visuo-motor organization, memory, thinking, operations, executive functions, problem solving, planning, reasoning, and judgement. (p xii)

Perception and cognition cannot be entirely differentiated from each other; no borderline between the two has been clearly defined in the literature.[3] Perception and cognition may be conceived as two ends of a continuum. On the perceptual end, action and awareness are more immediate and are related to the concrete features of the environment and of experience. Perception involves immediate apprehension and appreciation of sensory data. Recognizing the smell of coffee, the taste of ice cream, or the sight of a flower are examples of perception. Yet perception is not merely a passive process of receiving sensory information. Rather, it is an active process of searching and judging the environment and recognizing its features.[1]

In contrast, cognitive action and awareness are more abstract and reflective, involving the formulation of intentions and action plans. Hence, processes normally termed "cognitive" involve more abstract and conscious reflection or anticipation not tied to immediate sensory data. Thus, cognition is involved in making coffee, in deciding between chocolate and strawberry ice cream, and in arranging flowers in a bouquet.

Abreu and Toglia[3] make another important distinction. Some perceptual abilities are related to a particular sensory system, but cognition interfaces with all forms of sensory information. Perception can guide a range of action (e.g., driving and walking) at the same time that cognitive processes are actively involved in such unrelated acts as talking or planning ahead. Moreover, perception may guide actions (e.g., typing) that are in the service of higher cognitive processes (e.g., writing this book).

Thus, the continuum from perception to cognition extends from few to many sensory modalities, and from spontaneous to reflective processes. The relationship between perception and cognition may also be thought of in the following way: Perceptual processes represent lower-level operations that are part of a broader set of processes referred to as cognition. The tendency for the literature to refer to cognitive processes and cognitive rehabilitation as incorporating elements of perception (as does, e.g., Katz's quotation above) suggests that perception may be increasingly seen as a component of cognition.*

Interdisciplinary Base

The perceptual and cognitive concepts and related interventions used in occupational therapy are based on the work of neuroscience and neuropsychology.[1] One important influence has been the work of scientists who have studied the effects of traumatic brain lesions on cognition and perception; another has been research in the field of ecological perception.[2] The researchers who created measures of specific perceptual and cognitive performances have also influenced occupational therapists' views of these phenomena. Theories from psychology have been incorporated into this model, especially from learning theory, which stresses information processing. A more recent influence is dynamical systems theory, which is resulting in a move toward more process-oriented and occupationally contexted views of perception and cognition.

---

*Nonetheless, there are certainly exceptions to the use of cognition as an umbrella concept encompassing perception. For example, Warren[37] includes visual cognition as a subconcept within her discussion of visual perception. In part, the inconsistency in terminology and concepts related to perception and cognition reflects the fact that occupational therapists who are working toward an articulation of theoretical arguments and their application are building on different areas of interdisciplinary literature, each of which has its own terminology and concepts that do not coincide with those in other bodies of literature.

Theoretical Arguments

Since this model is in an early stage of development, no comprehensive, widely accepted theoretical explanation of the cognitive-perceptive processes in occupational performance has been articulated. However, definite themes are emerging, so that it is possible to identify preliminary theoretical arguments concerning order, disorder, and therapeutic intervention.

Order

Underlying this model is the assumption that performance in occupations is based on the ability of persons to perceive and evaluate sensory information and on their ability to conceive of, plan, and execute purposeful action. These cognitive-perceptual abilities are the basis for interaction with the environment in work, play, and daily living tasks.

The earlier efforts to explain cognition, perception, and their role in everyday performance focused on specifying taxonomies of perceptual and cognitive abilities. While such taxonomies are still a component of this model, more recent literature emphasizes explaining the cognitive and perceptual processes manifested in occupational performance.

Taxonomies of Cognitive and Perceptual Abilities. Understanding of cognitive and perceptual abilities used in occupational performance first emerged from clinical observations of specific performance problems and from development of standardized tests designed to capture some component(s) of perception and/or cognition. For example, Quintana[28] offers the following list of cognitive-perceptual functions:

- Body scheme (i.e., spatial arrangement of one's body parts)
- Discrimination of right from left
- Identification of one's body parts
- Being able to name which finger is being touched (finger gnosia)
- Recognition of both sides of the body (the corresponding deficit is ignorance of one side of the body)
- Recognition of one's deficits
- Realizing the position of one's body in space
- Recognition of the relation of self to other objects
- Awareness of spatial relations
- Being able to find one's way from one place to another (topographical orientation)
- Distinguishing foreground from background (figure-ground)
- Carrying out purposeful movement (praxis)
- Carrying out drawing and constructional tasks (constructional praxis)

- The ability to get dressed (dressing praxis)
- Attention
- Orientation to person, place, and time
- Memory
- Problem solving

Zoltan, Seiv, and Freishtat[40] offer a similar collection of cognitive-perceptual areas of performance. Their taxonomy also includes such abilities as:

- Visual attention and scanning of the field of vision
- The ability to recognize faces
- The ability to initiate, plan, and organize performance
- Mental flexibility
- Abstraction

As these two examples show, there is no universally accepted taxonomy of perceptual and cognitive abilities. Moreover, these categories have a number of important limitations. They are not mutually exclusive, nor do they reflect a consistent approach to classification.

Because there is a great deal of overlap between these areas of cognitive-perceptual function, some authors have questioned just how useful they are.[32] In fact, Toglia[33] suggests focusing instead on the "underlying conditions and processing strategies that influence performance." It appears that the trend in this model is to de-emphasize taxonomies of cognitive-perceptual abilities and focus on explanations of the processes involved across cognitive and perceptual domains.

Explaining the Cognitive-Perceptual Process. Just as with the taxonomical approach, there is no single formulation of the processes involved in perception and cognition. Four themes seem to be important in theoretical modeling of cognitive and perceptual processes:

1. Steps or stages in the organization of information
2. Cognitive strategies
3. The process of learning
4. The dynamic interaction between person, task, and environment

Cognitive-Perceptual Stages. Abreu and Toglia[2,3] offered one of the earliest conceptual schemes for explaining both perceptual and cognitive processes. Their schema, later elaborated by Abreu and Hinajosa,[4] identified three stages of information processing:

1. Detecting relevant stimuli
2. Discriminating and analyzing stimuli
3. Formulating responses based on hypotheses derived from comparing current sensory stimuli and past experiences

The importance of identifying stages of information processing is that it allows therapists to identify where, along the process, individuals may be having difficulty and may need remediation and/or support.

Cognitive Strategies. Abreu and Toglia[3] point out that *cognitive strategies* affect how efficiently a person can process information. Cognitive strategies are the tactics that a person employs in occupational performance. Such strategies include planning ahead, choosing where to begin, varying one's speed, systematically searching for information, and generating alternatives. While the stages of cognitive-perceptual processing are universal and closely linked to organization of the human brain, cognitive strategies are learned methods of acquiring and dealing with information. Since these strategies affect how efficiently a person processes information, they have the ability to either limit or enhance cognitive-perceptual functioning.

Learning.   An important concept in this model is learning. *Learning* refers to a change in behavior[23] or in the capacity to respond to the environment that results from practice or experience. All learning reflects changes in the brain that result from interactions with the environment.[3,23]

Closely related to the concept of learning is the idea of generalization or *transfer of learning*. Depending on the level of learning of which persons are capable, they may be variously able to transfer a cognitive-perceptual strategy from the activity in which it was learned to another activity or situation. Authors speak of the degree of learning transfer of which a person is capable.

Neistadt[23] incorporates the idea of transfer of learning into a conceptualization of the levels of information processing and learning of which persons are capable. She discusses three levels of learning:

1. *Association learning,* in which a person learns a connection between two events
2. *Representational learning,* which involves forming internal representations or images of events and their spatio-temporal organization
3. *Abstract learning,* which involves acquiring rules, knowledge, and facts that are not context-dependent

Persons capable of abstract learning will be able to generalize learning of conceptual and perceptual strategies to tasks and situations that are significantly different from the learning context, whereas persons restricted to association learning will not be able to generalize widely. Hence, persons in the latter group need to learn each task required for their occupational life individually, whereas those in the former group will learn strategies and apply them to a range of occupations.

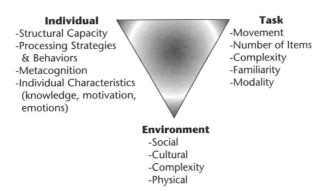

Individual
-Structural Capacity
-Processing Strategies
& Behaviors
-Metacognition
-Individual Characteristics
(knowledge, motivation,
emotions)

Task
-Movement
-Number of Items
-Complexity
-Familiarity
-Modality

Environment
-Social
-Cultural
-Complexity
-Physical

Figure 8–1. Dynamic interactional model of cognition. (From Toglia,[32] p 108, with permission.)

Dynamic Interactional View. Toglia[23] offers a dynamic interactional view that not only builds on information processing ideas but also incorporates a dynamical systems perceptive (Fig. 8–1). According to her approach, cognition should be seen as the ongoing product of a dynamic process of interaction between an individual, the task being performed, and the environment.[32] Within the individual she includes:

1. Structural capacity, which is the physical (e.g., neurological) capacity for information processing
2. Cognitive processing strategies* and behaviors, which are the approaches, routines, and tactics that the person uses to select and guide information processing (examples include prioritizing versus clustering information, discriminating between important versus unimportant information)
3. *Metacognition,* which refers to awareness and control of one's cognitive processes and capacities
4. Individual characteristics, which include knowledge based on experience, motivation, and emotions

The environment includes social, physical, and cultural elements that may influence the person's ability to process information. For example, social interaction can be an important influence on the kind of strategies persons learn for processing information. Moreover, the degree of physical, social, and cultural familiarity of an environment can also influence information processing.

The task refers to the occupation the person is performing; it can be characterized through two parameters: surface characteristics and concep-

---

*While Toglia uses the term, cognitive processing strategies, a reading of her work suggests that she means essentially the same thing as authors who refer to cognitive strategies. She gives a very strong emphasis to them and has offered a much more comprehensive cataloguing of these strategies than other occupational therapy authors.

tual characteristics.[32,33] *Surface characteristics* refer to such things as the number, qualities, and arrangement of objects; types of stimuli; task directions; and movement demands. Surface characteristics are, therefore, readily observable features of a task. *Conceptual characteristics* are not directly observable; they include the kinds of skills and strategies the task demands based on its complexity and familiarity, as well as the meaning it evokes.

According to Toglia,[32] cognition involves dynamic interaction of all these elements:

> The environment can mediate processing between the task and the individual. In some situations the task parameters may be the primary influence on information processing, in other situations the environment or the individual characteristics may be the most influential.

Understanding cognitive processes requires attention to the interaction between the three components. Cognitive processing involves receiving, elaborating, and monitoring incoming information and using this information flexibly across tasks. Cognition also involves using efficient information processing strategies, evoking previous knowledge, and using metacognition.

Cognitive processing, cognitive strategies, and metacognition are all emergent phenomena that are influenced by environmental and task parameters. When those parameters change, cognitive processes and strategies may shift into different modes of operation. For example, a person may use one cognitive strategy until a task reaches a certain level of complexity and then shift to another strategy.

Toglia's framework based on dynamical systems appears to be the most comprehensive formulation of cognitive processes, and it shares features with other important occupational therapy conceptualizations. In addition, it is the approach that most clearly embraces dynamical systems ideas (which, as we noted in Chapter 4, are central to the focal viewpoint of the field's current paradigm). As such, it appears to be the kind of theoretical articulation of cognitive-perceptual processes that will emerge in this model.

Disorder

Perceptual and cognitive dysfunction result from brain damage and disorganization. One of the major diagnoses that involves cognitive-perceptual problems is cerebrovascular accident (CVA). CVA is among the most frequently represented diagnoses in occupational therapy practice. This model is also applied to persons with traumatic brain injury, persons with CNS disorders (e.g., cerebral palsy), and persons who have developmental and learning disabilities.

Individuals with brain damage are left with reduced information processing capacity:

> This reduction in information processing capacity can result in global or specific deficits depending on the nature of the brain damage. . . . The brain-damaged person has difficulty structuring and organizing information. . . . Clinically, the patient may not automatically attend to the relevant feature of a task, group similar items together, formulate a plan, or break the task down into steps.[3]

The breakdown in information capacity can be seen at each the three stages of sensory information. For example, a person may have a problem with attention that impairs the ability to detect stimuli.[4] Thus, a disorganization of one or more information-processing components contributes to recognizable cognitive-perceptual dysfunctions.

Toglia[33] also observes that cognitive dysfunction "represents a decrease in the use of efficient processing strategies to select, discriminate, organize, and structure incoming information. Neistadt[23] points out that brain damage can variously impact the ability for leaning. Metacognition can also be impaired, as when persons are unaware of their cognitive-perceptual problems.

The basic view of this model is that when persons have CNS damage, a combination of information-processing abilities, learning abilities, and metacognition can be impaired.[23,32] Hence patient problems are conceptualized in terms of the specific kinds of information-processing difficulties they have, the degree of limitation in learning they experience, and their metacognitive status.

The cognitive-perceptual problems that persons demonstrate depend on the nature of insult to the central nervous system. It is being recognized now that these problems are also dependent on task and environmental context.[23,32] For example, persons with cognitive-perceptual problems may not have difficulty processing information in simple tasks but may show problems when task parameters change. The kinds of cognitive-perceptual problems a person demonstrates may be global, or they may be manifest in specific areas of cognitive-perceptual functioning, such as visual processing. For this reason, attention is still paid to specific areas of cognitive-perceptual dysfunction.

Classifying Specific Areas of Dysfunction. A number of specific areas of dysfunction are defined in this model. Some of these dysfunctions are based on readily observable deficits such as memory loss. Others are identified with specific assessments that identify a type of disorder.

Some examples of common areas of cognitive-perceptual dysfunction are disruption of body scheme, lack of left/right discrimination, difficulty with body part identification, unilateral neglect (i.e., neglect of one side of the body), dyspraxia, attention deficits, problems with visual scanning, disorientation, and memory loss.

Disruption of Occupational Performance. Because the brain is less capable of processing sensory information and is consequently unable to interpret and translate it into appropriate plans of action, the individual's occupational performance is impaired. Hence, difficulties in work, play or leisure, and self-care result from significant impairment of perceptual and cognitive capacities. In some cases, specific kinds of occupational performance difficulties have been shown to be associated with a given perceptual impairment. For example, persons with unilateral neglect have difficulty dressing because they do not recognize the affected side of the body. In other cases, the dysfunction is defined by its functional implication (e.g., dressing apraxia). A more global perceptual or cognitive disorder may have effects on all areas of performance. For example, memory loss or poor problem solving may impair function through a whole range of occupational tasks. As will be noted later, there is a growing research literature that seeks to demonstrate the relationship between perceptual and cognitive deficits and functional performance problems.

Therapeutic Intervention

Traditionally, the rationale for cognitive-perceptual intervention has been divided into remedial approaches, which seek to restore specific cognitive-perceptual abilities, and adaptive approaches, which emphasize enabling patients to use remaining abilities and to compensate for deficits.[29] Treatment aimed at remediating perceptual and cognitive problems uses tasks that require the brain to process information—in particular tasks that target impaired information-processing capacities.[20] The remedial approach is based on the idea that the brain has capacity to reorganize and, therefore, reclaim its informational processing capacity to an extent. Adaptive approaches help persons learn to capitalize on their existing potentials and to use strategies to substitute or compensate for limitations. The adaptive approach also stresses making the individual aware of his or her own perceptual and cognitive limitations in order to compensate for his or her problems. Finally, this approach recognizes that performance will be enhanced if the environment or the task is modified to accommodate the particular limitations of the individual.

As Neistadt[23] recently argued, both remedial and compensatory cognitive-perceptual interventions involve learning, which depends on plasticity of the brain. This means that appropriate treatment approaches for persons with a brain injury depend upon both the individual's potential for recovery of information processing capacities and the potential for learning.[27] This potential for learning and recovery is influenced by "the person's general mental and physical health, the severity of the injury, and the amount and quality of environmental stimuli in that person's life."[23] Occupational therapy enables learning and recovery by manipulating the environmental stimuli in the form of presenting occupational tasks and modifying the social context. How this is best done and what it can achieve depends on the other factors noted above.

Neistadt[23] suggests that therapy should be undertaken according to the levels of information processing and learning of which persons are capable (referring to the three levels of learning noted earlier). The success of different treatment approaches depend on the kind of learning of which a person is capable. For example, a person who relies on associative learning will have difficulty transferring learning to tasks that differ considerably from the learned task or to new contexts. Representational learners transfer learning more readily (i.e., they are able to perform learned tasks under different conditions), but they have difficulty in transferring learning to new tasks or totally new situations. According to Neistadt,[23] clients with the most ability to transfer learning benefit from a remedial approach, which assumes transfer of learning, whereas those with less ability to transfer learning benefit from an adaptive approach, which emphasizes learning specific functional tasks.

Toglia[31] also argues that transfer of learning exists on a continuum from near to far. Transfer is considered to be near when only one or two surface characteristics (e.g., physical features or arrangement of objects used, context, rules or directions) of the task are altered. Transfer is considered far when most or all surface characteristics are different. Like Neistadt, Toglia[31] argues that treatment should be graded as to how much transfer of learning a patient is capable of. As a patient improves, tasks can be varied to further enhance transfer of learning.

Metacognition also determines the patient's ability to transfer learning and benefit from remedial and compensatory approaches. Metacognition includes knowledge of one's cognitive capacities and process, ability to assess task difficulty, select cognitive strategies, and monitor one's performance.[32] When metacognition is impaired, the ability to transfer learning will also be impaired, and both remedial and compensatory strategies will have more limited success.[31]

Traditional cognitive-perceptual treatment approaches tended to be "deficit specific," that is, aimed at remediating or compensating for specific areas of deficits identified in testing. Such a targeted approach assumed that cognitive-perceptual deficits could be differentiated into discretely meaningful categories and that these deficits could be specifically addressed. Moreover, it was often assumed that cognitive-perceptual skills were hierarchically organized so that the simpler ones should be retrained first, proceeding on to more complex ones. Finally, it was assumed that once a particular area was improved, the patient would show improvement in all tasks and situations requiring that ability (referred to as generalization or transfer of training).

Recent approaches have adopted more holistic, process-oriented, or dynamical systems approaches. Holistic approaches emphasize a top-down strategy that focuses on the highest level of cognitive-perceptual functioning and its role in integrating lower level or component functions.[13,21,22,38] The process view emphasizes that activities should be selected to:

involve specific processing at particular levels of the central nervous system. If the client attends to the stimulus events of the activities, then registering the stimulus event is feasible. If the client detects the information then their ability to analyze information for use is feasible. If the client is able to analyze the information, then the client can compare the stimulus events with long-term memories and relate the stimulus to the overall purpose and goal of the activities.[4]

Hence, activities should be chosen to elicit and challenge these information processing capacities.

The dynamical approach emphasizes understanding how cognitive-perceptual behavior emerges under different task and contextual conditions.[32] This approach examines how and under what conditions a patient shows a problem. For example, a patient may have no difficulty in a cognitive-perceptual area until a task exceeds a certain threshold of complexity (number of component parts or steps) or until the environment is changed. Hence the therapist simultaneously examines how the patient processes information and how such strategies succeed and fail under different task and environmental conditions. In this way the therapist can identify task and environmental dimensions that create difficulty for the patient, as well as difficulties in patient information processing that create problems across different kinds of tasks. Next, individualized treatment, which takes this information into consideration, is developed.

Basic to the individualized treatment is estimating the patient's potential for change. Persons who are aware of errors, and who respond to cues and to modifications in tasks, will benefit from a multicontext approach, in which a patient's ability to process information across different situations is enhanced.[32] Patients without such awareness and responsiveness will most likely receive a functional approach, which does not assume improvement of underlying abilities and transfer of training.

Technology for Application

Assessment

To determine whether perceptual or cognitive deficits exist, the therapist must rule out other, more basic problems. For example, apraxia is defined as the inability to carry out purposeful movement when sensation is intact and the person has capacity for coordinated voluntary movement. Only when assessment determines that those sensory and coordination abilities are intact can the dysfunction be considered to be due to the inability to organize sensory information and plan and execute coordinated movement in order to accomplish tasks.

A wide range of standardized tests and informal procedures is available for evaluating cognitive and perceptual deficits. Many of the standard tests in use by occupational therapists have been developed by neuropsychologists. Some tests have now been developed by occupational therapists. For example, the A-One is an assessment that links functional performance in occupations to neurobehavioral deficits.[5] It identifies both the level of independence in five activities of daily living (ADL) and the presence and severity of specific neurobehavioral impairments through analysis of how the impairments affect ADL tasks.

Another example is the Loewenstein Occupational Therapy Cognitive Assessment (LOTCA).[12,14] Originally developed in Israel, it is now widely used worldwide. It consists of four major areas (orientation, perception, visuomotor organization, and thinking operations) represented by a total of 20 subtests. The LOTCA is designed to capture both patient abilities and limitations and to determine the capacity to cope with routine occupational tasks.

Therapists usually employ a battery of standardized tests in association with this model.[3,40] Nonetheless, other methods of assessment are also considered important. Abreu and Toglia[3] note that standardized tests may provide only limited information about the patient's functioning because there is not a perfect relationship between perceptual and cognitive deficits and occupational performance. Consequently, Abreu and Toglia[3] and Neistadt[20] note the importance of going beyond standardized tests to gather qualitative information and to observe how the deficits affect persons' performance in their occupational tasks. As Abreu and Toglia[3] point out, the occupational therapist's role is to evaluate function and dysfunction, and therefore cognitive-perceptual data must be viewed in terms of its implications for occupational performance.

A new approach to assessment based on dynamical principles emphasizes simultaneously examining the cognitive and perceptual processing of a person, along with noting the impact of variation of task parameters and environmental conditions.[33] For example, Toglia and Finkelstein[33] developed the Dynamic Visual Processing Assessment, which examines scanning, object perception, unilateral inattention, and keeping track of visual information. This assessment determines how such parameters as number of items and their arrangement affect performance in these areas. It also examines the impact of environmental cuing and self-awareness of errors.

Treatment

As the earlier discussion of theoretical arguments about intervention pointed out, there are essentially two different approaches to remediating cognitive and perceptual problems; that is, intervention aims either at improving or compensating for limitations of cognitive-perceptual abilities. These two approaches to the treatment of cognitive-perceptual deficits are referred to as remedial and functional training (sometimes referred to as adaptive training).[3,20,40]

According to Neistadt,[20] remedial training "seeks to promote the recovery or reorganization of impaired CNS functions." Remedial training is based on the premise that task training results not only in learning the specific task but also in increasing the cognitive or perceptual skill used in the task.[40] Thus, training is expected to transfer to other situations and tasks in which the perceptual or cognitive skills are required. As noted earlier, use of this approach should depend on a determination that the patient is capable of learning in such a way as to effectively transfer training.

Functional (or adaptive) training does not rely on changing disordered cognitive-perceptual capabilities, but seeks to enable individuals to perform optimally despite such limitations. Neistadt[20] refers to this approach as adaptive, pointing out that therapy provides "training not in the perceptual skills of functional behavior, but in the activity of daily living behaviors themselves." Consequently, this approach emphasizes finding and using means for the person to accomplish necessary tasks and routines despite the presence of cognitive-perceptual deficits.

The functional approach has two categories:

1. Compensation, in which the patient is made aware of his or her problems and taught to make allowances for them
2. Adaptation, or changing the environment to make up for the person's deficits

An example of the compensation approach to functional training is training to overcome visual scanning deficits. Usually, visual scanning occurs automatically in response to novel stimuli (i.e., something new or a change in the stimulus field), and when persons consciously search for information in the visual field. When deficits in visual scanning occur, patients can learn to override them. Once they are shown how visual scanning normally functions and how their own is not functioning, they can be taught new, conscious visual behaviors that compensate for the lack of automatic visual scanning in situations such as reading and driving.[37]

Environmental adaptation often involves establishing a particular set of circumstances in which the person performs tasks (e.g., an invariant routine, the use of sensory and cognitive cues to support the task process, or changing the materials needed to complete a task). Some environmental adaptations also require a family member or caretaker to supervise and provide cues and other necessary support.[1]

In the past, it was believed that the sequence of treatment should recapitulate (repeat the stages of) developmental states.[15] It was argued that, following brain injury and the disorganization of perceptual and cognitive abilities, persons best relearn and reorganize if they follow the developmental sequence with which the skills were first learned. Abreu and Toglia[3] disagree. They argue that because of the store of knowledge in the adult brain, the circumstances for relearning perceptual and cognitive tasks after brain damage are very different from the conditions of initial developmental learning. Most approaches currently described in the literature do not recommend a developmentally sequenced approach. Rather, they argue for an approach tailored to the remaining capacities, nature of processing impairments, and learning potential of the patient or client.

Finally, since metacognition affects patients' abilities to transfer learning and make use of adaptive strategies to compensate for problems, therapists seek to improve metacognition. This can include helping the patient gain insight into problems, evaluate task demands, and assess outcomes of performance.[32]

Modalities Used in Therapy

The range of activities used in the remedial approach is wide. In many cases, therapists use testing materials to train cognitive-perceptual skills; that is, the tasks used to test perceptual and cognitive abilities are used as drills to exercise and develop these skills.[20,40] For example, a patient may practice connecting a series of dots or copying a simple design in order to overcome visual scanning deficits. Zoltan, Seiv, and Freishtat[40] note that patients sometimes object to cognitive training as childish, degrading, and irrelevant. For this reason, training tasks based on normal occupation performance may be preferable.

One challenge with using occupational tasks is the need to analyze an activity to determine which perceptual and cognitive skills the activity calls for.[11] Development of protocols for training persons in the contexts of occupations is one way to standardize how patients are presented with perceptual and cognitive demands. An example of such an approach is a meal preparation treatment protocol developed by Neistadt.[24] With the increase of dynamical systems concepts that stress the importance of task parameters in determining performance, and with improved methods of identifying task parameters, the use of occupational tasks for remediation will likely increase, while training drills will decrease.

The use of computers for retraining many perceptual skills is increasing because of their greater acceptability to many patients and clients and because of the wide range of available, relevant software. When computer retraining was first introduced, enthusiasm was great, but clinical observation suggests that this type of training does not generalize well into other areas of activity. Such computer exercises appear to be most useful in the early stages of recovery, when the most basic capacities are returning. Later, activities more nearly matched to desired life tasks appear more useful.

As this model is further developed, the modalities will be further refined and tested for their relevance and efficacy. It does appear, however, that occupational tasks that both demand cognitive-perceptual abilities and reveal deficits may be the most useful context for both remedial and adaptive intervention strategies.

Research

Research related to this model is varied. One active area of research is the development and testing of assessment tools.[7,9,11,35,36] Other studies have evaluated the incidence of cognitive-perceptual deficits in persons with various kinds of neurological impairments. One such project was a study of the patterns of dysfunction in motor planning, language, and memory in persons with Alzheimer's disease.[6] Another study demonstrated that children with cerebral palsy lagged behind normal children in the development of visual-perceptual skills.[18] Other examples of this type of research are a study that investigated relationships between visual-perceptual motor abilities and clumsiness in normal and learning-disabled children;[26] and studies of visuospatial, visual perception, and praxis deficits in persons who have experienced a stroke.[15,39]

Other studies have sought to demonstrate the impact of cognitive-perceptual deficits on occupational performance. One study of persons 4 to 6 years after their strokes documented that perceptual deficits not only endured but also had as much impact on self-care performance as did motor impairments.[4] Four other studies found that deficits in perception were correlated with self-care problems[15,25,30] and two other studies of stroke patients found that cognitive skills correlated with self-care skills, and cognitive improvement correlated with improvement in self-care skills.[10] However, findings of these and other studies suggest that the relationship of perception and cognition to functional performance is not strong.

If measures of perceptual and cognitive ability that factor in occupational task and context are developed and used in such research, it is likely that stronger relationships will be demonstrated. Future research should certainly include efforts to show more clearly how perceptual and cognitive deficits relate to performance problems in daily occupations. Also needed are studies to evaluate the outcomes of different treatment approaches.[20,34,35] Neistadt[20] has identified a number of research questions that could be posed to investigate the assumptions underlying treatment aimed at improving perceptual and cognitive deficits. One vital question is whether occupational therapy aimed at cognitive and perceptual skills enhances functional performance.

Discussion

The cognitive-perceptual model is in the early stages of development. Its future development appears inevitable, given the pervasiveness of cognitive and perceptual deficits in occupational therapy patients and clients, and given the wide range of techniques occupational therapists employ to remediate such deficits.

One interesting aspect of this model is that research, as much as clinical application, has advanced interest in the whole area. The research literature is beginning to document both the extent of cognitive-perceptual deficits in persons with brain damage and the impact of these deficits on occupational performance. As this model is more clearly articulated, research is likely to lead to a cumulative and authoritative body of knowledge.

At this point, two of the major tasks for development of this model are to achieve more consistency in terminology and concepts and to synthesize these concepts into a coherent set of theoretical arguments. This model clearly seems to be moving in consistent directions and some very well articulated literature has been published. This suggests that such a synthesis will be accomplished in the future.

TERMS OF THE MODEL

association learning	Learning a connection between two events.
abstract learning	Acquiring rules, knowledge, and facts that are not context-dependent.
cognition	The ability to attend to, process, store, retrieve, and manipulate and assimilate information.
cognitive strategies	Tactics for processing information, including planning ahead, choosing where to begin, varying one's speed, systematically searching for information, and generating alternatives.
conceptual characteristics	The kinds of skill and strategies a task demands and the meaning it evokes.
learning	Change in behavior or in the capacity to respond to the environment that results from practice or experience.
metacognition	Awareness of one's own cognitive processes.
perception	Integration of sensory impressions into psychologically meaningful information.
representational learning	Forming internal representations or images of events and their spatiotemporal organization.
surface characteristics	Readily observable features of a task including number, qualities, and arrangement of objects, types of stimuli, task directions, and movement demands.
transfer of learning	The ability to apply strategies learned in a task and situation to other tasks and situations.

SUMMARY

The Cognitive-Perceptual Model

FOCUS
- The model addresses persons with damage to the central nervous system.
- Instead of a single, widely accepted formulation, there are a number of related conceptual schemes for understanding and remediating cognitive and perceptual problems.
- Built upon an understanding of the brain's information-processing ability and its impairment in cases of brain injury, the model is concerned with how impaired cognitive and perceptual processes restrict occupational performance.

DEFINITIONS OF PERCEPTION AND COGNITION
- Perception is:
  - The integration of sensory impressions into meaningful information
  - A dynamic process involving detection and analysis, hypothesis formation, and response to sensation
- Cognition is:
  - The ability to attend to, process, organize, store, retrieve, and manipulate information
  - A process of using hindsight, foresight, and insight to select action
  - A composite of attention, memory, initiation, planning, reflection, and adaptive problem solving
- Perception and cognition can be conceived as two ends on a continuum:
  - Perception involves immediate action and awareness related to the concrete features of the environment.
  - Cognition involves abstract and reflective action and awareness.
- Perception is increasingly seen as a component of cognition.

INTERDISCIPLINARY BASE
- Neuroscience, neuropsychology, ecological perception, and learning theory are traditional influences.
- A more recent influence is dynamical systems theory.

THEORETICAL ARGUMENTS
- No comprehensive theoretical explanation of the cognitive-perceptive processes in occupational performance has been articulated, but definite themes are emerging.

Order
- Performance in occupations is based on the ability of persons to perceive and evaluate sensory information and the ability to conceive of, plan, and execute purposeful action.

- Early efforts to explain cognition, perception, and their role in performance specified taxonomies, while more recent literature emphasizes explaining cognitive and perceptual processes.
- There is no universally accepted taxonomy of perceptual and cognitive abilities.
- Existing taxonomies do not reflect a consistent approach to classification.
- Some authors have questioned just how useful the taxonomies are.
- Four themes appear important in theoretical modeling of cognitive and perceptual processes:
  - Steps or stages in the organization of information
  - Cognitive strategies
  - The process of learning
  - The dynamic interaction between person, task, and environment
- Three stages of information processing:
  - Detecting relevant stimuli
  - Discriminating and analyzing stimuli
  - Formulating responses based on comparing current sensory stimuli and past experiences
- Cognitive strategies:
  - Affect efficiency of information processing
  - Include tactics of planning ahead, choosing where to begin, varying speed, searching for information, and generating alternatives
- Learning refers to a change in behavior or in the capacity to respond to the environment resulting from practice or experience, reflecting changes in the brain.
- Three levels of learning:
  - Association learning (learning a connection between events)
  - Representational learning (forming internal representations or images of events)
  - Abstract learning (acquiring rules, knowledge, and facts that are not context-dependent)
- Dynamic interactional view sees cognition as the ongoing product of interactions between individual, task, and environment.

Disorder

- Perceptual and cognitive dysfunction result from brain damage and disorganization.
- Individuals with brain damage are left with reduced information-processing capacity that can affect all three stages of sensory information processing.
- Cognitive dysfunction reflects decreased efficiency for selecting, discriminating, organizing, and structuring information.
- Patient problems are conceptualized in terms of specific kinds of information-processing difficulties, degree of limitation in learning, and their metacognitive status.

- The cognitive-perceptual problems that persons demonstrate depend on:
  - The nature of the insult to the central nervous system
  - The task and environmental context
- Reduction of brain capacity for processing, interpreting, and translating sensory information into appropriate plans of action, impairs occupational performance.

Therapeutic intervention

- Remedial approaches seek to restore specific cognitive-perceptual abilities.
- Adaptive approaches emphasize enabling patients to use remaining abilities and compensate for deficits.
- Therapy enables learning and recovery by presenting occupational tasks and modifying the physical and social context according to the information processing and learning of which persons are capable.
- Traditional cognitive-perceptual treatment approaches are aimed at remediating or compensating for specific areas of deficits, but recent approaches adopt a more holistic, process-oriented and/or dynamical systems approach.
- Holistic approaches focus on the highest level of cognitive-perceptual functioning and its role in integrating lower level or component functions.
- The process view emphasizes selecting activities to involve specific processing at particular levels of the central nervous system.
- The dynamical approach emphasizes understanding how cognitive-perceptual behavior emerges under different task and contextual conditions.

TECHNOLOGY FOR APPLICATION

- A wide range of standardized tests and informal procedures exists for evaluating cognitive and perceptual deficits. Tests developed by occupational therapists include:
  - A-One (an assessment that links functional performance in occupations to neurobehavioral deficits)
  - Loewenstein Occupational Therapy Cognitive Assessment (consisting of orientation, perception, visuomotor organization, and thinking operations); designed to capture abilities and limitations and determine the capacity to cope with routine occupational tasks
- Standardized tests may provide only limited information about functioning, since there is not a perfect relationship between perceptual and cognitive deficits and occupational performance.
- Qualitative information and observation of how deficits affect occupational performance is important.
- Assessment based on dynamical principles emphasizes examining cognitive and perceptual processing along with the impact of variation of task parameters and environment.

Treatment

- Remedial training promotes recovery or reorganization of impaired CNS functions and is expected to transfer to other situations and tasks in which these perceptual or cognitive skills are required.
- Functional (adaptive) training enables individuals to perform optimally despite limitations and includes:
  - Compensation, in which the person is made aware of problems and taught to make allowances
  - Adaptation, or changing the environment to make up for deficits
- Current approaches do not recommend a developmental sequence, but rather one tailored to the remaining capacities, nature of processing impairments, and learning potential of the patient or client.

RESEARCH

- Research areas include:
  - Development and testing of assessment
  - Evaluating the incidence of cognitive-perceptual deficits
  - Demonstrating the impact of cognitive-perceptual deficits on occupational performance

References

1. Abreu, BC: Physical Disabilities Manual. Raven Press, New York, 1981.
2. Abreu, BC: Perceptual cognitive rehabilitation—an occupational therapy model. Physical Disabilities. Special Interest Section Newsletter 8:1, 1985.
3. Abreu, BC, and Toglia, JP: Cognitive rehabilitation: A model for occupational therapy. Am J Occup Ther 41:439, 1987.
4. Abreu, BC, and Hinajosa, J: The process approach for cognitive-perceptual and postural control dysfunction for adults with brain injuries. In Katz, N (ed) Cognitive Rehabilitation: Models for Intervention in Occupational Therapy. Andover Medical, Boston, 1992.
5. Arnadottir, G: The brain and behavior: Assessing cortical dysfunction through activities of daily living. CV Mosby, St Louis, 1990.
6. Baum, CM, et al: Performance components in senile dementia of the Alzheimer type: Motor planning, language, and memory. Occupational Therapy Journal of Research 8:356, 1988.
7. Baum, C, and Edwards, DF: Cognitive performance in senile dementia of the Alzheimer's type: The Kitchen Task Assessment. Am J Occup Ther 47:431–436, 1993.
8. Berspang, B, Viitanen, M, and Ericksson, S: Impairments of perceptual and motor functions: Their influence on self-care ability 4 to 6 years after stroke. Occupational Therapy Journal of Research 9:27, 1989.
9. Boys, M, et al: The OSOT perceptual evaluation: A research perspective. Am J Occup Ther 42:92, 1988.
10. Carter, LT, et al: The relationship of cognitive skills performance to activities of daily living in stroke patients. Am J Occup Ther 42:449, 1988.
11. Cermak, SA: Developmental dyspraxia. In Roy, EA (ed): Advances in Psychology: Vol 23: Neuropsychological Studies of Apraxia and Related Disorder. Elsevier Science, North Holland, New York, 1985.
12. Cermak, SA, Katz, N, McGuire, E, Greenbaum, S, Peralta, C, and Maser-Flanagan, V: Performance of Americans and Israelis with cerebrovascular accident on the Loewenstein Occupational Therapy Assessment (LOTCA). Am J Occup Ther 49:500–506, 1995.
13. Goodgold-Edwards, SA, and Cermak, S: Integrating motor control and motor learning concepts with neuropsychological perspectives on apraxia and developmental dyspraxia. Am J Occup Ther 44:431, 1990.

14. Izkovich, M, Elazar, B, Averbuch, S, and Katz, N: LOTCA Loewenstein Occupational Therapy Cognitive Assessment Manual. Maddak, Pequaalnnock, NJ, 1990.
15. Kaplan, J, and Hier, DE: Visuo-spatial deficits after right hemisphere stroke. Am J Occup Ther 36:314, 1982.
16. Katz, N: Introduction: Comparison of cognitive approaches in occupational therapy. In Katz, N (ed): Cognitive Rehabilitation: Models for Intervention in Occupational Therapy. Andover Medical, Boston, 1992.
17. Kunstaetter, D: Occupational therapy treatment in home health care. Am J Occup Ther 42:513, 1988.
18. Menken, C, Cermak, SA, and Fisher, A: Evaluating the visual-perceptual skills of children with cerebral palsy. Am J Occup Ther 41:646, 1987.
19. Neistadt, ME: Occupational therapy treatment goals for adults with developmental disabilities. Am J Occup Ther 40:672, 1986.
20. Neistadt, ME: A critical analysis of occupational therapy approaches for perceptual deficits in adults with brain injury. Am J Occup Ther 44:299, 1990.
21. Neistadt, ME: Perceptual retraining for adults with diffuse brain injury. Am J Occup Ther 48:225–233, 1993.
22. Neistadt, ME: Using research literature to develop a perceptual retraining treatment protocol. Am J Occup Ther 48:62–72, 1994.
23. Neistadt, ME: The neurobiology of learning: Implications for treatment of adults with brain injury. Am J Occup Ther 48:421–430, 1994.
24. Neistadt, ME: A meal preparation treatment protocol for adults with brain injury. Am J Occup Ther 48:431–438, 1994.
25. Nelle, D, Titus, M, Gall, NG, Yerxa, EJ, Roberson, TA, and Mack, W: Correlation of perceptual performance and activities of daily living in stroke patients. Am J Occup Ther 45:410–417, 1991.
26. O'Brien, V, Cermak, SA, and Murray, E: The relationship between visual-perceptual motor abilities and clumsiness in children with and without learning disabilities. Am J Occup Ther 42:359, 1988.
27. Poole, JL: Learning. In Trombly, C (ed) Occupational Therapy for Physical Dysfunction, ed 4. Williams & Wilkins, Baltimore, 1995.
28. Quintana, LA: Evaluation of perception and cognition. In Trombly, C (ed): Occupational Therapy for Physical Dysfunction. Williams & Wilkins, Baltimore, 1995, p 201.
29. Quintana, LA: Remediating cognitive impairments. In Trombly, C (ed): Occupational Therapy for Physical Dysfunction, ed 4. Williams & Wilkins, Baltimore, 1995.
30. Rubio, KB, and Van Deusen, J: Relation of perceptual and body image dysfunction to activities of daily living of persons after stroke. Am J Occup Ther 49:551–559, 1995.
31. Toglia, JP: Generalization of treatment: A multicontext approach to cognitive perceptual impairment in adults with brain injury. Am J Occup Ther 45:505–516, 1991.
32. Toglia, JP: A dynamic interactional approach to cognitive rehabilitation. In Katz, N (ed) Cognitive Rehabilitation: Models for Intervention in Occupational Therapy. Andover Medical, Boston, 1992, p. 113.
33. Toglia, JP, and Finkelstein, N: Test protocol: The dynamic visual processing assessment. New York Hospital-Cornell Medical Center, New York, 1991.
34. Van Deusen, J: Unilateral neglect: Suggestions for research by occupational therapists. Am J Occup Ther 42:441, 1988.
35. Van Deusen, J, and Harlowe, D: Continued construct validation of the St. Mary's CVA evaluation: Bilateral awareness scale. Am J Occup Ther 41:242, 1987.
36. Van Deusen Fox, J, and Harlowe, D: Construct validation of occupational therapy measures used in CVA evaluation: A beginning. Am J Occup Ther 38:101, 1984.
37. Warren, M: Identification of visual scanning deficits in adults after cerebrovascular accident. Am J Occup Ther 44:391, 1990.
38. Warren, M: A hierarchical model for evaluation and treatment of visual perceptual dysfunction in adult acquired brain injury, Part 1. Am J Occup Ther 47:42–54, 1993.
39. York, CD, and Cermak, SA: Visual perception and praxis in adults after stroke. Am J Occup Ther 49:543–550, 1995.
40. Zoltan, B, Seiv, E, and Freishtat, B. Perceptual and Cognitive Dysfunction in the Adult Stroke Patient. Slack, Thorofare, NJ, 1986.

CHAPTER 9

THE GROUP WORK
MODEL

O ther models presented in this book focus primarily on the person. This concern with the individual reflects the fact that, traditionally, occupational therapy services have aimed at maintaining or improving some facet of the person who has a disability. Consequently, the knowledge and practice of the field have been organized around an understanding of the individual's motives, habits, motor capacities, cognition, and so on.

Nonetheless, over the past couple of decades, occupational therapists have become increasingly aware that they must also be concerned with the families, schools, workplaces, and other social settings in which persons perform. As more attention is paid to these various social groups, two things have become increasingly apparent. First, persons with a disability are profoundly affected by and cannot be understood apart from the social contexts in which they perform. Second, persons with disabilities also affect the social groups to which they belong. For instance, occupational therapists working in the area of pediatrics have found not only that the family is the primary group within which the child must develop, but also that the family with a disabled child faces unique challenges to maintain an adaptive family life. Similar circumstances are found in families that must care for an older member with a disability. Moreover, when therapists seek to help workers with injuries or disabilities to adjust to the workplace, they must pay attention to how coworkers and supervisors affect the worker's productivity and satisfaction. Finally, they sometimes must consider not only the individual, but also the group to which the disabled individual belongs as the recipient of services.

169

In these and other situations, occupational therapists must carefully consider the interface of the individual and the social group. They must also appreciate how different characteristics of the group can either support or detract from the member's occupational behavior. Finally, therapists must often address how the group can be supported and/or changed so that its members are enabled to better perform and achieve satisfaction. In sum, occupational therapists increasingly must have both an understanding and a means of dealing with various groups to which persons with disabilities belong.

Occupational therapists also use groups of clients interacting together as a means of providing therapy. The use of groups in the context of therapy has always been part of occupational therapy. For example, groups were used during the era of the mechanistic paradigm to achieve psychodynamically oriented interactions between patients. More and more, however, occupational therapists are paying specific attention to how the dynamics of groups maintain or improve the occupational behavior of their participants. In this sense, group dynamics is being recognized as a factor influencing an individual's occupational adaptation.

Moreover, therapists recognize that there are distinct therapeutic advantages to addressing some client problems in the context of groups. Another factor augmenting the use of groups in occupational therapy is the emphasis on cost containment in health care. When services can be effectively offered in groups, they are less expensive than services offered on a one-to-one basis. Not surprisingly then, the extent to which groups are used in therapy is increasing steadily.[3,8] This growing use of groups as therapy has created a need for more knowledge in occupational therapy about how groups function and affect their members.*

A decade ago, Howe and Schwartzberg[3] first introduced the group work model. Their original intent was to provide a set of concepts and techniques specifically for the therapeutic use of groups. In a second edition of their book, *A Functional Approach to Group Work in Occupational Therapy*, they have paid somewhat more attention to naturally occurring groups. They observe that groups are essential to human experience:

> Group life has always played an important role in civilization, and throughout history people have considered groups to be essential to sur-

---

*The model of human occupation (see Chapter 10) addresses how social groups influence an individual's functioning; however, the focus of that model is still on the individual. Hence, it does not explicate the dynamics of groups sufficiently to guide practice where the primary concern is with the group. Kaplan,[9] in *Directive Group Therapy*, describes a way of using groups as a therapeutic method, based on the model of human occupation, suggesting that therapists wishing to develop group interventions may find it useful to combine the group work and human occupation models.

vival. We are born into a family group and later expand our social network to include work groups, social groups, recreational groups, and the like. It is through groups that we avoid isolation and learn about ourselves and other people.[7]

While the model has grown to more directly address naturally occurring groups, the main focus of this model is still on the use of groups as therapy.

Howe and Schwartzberg[8] have clearly stated their intention to propose a theory-based model for practice. Hence, they have sought to create an explanation of groups that reflects the unique concerns of the field. In this regard, they emphasize that occupational therapy is concerned with *functional groups*. The functional group is a social setting that enhances the occupational behavior of participants. Within the functional group, members engage in occupational behavior that is related to the overall purpose or goal of the group. The authors of this model extrapolate their ideas about the functional group from concepts about normal group dynamics and from concepts used to explain the workings of therapeutic groups. They are careful to distinguish functional groups, which involve members' participation in occupation, from psychodynamic groups, which focus on using discussion and group dynamics to resolve intrapersonal and interpersonal difficulties. In this regard, this model's authors have chosen, from an extensive literature on groups, those concepts that they believe are most useful for explaining the impact of group processes on occupation. Howe and Schwartzberg[8] also note that their concept of the functional group is not limited to therapy groups. They point out that naturally occurring groups such as family or work groups are also examples of functional groups.

Interdisciplinary Base

The primary interdisciplinary base for this model is the sociological and social psychological literature on group dynamics. The authors are also influenced by writings on the therapeutic properties of groups as articulated in psychiatry and other mental health professions. In addressing how individual needs are met in groups, they draw upon psychological theories of motivation (e.g., the concept that people have the intrinsic motive to engage in activity and the concept of a hierarchy of human needs).

From occupational therapy, the authors have drawn upon concepts of occupation and adaptation through participation in occupations. These concepts are used to understand how groups can meet occupational needs and how to create an "occupational context" in a group.

Theoretical Arguments

Schwartzberg and Howe[8] identify assumptions, concepts, and statements of principles that are central to this model.* Together these constitute the theoretical arguments of this model. The theoretical arguments of this model are twofold; that is, they address:

1. The nature and processes of functional groups
2. How the individual contributes to group dynamics and achieves need satisfaction and change within groups

Since this model deals both with the dynamics of groups and with the individual as a group participant, discussion of the theoretical arguments are divided into these two areas in the sections that follow.

Order: Individuals as Group Participants

According to this model, people are biopsychosocial beings with interrelated emotions and behaviors who grow and change over the course of life. The model also argues that people are fundamentally oriented toward "doing" and are motivated to be competent.[8]

Moreover, people are recognized as social beings who need to exist in groups. In groups, people communicate and interact with others and meet many of their basic needs, including the need to engage in action and be recognized as competent.[8] These are the characteristics that persons bring with them as participants in groups.

The authors also state that the individual's adaptation is promoted in groups. *Adaptation* refers to a person's adjustment to the environment. The authors argue that adaptive individual action within groups should be:

1. Purposeful, which means that both the individual and the group recognize the action as congruent with individual needs and group goals
2. Self-initiated, which means that individuals both choose to be a part of the group and have a desire to improve their skills or understanding within the group
3. Spontaneous, which means that action is centered on the here-and-now and emphasizes learning in the present
4. Group-centered, which means that action is interdependent and takes into consideration the needs of all members of a group

---

*While Howe and Schwartzberg[8] do acknowledge that their intention is to articulate a conceptual model of practice as it was outlined in the first edition of this book, they use a different approach to categorizing their theoretical statements. For purposes of consistency in this text, I have organized their arguments into the same format that I use to discuss other conceptual models of practice.

When an individual's behavior within a group has these features, individual participants are supported in adapting. Moreover, in functional groups, members are required to make choices and to perform work, play, and self-maintenance tasks. The act of participating in these occupations builds upon the natural health-maintaining and health-enhancing impact of occupations.

Order: Groups

The authors characterize groups as having their own organizational nature. A group generates a *psychological field*, which acts like an energy field, influencing the behavior of the group as a whole. The members of the group are each influenced by this psychological field to behave as a part of the group. This means that a group is viewed as more than the collection of its members; it has its own set of dynamics. As such, groups require goals related to the group as a whole.[8] These collective goals of the group allow the group to be self-directed, and they also cement together the dynamic interaction between members.

Groups also have a *group structure*. Howe and Schwartzberg[7] note that structure refers to a combination of interconnected and interdependent parts of a group. Many factors may influence group structure. Size, composition of members, group history, and setting are examples of factors that affect group structure. These and other features of group structure influence the ability of the group to reach its goals or achieve its purpose.

Groups also require individuals to fulfill roles necessary to the group's functioning. *Group roles* refer to all the positions that are necessary to a group's functioning and that must be filled by group members. Howe and Schwartzberg[8] acknowledge three types of roles within groups:

1. Group task roles, which assist the group to define and solve group problems
2. Group building and maintenance roles, which help the group function as a whole
3. Individual roles, which are concerned with individual needs

Members of a group may take on these roles at different points in time, and they may enact more than one of these roles. The most important role of any group is the role of the leader. An effective leader knows how to use group structure to influence group process.[7]

Finally, groups have a developmental history. Although the developmental course of a group is not always predictable, the developmental history of any group is important to its future. An effective group leader must have awareness of *group history*, the unfolding story of the group's past structure and functioning.

Since groups are made up of individuals, successful groups require members' attachments to people (as a basis for group cohesion) and attachment to objects (as a basis for task-oriented functions within groups). Groups also build on the strengths of participants, and they require that persons use their strengths to perform as group members.

Since groups take their nature from the larger social context, they model social behavior patterns from the larger society. Thus, each group provides a structure that guides individual participation. Further, by building cohesiveness among members, groups provide a supportive milieu in which members both give and receive assistance and feedback.

Since group order is built on and requires commitment and performance from members, and because groups are carriers of the activities, expectations, and norms of the larger society, groups are an ideal context for engaging individuals in transforming experiences. Moreover, groups can provide structure and support for individuals as they are going through change.

Disorder

The authors of this model focus on the characteristics of therapeutic groups and, therefore, do not give extensive consideration to the kinds of problems that can arise in groups and that make groups dysfunctional in themselves.[8] However, they do note that groups that lack purposeful activity will threaten the health of their individual members.

When groups lack purposeful activity, their members become idle. This, in turn, leads to individual disorientation (e.g., lack of self-esteem, alienation from others, and poor interpersonal skills) and loss of habits. While the positive influence of groups on participants is to engage them in occupational tasks relevant to the group's purpose or goals, the absence of this opportunity can have a deleterious effect on members of the group.

This model also does not address the kinds of dysfunction that individuals might bring to groups and that might affect group function. The authors of the model do note that functional groups are appropriate for persons who experience a variety of emotional, cognitive, or physical problems that reduce or prevent purposeful activity.[8]

Therapeutic Intervention

The themes of preservation and change in this model concern the influence of occupationally oriented groups on individuals. As the authors state, the "functional group seeks to enhance occupational behavior and thus adaptation."[8] They argue that groups mobilize a variety of forces that shape people. First, groups provide persons with choices for activity and encourage people to assume responsibility for meeting their needs. Groups can provide a sense of identity and self-worth to their members. Further, they offer social positions (roles) that can meet a variety of individual needs and, at the same time, require persons to respond to environmental expectations. Groups also provide a structure that guides individual participation, along with socializing influences that are necessary for learning of adaptive occupational behavior; that is, the group provides norms and expectations that channel learning toward socially acceptable and valued behaviors.

Thus, groups elicit adaptive responses from members and influence the individual to participate positively and, thereby, change. Howe and Schwartzberg[8] identify three types of impacts that groups can have on their members:

1. They motivate members to engage in purposeful and meaningful action.
2. They provide realistic experiences to members in a supportive environment where skills can be learned.
3. They move dependent and maladaptive members toward independence and adaptation.

Technology for Application

An important part of the technology of this model is the role of the therapist as group leader. Leadership is a function of the leader's ability to use leadership styles and strategies effectively. Howe and Schwartzberg[6] define *leadership* as the "ability to promote those behaviors that lead to the satisfaction of group needs." They note that leadership involves guiding both task functions and maintenance functions. *Task functions* enable the group members to work together to complete tasks. *Maintenance functions* strengthen group cohesion and group effectiveness.

Howe and Schwartzberg[6] provide a detailed examination of the traits and behaviors that therapists must employ to be effective group leaders. Traits include genuineness and empathy. Behaviors include modeling behavior for members, facilitating communication between members, and giving feedback to members. In addition, the therapist needs to know the effects of tasks and processes used in groups and to be able to plan and use them. These skills are required to facilitate group process and to meet a range of group members' needs.

Assessment

The authors identify a number of methods for assessing the group process and group-oriented individual behavior. These include observational methods for analyzing group communication patterns, members' roles and interactions, group content and process, and group behavior. Howe and Schwartzberg[8] also suggest how the group can be led to engage in the self-evaluation of their meetings. They also offer a method for evaluating group history to determine how a group has progressed.

Suggested tools for individual evaluation include a group interview for evaluating prospective group members and a method of assessing the individual members' performance in the group. The authors note that the group can be used as an arena for evaluation of individual occupational behaviors that are necessary for function in life roles.

Treatment

This model's treatment approach focuses on group process, stages of groups, task orientation, and group influence on individual adaptation. The authors discuss how therapists can use these four aspects of groups to make them therapeutic.

Group Process. The ways in which a group functions and communicates is referred to as *group process.* The leader of a group influences the group process by considering and using five factors:[7,8]

1. Maximal involvement through group-centered action
2. A maximal sense of individual and group identity
3. Flow experience
4. Spontaneous involvement of members
5. Member support and feedback

Involvement of group members can be maximized by appropriate orientation to the group, explanations of procedures, and task organization. These procedures must be at the appropriate level of challenge for group members. The leader can enhance individual and group identity by creating a safe (i.e., not too challenging or complicated) and stable (i.e., predictable) group environment and by clearly identifying the nature and purpose of the group for the members. Individual identity can be enhanced through assigned roles in the group.

Flow experience refers to an ease and pleasure in action that occurs when an individual's capacities are matched to the opportunities provided in the group. Spontaneity can be modeled by the leader and supported by interpersonal acceptance of behaviors that fall within group norms, values, and boundaries. Finally, each group leader should encourage members to provide emotional support and feedback on the behavior of other members. Appropriate communication skills for this can be modeled and taught in the group.

Stages of Group Process. Conducting a group is conceptualized as including four stages: design, formation, development, and termination. During the design phase, the therapist defines tentative group goals, develops general plans for the group as a whole and for specific sessions, selects the members, and initially structures the group and the tasks to be undertaken in the group. The therapist balances structure and openness so that the group can be as self-structuring as possible (i.e., not overly dependent on the therapist as leader).

During the formation stage, the leader selects and facilitates purposeful, self-initiated, spontaneous, group-centered action. In this phase the group leader is also responsible for setting the group climate and clarifying group norms and goals. In the development stage, the leader assesses the group's progress and problems and develops strategies for managing the latter. Leadership at this stage requires the therapist to involve members in goal setting and making adaptations of tasks. The therapist also must facilitate the assumption of various roles in the group by its members. The final phase, termination, involves dealing with members' emotional reactions, facilitating the communication of concerns and feelings among members, reviewing the group process, reviewing individual progress, dealing with unfinished business, and focusing on the transfer of learning to outside the group.

Howe and Schwartzberg[8] offer detailed discussions of each phase of group process, providing strategies and guidelines for implementing a functional group. They also provide case studies that illustrate the implementation of groups in different stages.

Task Orientation. Howe and Schwartzberg[6] state specifically that functional groups focus on action, or doing. The core of the functional group in occupational therapy is the "use of directed, purposeful occupations, or activities, to positively influence a person's sense of well-being or state of health." The model sees the purpose of group process as supporting and providing a special social milieu for task behavior.

Influence of Groups on Individual Adaptation. Group process, including the task orientation of groups and the dynamics of group interaction, has an impact on the experience and behavior of each group member. Each member brings his or her own goals, interests, strengths, and weaknesses to the group context. By interacting with the group and by performing occupations in the group context, each member is enabled to adapt in daily life occupations. This process, as illustrated in Figure 9–1, is the core of the group work model. As the figure illustrates, the leader is at the center of the group and influences group processes. The functional group always involves individual action or doing, in addition to the interaction between members. Both the doing and social interaction are influenced by the composition of the group (i.e., the level of function and nature of problems of the group members; the role of members; members' demographic characteristics, resources, and leadership). Doing and social interaction are also influenced by metacharacteristics of the group, including the climate, phases, and structure of the group. Finally, each individual's participation in the group is influenced by intrapersonal factors, including goals, interests, strengths, and weaknesses.

Composition

LEVEL OF FUNCTION
PROBLEM/DIAGNOSIS
ROLE
AGE, SEX, SOCIO-ECONOMIC STATUS
FINANCIAL RESOURCES
LEADER

Meta-Characteristics

group climate-setting
phases (group course)
structure of group:
    size
    open vs. closed
    duration, etc.

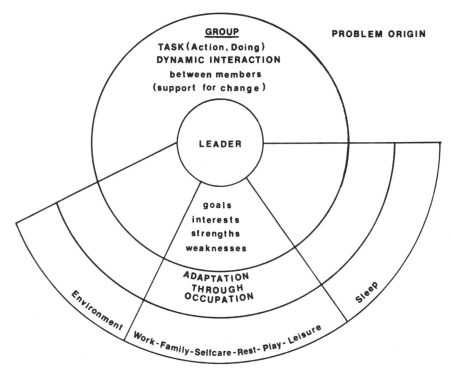

Figure 9–1. The functional group model. (From Howe, MC and Schwartzberg, SL, p 98, with permission.)

Ultimately, the individual's doing and interaction facilitates a process of occupational adaptation through which the person is enabled to more effectively participate in the environments that surround occupational life.

Research

The authors acknowledge that relatively few studies on group work have been completed. They indicate that existing research is related to the following two questions:

1. What is the impact of group format on the quantity and meaning of action and on members' functioning?
2. What influence does group format have on the cost-effectiveness of treatment?

In reference to the first question, two studies found that activity-based groups were more effective than a verbal group in improving clients' independent functioning and perceptions of their social skills.[2,10] Another study examined the impact of three different group formats (parallel task group, process-oriented verbal group, and process-oriented activity group) on social interaction.[13] This study identified differences in the quality and quantity of verbal communication exhibited by members in the different groups. Yet another study examined the variations in affective response between activities done alone and activities done in groups, and between activities chosen by members and activities assigned.[5] Studies such as these can identify the kind of impact that group characteristics have on group process and individual behavior and change within groups.

The following are representative of studies that have addressed the question of effectiveness. One study found that group treatment of patients who had received hip replacements was more cost-effective than individually oriented treatment.[15] Another study found that group-based occupational therapy had a positive impact on the functional status of persons with Parkinson's disease, while being less labor-intensive than services offered individually.[4] While such studies do not add a great deal to the understanding of how groups function, they are, nevertheless, important since they can be used to demonstrate the value of using group approaches to solving patient/client problems.

A third type of research is reflected in two recent qualitative studies that identified helping factors in a support group for persons with head injury.[12,14] Such studies will be critical to revealing what elements of groups are most important for achieving positive outcomes. Such studies will also contribute to the development of a sounder theoretical conceptualization of the group dynamics that influence occupational behavior.

Discussion

Some persons have argued that groups are a tool of occupational therapy practice and not a model of practice per se. For example, Borg and Bruce[1] published *The Group System: The Therapeutic Activity Group in Occupational Therapy*, which mainly discusses group work as a tool of therapy. Mosey[11] has also discussed group dynamics and the use of therapeutic groups. She views the use of groups as a therapeutic tool, not as a frame of reference or a model. Howe and Schwartzberg[8] disagree, arguing that the group work model is a conceptual practice model combining theory, research, and practice. In this respect, the authors of the group work model have made an important contribution to developing a conceptual model of practice.

Nonetheless, Howe and Schwartzberg have developed this model with a much stronger focus on the therapeutic use of groups than on how naturally existing groups influence occupational behavior. As noted earlier, they also point out that the concept of the functional group applies not only the therapy groups, but also to naturally occurring groups such as the family and work units. If this model is to be applied more broadly—that is, to be used as a means of understanding the kinds of functional groups that occupational therapists encounter (families, coworkers, classrooms of students, and so on)—the theoretical arguments will need to be significantly broadened. The authors of the model will have to pay more attention to group dynamics within naturally occurring groups, and they will have to address dysfunction in these groups.

The technology for application of this model (e.g., assessments and strategies for intervention) for naturally occurring groups will also need to be developed. For instance, additional concepts and technology appear to be necessary before therapists can readily apply the theory of functional groups to the family. If this model does not develop in the direction of further addressing naturally occurring groups, there will likely emerge another model of practice that does focus on work, family, and other societal groups within which persons carry out their occupational behavior.

The group work model is relatively new, and it remains to be seen in which direction it will develop. If this model continues to focus primarily on the use of therapeutic groups, it is likely that other models that address such groups as the family will emerge in occupational therapy. Addressing naturally occurring groups would appear a natural extension of this model. Such application would greatly increase the model's scope of usefulness for occupational therapy.

TERMS OF THE MODEL

adaptation	A person's adjustment to the environment.
functional group	A gathering of people that focuses on enhancing its participants' occupational behavior.
group dynamics	Properties of a group that emerge from the interactions among group members.
group history	The story of the group's past structure and functioning.
group process	Ways in which the group functions and communicates.
group roles	The social position members assume within the group.
group structure	The group form; the combination of mutually connected and dependent parts of a group.
leadership	The ability to promote those behaviors that lead to the satisfaction of group needs.
maintenance functions	Processes that strengthen group effectiveness and cohesion.
psychological field	A property of groups that acts like an energy field, influencing the behavior of the group as a whole and the behavior of individual members of the group.

SUMMARY

The Group Work Model

FOCUS

- The original intent was to provide concepts and techniques for therapeutic use of groups.
- While the model has grown to more directly address naturally occurring groups, the main focus of this model is still on the use of groups as therapy.
- Occupational therapy is concerned with functional groups (social settings in which members engage in occupational behavior related to the purpose of the group); both therapeutic groups and groups such as family are examples of functional groups.

INTERDISCIPLINARY BASE

- Sociological and social psychological literature on group dynamics, writings on the therapeutic properties of groups, and occupational therapy concepts of occupation and adaptation are used to understand group processes and their therapeutic potential.
- Psychological theories of motivation are used for understanding how individual needs are met in groups.

THEORETICAL ARGUMENTS

- The theoretical arguments of this model are twofold and address:
  - The nature and processes of groups
  - How the individual contributes to group dynamics and achieves need satisfaction and change in groups

Order: Individuals as Group Participants

- Persons have the following characteristics as participants in groups:
  - Biopsychosocial nature with interrelated emotions and behaviors
  - Growth and change over the course of life
  - Fundamental orientation toward "doing" and motivation to be competent
  - Need to exist in groups (to engage in social action and be recognized as competent)
- Individual adaptation (adjustment to the environment) is promoted in groups when individual action within groups is:
  - Purposeful (individual and the group recognize the action as congruent with needs and goals)
  - Self-initiated (individuals choose to belong to group and desire to improve skills or understanding)
  - Spontaneous (action is centered on here-and-now and emphasizes learning in the present)

- ○ Group-centered (action is interdependent and considers needs of all group members)
- In functional groups, members make choices and participate in occupations, evoking the natural health-maintaining/enhancing impact of occupations.

Order: Groups

- Groups generate a psychological field that influences:
  - ○ The behavior of the group as a whole
  - ○ Members to behave as a part of the group
- Groups:
  - ○ Have dynamics unique to the group as a whole
  - ○ Require goals related to the group as a whole (goals that allow the group to be self-directed and cement the dynamic interaction between members)
- Group structure (composed of mutually connected and dependent parts) influences the ability of the group to reach its goals and is influenced by such factors as:
  - ○ Size
  - ○ Composition of members
  - ○ Group history
  - ○ Setting
- Group roles (positions necessary to a group's functioning) must be filled by group members. There are three types of roles:
  - ○ Group task roles, which assist the group to define and solve group problems
  - ○ Group building and maintenance roles, which help the group function as a whole
  - ○ Individual roles concerned with individual needs
- The most important role of any group is that of the leader, who uses group structure to influence group process.
- Developmental history (the unfolding story of the group's past structure and functioning) is important to any group's future.
- Successful groups require attachments to:
  - ○ People (as a basis for group cohesion)
  - ○ Objects (as a basis for task-oriented functions within groups)
- Groups:
  - ○ Take their nature from the larger social context
  - ○ Model social behavior patterns from the larger society
  - ○ Provide a structure that guides individual participation
  - ○ Provide a supportive milieu in which members both give and receive assistance and feedback
  - ○ Provide structure and support for individuals as they are going through change

Disorder

- Groups that lack purposeful activity will threaten the health of their individual members.

Therapeutic Intervention

- Groups mobilize forces that shape people toward adaptive occupational behavior. Thus, groups:
  - Provide persons with choices for activity
  - Encourage people to assume responsibility for meeting their needs
  - Provide a sense of identity and self-worth to members
  - Offer social positions (roles) that meet individual needs
  - Require persons to respond to environmental expectations
  - Provide a structure that guides individual participation
  - Provide socializing influences (norms and expectations) that channel learning toward socially acceptable and valued occupational behaviors
  - Elicit adaptive responses from members and influence the individual to participate and change
- A group can influence members in three ways:
  - By motivating engagement in purposeful and meaningful action
  - By providing realistic experiences in a supportive environment where skills can be learned
  - By moving dependent and maladaptive members toward independence and adaptation

TECHNOLOGY FOR APPLICATION

- Role of the therapist as group leader:
  - Use of leadership styles and strategies
  - Promotion of behaviors to satisfy group needs
- Leadership involves guiding:
  - Task functions that enable the group members to work together to complete tasks
  - Maintenance functions that strengthen group cohesion and group effectiveness
- Traits and behaviors of effective group leaders:
  - Genuineness and empathy
  - Modeling behavior for members
  - Facilitating communication
  - Giving feedback
  - Knowing and using the effects of tasks and processes to facilitate group process and meet members' needs
- Methods for assessing the group process and group-oriented individual behavior:
  - Observe/analyze group communication patterns, members' roles and interactions, group content and process, and group behavior

- Self-evaluate group meetings
- Evaluate group history to determine how a group has progressed
- Interview to evaluate prospective group members
- Assess individual members' group performance
- Use the group as an arena for evaluating individual occupational behaviors
- Treatment approach focuses on:
  - Group process
  - Stages of groups
  - Task orientation
  - Group influence on individual adaptation
- The leader of a group influences the group process by considering and using five factors:
  - Maximal involvement through group-centered action
  - A maximal sense of individual and group identity
  - Flow experience (ease and pleasure in action when an individual's capacities are matched to the opportunities provided in the group)
  - Spontaneous involvement of members (supported by interpersonal acceptance of behaviors that fall within group norms, values, and boundaries)
  - Member support and feedback
- Conducting a group involves four stages:
  - Design (define tentative group goals, develop general plans for group, select members, initially structure group and tasks)
  - Formation (select/facilitate purposeful, self-initiated, spontaneous, group-centered action, set group climate, clarify group norms and goals)
  - Development (assess group's progress and problems, develop strategies)
  - Termination (deal with members' emotions, facilitate communication, review group/individual progress, deal with unfinished business, focus on the transfer of learning)
- The core of the functional group is use of directed, purposeful occupations to influence a person's well-being.
- Group process (task orientation and dynamics of group interaction) has an impact on the experience and behavior of each member. By interacting with the group and by performing occupations in the group context, each member is enabled to adapt in daily life occupations.

RESEARCH

- Existing research is related to the following questions:
  - What is the impact of group format on the quantity and meaning of action and on members' functioning?
  - What influence does group format have on cost-effectiveness of treatment?

References

1. Borg, B, and Bruce, MS: The Group System: The Therapeutic Activity Group in Occupational Therapy. Slack, Thorofare, NJ, 1991.
2. DeCarlo, JJ, and Mann, WC: The effectiveness of verbal versus activity groups in improving self-perceptions of interpersonal communication skills. Am J Occup Ther 39:20–27, 1985.
3. Duncombe, LW, and Howe, MC: Group work in occupational therapy: A survey of practice. Am J Occup Ther 39:163, 1985.
4. Gauthier, L, Dalziel, S, and Gauthier, S: The benefits of group occupational therapy for patients with Parkinson's disease. Am J Occup Ther 41:360–365, 1987.
5. Henry, AD, Nelson, DL, and Duncombe, LW: Choice making in group and individual activity. Am J Occup Ther 38:245, 1984.
6. Howe, MC, and Schwartzberg, SL: A Functional Approach to Group Work in Occupational Therapy. JB Lippincott, Philadelphia, 1986, pp 89, 94, and 111.
7. Howe, MC, and Schwartzberg, SL: Structure and process in designing a functional group. Occupational Therapy in Mental Health 8:1, 1988.
8. Howe, MC, and Schwartzberg, SL: A Functional Approach to Group Work in Occupational Therapy, ed 2. JB Lippincott, Philadelphia, 1995.
9. Kaplan, KL: Directive Group Therapy: Innovative Mental Health Treatment. Slack, Thorofare, NJ, 1988.
10. Klyczek, JP, and Mann, WC: Therapeutic modality comparisons in day treatment. Am J Occup Ther 40:606–611, 1986.
11. Mosey, AC: Psychosocial Components of Occupational Therapy. Raven Press, New York, 1986.
12. Schwartzberg, SL: Helping factors in a peer-developed support group for persons with head injury, Part 1: Participant observer perspective. Am J Occup Ther 48:297–304, 1994.
13. Schwartzberg, SL, Howe, MC, and McDermott, A: A comparison of three treatment group formats for facilitating social interaction. Occupational Therapy in Mental Health 2:1, 1982.
14. Shulz, CH: Helping factors in a peer-developed support group for persons with head injury, Part 2: Survivor interview perspective. Am J Occup Ther 48:305–309, 1994.
15. Trahey, PJ: A comparison of the cost-effectiveness of two types of occupational therapy services. Am J Occup Ther 45:397–400, 1991.

CHAPTER 10

THE MODEL OF
HUMAN OCCUPATION

The model of human occupation is concerned with a broader range of phenomena than most other models. This model addresses the motivation for occupation, the patterning of occupational behavior into routines and lifestyles, the nature of skilled performance, and the influence of environment on occupational behavior. Unlike most models, which are designed for specific populations, this model is intended for use with any person experiencing occupational dysfunction. Consequently, the model of human occupation is applied across the age span and across a wide range of diagnoses.

This model grew from efforts to refine and apply concepts developed in the occupational behavior tradition.* The model was introduced in the 1980s[48,49,59,60] and has been more fully articulated in two editions of *A Model of Human Occupation: Theory and Application*.[50,51] While the model was introduced in the United States, scholars and clinicians worldwide now contribute to its development and application.

Interdisciplinary Base

Since this model attempts to conceptualize a wide range of phenomena, it draws upon a broad scope of interdisciplinary concepts. The model was orig-

---

*Readers will recall from Chapter 3 that occupational behavior was a theoretical tradition that arose in the late 1950s and continued through the 1970s. It was represented in the work of a number of scholars who were attempting to go beyond the narrow focus of the mechanistic paradigm and return the field to concern for occupation. The original authors of this model were trained within the occupational behavior tradition and sought to integrate a wide range of concepts from that tradition into a single, coherent model for practice.

inally based on concepts of general and open systems theory. More recently, this model has incorporated dynamical systems concepts. The model also uses concepts from ego psychology concerning human needs and motives. Interdisciplinary concepts of narrative have influenced the current formulation of motivation in this model. Concepts from sociology, social psychology and philosophy, and from early occupational therapy literature have been incorporated in an effort to understand how occupational behavior is organized into everyday patterns. The view of the environment in this model is influenced by literature from environmental psychology and anthropology.

Theoretical Arguments

The model of human occupation seeks to account for the motivation, performance, and organization of occupational behavior in everyday life. Hence, the theoretical arguments of this model address these aspects of occupation, explain what happens to them in states of dysfunction, and point to how they can be remediated.

Order

The model makes the following arguments (Fig. 10–1) about humans' occupational behavior:

1. The human being is a complex organization of three subsystems (volition, habituation, and mind-brain-body performance) that motivate, organize, and make possible performance of occupation.
2. Occupational behavior emerges from interaction of the human system with the environment. Further, occupational behavior shapes the subsequent organization of the human system.
3. The volition subsystem arises from a need for action and is composed of personal causation (beliefs and feelings about one's capacity and control), values, and interests. This subsystem anticipates, chooses, experiences, and interprets occupational behavior.
4. Occupational behavior demonstrates a pattern that is influenced by one's habituation subsystem; this subsystem is composed of habits and internalized roles.
5. Occupational performance is composed of motor, process, and communication/interaction skills that emerge from the interaction of one's mind-brain-body performance subsystem with the environment.
6. The social environment (including occupational forms and social groups) and the physical environment (including objects and spaces) provide both opportunities and constraints that shape occupational behavior.

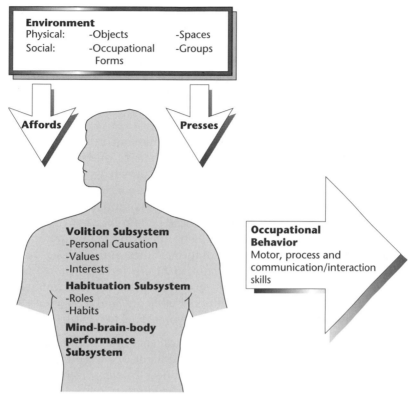

Figure 10–1. The human open system.

Each of these arguments is examined further in the following subsections.

The Human as a Dynamic System. According to this model, occupational behavior emerges from a cooperation of the three subsystems with conditions in the environment.[55] Consequently, the occupation a person is performing and the context in which he or she is performing are as important as underlying motives and capacity in determining how a person will perform.

A second systems theme in the model is that the action or occupational behavior of the human system is a central force in health, well-being, development, and change.[55] This idea begins with the recognition that humans are dynamic, self-organizing systems always unfolding and changing in time. Ongoing occupational behavior underlies this self-organization; that is, as human beings engage in work, play, and daily living tasks, they maintain and change their own capacities, beliefs, and dispositions.

The Volition Subsystem. This model asserts that all humans have a need to act that is uniquely expressed in each person's occupational behavior. Through their behavior, persons acquire individual dispositions toward acting in the world. Moreover, they accumulate a sense of their own effectiveness, an awareness of potentials for enjoyment and satisfaction, and a view of life that commits them to behave in certain ways. These dispositions and images are referred to as volition. Together, they constitute a person's motives for engaging in occupational behavior.

Volition is defined as a system of dispositions and self-knowledge that predisposes and enables persons to anticipate, choose, experience, and interpret occupational behavior.[57] *Dispositions* refer to cognitive and emotive orientations toward occupations, such as enjoying, valuing, and feeling competent to perform them. *Self-knowledge* refers to one's commonsense awareness of acting in the world; it is a store of knowledge about what one experiences and accomplishes when performing an occupation.

Volitional dispositions and self-knowledge comprise three areas: personal causation, values, and interests. These pertain to what one holds as important, how effective one is in acting on the world, and what one finds enjoyable and satisfying. Personal causation, values, and interests are interrelated and together constitute the content of our feelings, thoughts, and decisions about engaging in occupations.[57] The personal causation, values, and interests that make up one's volition enable one and lead one to anticipate, experience, choose, and interpret occupational behavior.

Personal Causation. Experience teaches what one can and cannot do well and engenders dispositions to feel confident or insecure about one's physical, intellectual, or interpersonal abilities. This experience results in one's *knowledge of capacity*, an awareness of and attitude toward one's present and potential abilities. Experience also reveals how effectively one uses capacities. The resulting *sense of efficacy* includes the perception of whether and how one controls one's own behavior (and underlying thoughts and emotions) as well as the sense of one's effectiveness in achieving desired outcomes of behavior. *Personal causation* is the composite of these two elements; it is defined as a collection of dispositions and self-knowledge concerning one's capacities for and efficacy in occupations.

Values. One's values define what is worth doing, how one ought to perform, and what goals or aspirations deserve one's commitment. Values are expressed in the common sense that guides the kind of life persons strive for in a particular culture. Values elicit strong emotions concerning how life should be and how one should behave. Consequently, one does not act contrary to one's values without feeling shame, guilt, failure, or inadequacy.

Values are defined as a coherent set of convictions that assign significance or standards to occupations, creating a strong disposition to perform accordingly. The concept of *personal convictions* refers to one's way of viewing life and the goals to be pursued in life. Personal convictions are simply one's commonsense beliefs about what matters in life. Hence, values locate one within a taken-for-granted world that makes sense of and gives worth to certain behaviors. How one sees life is secured in place by powerful emotions (e.g., feelings of importance, security, worthiness, belonging, and purpose). These emotions create *commitments*, which are strong emotional dispositions to follow what are perceived as right ways to behave.

Interests. Interests are generated from the experience of pleasure and satisfaction in occupational behavior. They reflect both natural dispositions (e.g., the tendency to enjoy physical or intellectual activity) and acquired tastes. The experience and awareness of enjoying an occupation creates a disposition or anticipation of future pleasure. Consequently, interests are felt as desires for participating in certain occupations.

Interests are defined as dispositions to find pleasure and satisfaction in occupations, and the self-knowledge of our enjoyment of occupations. The disposition to enjoy certain occupations or certain aspects of performance is referred to as *attraction*. The positive feelings associated with engaging in an occupation generates attraction. This attraction may be related to many different aspects of doing an occupation. Hence, attraction to any particular occupation most likely represents a confluence of several factors, such as enjoying the challenge, aesthetics, products, and human interaction provided by the activity.

Experience from doing results in the awareness that some occupations provide one with a sense of satisfaction and pleasure, while others bore, threaten, or fail to stimulate us. From such experience emerges *preference*, which is the knowledge that one enjoys particular ways of performing or particular activities over others.

Choices in Everyday Life. Personal causation, values, and interests together form a commonsense apprehension of one's self and one's world. They influence what one is likely to feel or think about the prospects for involvement in occupations and how one experiences and interprets occupational activities. In turn, the process of choosing, experiencing, and interpreting occupational behavior represents an ongoing cycle that sustains and transforms volition. In this way, personal causation, values, and interests are both the motive for and the product of one's occupational behavior.[57]

People consciously select many of the occupational activities that fill their days. These *activity choices* are defined as short-term, deliberate decisions to enter and exit occupational activities. Deciding to have lunch with a friend, watch a movie, wash the car, mow the lawn, take a walk, bake a cake, or read a newspaper are examples of activity choices.

Individuals also decide to make certain occupations an extended or permanent part of their lives. They make these kinds of decisions when they choose to enter a new role (e.g., becoming a marital partner, parent, or student), acquire a new habit (e.g., take up regular exercise), or undertake a project (e.g., planting and caring for a garden, writing a book, or building a fence around the yard). Such decisions require commitment to enter into a course of action or to sustain regular performance over time. These occupational choices ordinarily result from considerable deliberation and may involve an extended process of information-gathering, reflection, and imagination. Consequently, *occupational choices* are defined as deliberate commitments to enter an occupational role, acquire a new habit, or undertake a personal project.

Volitional Narrative. The volitional process of anticipating, choosing, experiencing, and interpreting one's occupational behavior is nested in ongoing life. Volitional thoughts, feelings, and choices reverberate with present circumstances, past memories, and images of a possible future. People integrate past, present, and future into a coherent whole through highly personal life stories that are called *volitional narratives*.[36,37,57] While volitional narratives may be told to others, they are primarily a personal process of making sense of one's occupational life. Human beings naturally make sense of things in the form of a story, perceiving themselves as the central character in the unfolding drama of life.

Volitional narratives integrate each person's values, personal causation, and interests. These stories make sense of how one performs and finds satisfaction and value in life. Volitional narratives embed the issues, concerns, hopes, and fears related to personal causation, values, and interests in the events and circumstances of one's life. Since stories both animate and anticipate the future (as when they project the fear that things may become worse or the hope that things will get better), they can energize or paralyze one's volitional choices. Consequently, volitional narratives are conceptualized to be powerful motivators. Helfrich et al.,[37] Mallinson et al.,[72] and Jonsson et al.[43] have studied volitional narratives in a range of persons and offer detailed examples of how these persons construct and use narratives to make sense of their lives.

People experience unfolding life as a continuation of their volitional narratives. Hence, through their occupational behavior, people strive to continue the story in ways that they believe are important, that bring satisfaction, and that they can achieve. People not only tell themselves (and others) where their lives are headed through their volitional narratives; they also seek to live out those narratives.

The Habituation Subsystem. To be competent, people must be integrated into the rhythms and customs that make up their physical, social, and temporal worlds. Moreover, people move through life occupying a sequence of social positions as family members, students, parents, workers, and so on. They are expected to behave and learn to behave in certain ways because of these roles. As a result, people acquire and exhibit recurring patterns of occupational behavior that make up much of their everyday lives.[20,54]

In the model of human occupation, the process of acquiring and repeating these patterns of occupational behavior is referred to as habituation.[54] The *habituation subsystem* is defined as an internal organization of information that disposes one to exhibit recurrent patterns of behavior. This habituation subsystem allows people to efficiently and automatically behave in their familiar physical, temporal, and social environments.

Habituation operates from appreciative tendencies that enable one, without deliberation or attention, to improvise consistent ways of behaving. The concept of appreciative tendency refers to the process by which one automatically recognizes a circumstance for what it is and also knows without reflection how to act in that circumstance. For example, people in Western cultures automatically recognize that when persons extend their hands they are offering a greeting, and they instinctively know how to reciprocate the behavior for producing a handshake. This model classifies the internalized appreciative tendencies of habituation into habits and roles.

Habits. As people go about the routines of daily life, they are guided by habits. Because of habits, one knows that it is time for breakfast, what route to take while driving to work, or what step comes next in a job task. Hence, habits allow one to comprehend and to behave in one's familiar world.

Habits preserve a way of doing something learned from earlier performance. Once in place, habits allow behavior to unfold automatically. Moreover, habits organize occupational behavior by (a) influencing how one performs routine activities, (b) regulating how time is typically used, and (c) generating styles of behavior (e.g., being meticulous versus nonchalant, or slow-paced versus fast-paced). Consequently, *habits* are defined as latent appreciative tendencies acquired from previous repetitions, operating at a preconscious, automatic level and influencing a wide range of behavioral patterns.[54]

Habits do not function as instructions for specific behaviors. Rather, habits serve as maps for keeping one's bearings and for steering one's behavior within unfolding events. Thus the concept of a *habit map* is used to refer to an internalized appreciative capacity that allows one to recognize familiar events and contexts, and to construct action for accomplishing a process or reaching a goal.

Internalized Roles. Occupational behavior reflects the roles one has internalized. Thus, people act as spouses, parents, workers, students, and so on. People also see themselves as spouses, parents, workers, or students when they are in these roles; their identity is shaped by their roles. Hence, the *internalized role* is defined as a broad awareness of a particular social identity and related obligations that together provide a framework for appreciating relevant situations and constructing appropriate behavior.[54]

When people perform role-related behavior they employ role scripts. These *role scripts* are appreciative tendencies that allow one to comprehend social situations and expectations and to construct behavior that enacts a given role. For example, one's role scripts allow one to automatically know how to differentially greet one's boss in a meeting or a close friend in a restaurant. Role scripts allow one to appreciate the role and context one is in and to automatically assemble the appropriate behavior for the role and the situation.

The roles one inhabits also create expectations for certain kinds of occupational performance. For example, the parent role requires one to do certain caretaking tasks, while the student role requires studying. People ordinarily have several roles that occupy routine times and spaces. For example, people generally are in the worker role during the work week and in the workplace; they are in the role of a spouse primarily at home and outside work hours. Consequently, roles organize occupational behavior by (a) influencing the manner and content of interactions with others, (b) requiring routine tasks, and (c) partitioning daily and weekly cycles into times when one ordinarily inhabits different roles. Having a complement of roles gives one rhythm and change between these different identities and modes of doing.

Interweaving of Habits and Roles. Together, habits and roles contribute to one's ability to recognize features and situations in the environment and to behave automatically. Roles guide how one performs within social positions; habits regulate other aspects of an individual's routine and ways of performing occupations. Habits and roles are interwoven in daily life and together organize routine behavior.

Much of one's occupational behavior belongs to a familiar round of daily life. For example, most people repeat the same morning scenario of getting up, grooming, and going to work or school 5 days a week. Because of roles and habits, these routines unfold with regularity and ease. Habituation plants one in the familiar territory of everyday life ready to appreciate its circumstances and poised to behave in customary ways.

Occupational Performance and Skill. The third subsystem makes possible performance in daily occupations. Performance refers to spontaneously doing those actions required to accomplish an occupation. Performance involves a complex interplay of musculoskeletal, neurological, perceptual, and cognitive phenomena. These musculoskeletal, neurological, cardiopulmonary, and symbolic constituents are organized into the *mind-brain-body performance* subsystem.*[26] This subsystem functions as an integrated whole; that is, the mus-

---

*The model of human occupation does not attempt to explain the inner workings of the musculoskeletal, neurological, or cognitive process. The authors of the model recognize that these explanations are found in other conceptual practice models. Rather, the model underscores the importance of seeing these musculoskeletal, neurological, and cognitive processes as part of an integrated subsystem and as part of a total human system. The model also emphasizes that while the mind-brain-body performance subsystem gives persons the capacity for performance, everyday occupational behavior requires more than capacity; it requires the collaboration of volition and habituation subsystems, which together provide the motives for choosing behavior and the maps and scripts for organizing behavior into patterns. Finally, the model emphasizes that these three subsystems operate in collaboration with the environment. Hence, the main contribution of the model to understanding performance capacity is to point out how it is embedded in a larger system and environmental context.

culoskeletal, neurological, cardiopulmonary, and symbolic constituents are interdependent. Occupational performance is the result of the unified action of all constituents of the mind-brain-body performance subsystem as they collaborate with unfolding circumstances and environmental conditions.

In the model of human occupation, skill is conceptualized as distinct from capacity. Whereas capacity refers to the underlying potential for behavior, skill refers to the characteristics of actual performance. Consequently, skill is defined as "observable elements of action which have implicit functional purposes."[26] The model identifies three areas of skill:

1. Motor skills, which refer to moving oneself and objects in space
2. Process skills, which refer to the management and modification of procedures
3. Communication/interaction skills, which refer to dealing with and sharing information with others

Within each of these three areas, discrete skills are identified. Hence, reaching, sequencing, and gesturing are examples of motor, process, and communication/interaction skills, respectively.

The Environment. According to this model, the environment influences occupational behavior in two ways:

1. It *affords* or gives opportunities for performance.
2. It *presses*, which means to recruit or require particular behavior.[53]

Environments simultaneously afford and press for occupational behaviors. By concurrently providing opportunity and constraint, environments create pathways for behavior. Moreover, environments have physical and social dimensions. Occupation involves encountering an interwoven physical and social environment.

The physical environment consists of spaces and the objects within them. *Spaces* refer to physical contexts in which persons may engage in occupational behavior. They include both naturally occurring spaces, such as an open field, a beach, or a lake and fabricated spaces, such as a lobby, kitchen, classroom, office, or factory. *Objects* refer to both natural and fabricated things with which persons may interact. Consequently, objects include books, trees, cars, rocks, chairs, clothes, and so on. Together, the spaces we inhabit and the objects we use influence behavior. They compel occupational behavior not only because of their physical properties and utilitarian value, but also because of the social meanings attached to them.

The social environment includes groupings of persons and occupational forms that persons perform.[53,76] *Social groups* refer to collections of persons that occur with regularity. Social groups provide and define expectations for roles, and they constitute a milieu or social space in which those roles are enacted. The ambience, norms, and climate of a group give opportunities for and demand certain kinds of occupational behavior. Contrast, for example, groups gathered for playing a game of poker, worshiping in church, working on a quilt, having Sunday dinner, and building a house. In each of these situations the attitudes and behaviors that are expected and allowed are quite different. Hence, the same person may exhibit a wide variation in behavior in each of these contexts.

Occupational forms are rule-bound sequences of action that are at once coherent, oriented to a purpose, sustained in collective knowledge, culturally recognizable, and named. An occupational form that is part of a group's typical behavior is something members will recognize and have language to describe. To say that occupational forms are rule-bound means that there is a conventional or correct way of performing them. The procedures, outcomes, and standards for occupational forms are maintained within cultural and social groups and passed on when one learns an occupational form. Hence, to learn how to square dance, play a game of football, give a lecture, write a term paper, bake a cake, or ride a horse is to learn a way of doing things that has expected outcomes or processes and conventional ways of getting the job done or rules to follow. Learning to perform means learning to reproduce a particular occupational form.

The environments in which one performs occupations are combinations of physical and social elements. These *occupational behavior settings* are composites of spaces, objects, occupational forms, and/or social groups that cohere and constitute a meaningful context for performance. Occupational behavior settings are places of being and acting in life, and they envelop us and become part of whatever we are doing. Occupational behavior settings include home, neighborhood, school or workplace, and sites for gathering, recreation, or resources (e.g., theaters, churches, clubs, libraries, museums, restaurants, and stores). Persons' occupational behavior is invited and shaped by these occupational behavior settings.

Disorder

According to the model, occupational dysfunction can be recognized when a person has problems performing, organizing, and/or choosing occupations, and when one's environment fails to support and expect adaptive behavior.[56] The volition, habituation, mind-brain-body performance subsystems, and the environment may all contribute to occupational dysfunction, which ordinarily involves some combination of these factors.

Dysfunction in Volition. When persons experience dysfunction, their volition can be affected in many ways.[56] Sometimes volitional dispositions, self-knowledge, and narratives lead to activity and occupational choices that are maladaptive. On the other hand, acquired physical, emotional, or cognitive impairments can threaten or disrupt previously adaptive volition.

Personal Causation. Persons with disability may have to deal with the knowledge that they have severely restricted capacity or that their former abilities are no longer available. They may find themselves unable to achieve what they desire and compare themselves unfavorably with others. As a consequence, feelings of inadequacy, shame, fear of failure can come to dominate personal causation.

Sometimes it is extremely difficult for persons to know what their capacities will be in the face of progressive diseases or changing environments. Persons may also under- or overestimate their capacities and likelihood of success, making decisions that unnecessarily restrict performance or expose them to danger or failure. Knowing one's loss or lack of capacity can be very painful, leading to depression and demoralization.

When personal causation is negatively affected, persons may make choices that restrict behavior and avoid opportunities for development. They also may make choices that result in further maladaptive behavior. Feelings of inefficacy often lie at the core of a cycle of dysfunction, locking persons into a cycle of acting and feeling ineffective.

Values. The interface of dysfunction and value is complex. Some dysfunctions may be precipitated by holding values that are deviant, internally conflicted, or lead to maladaptive occupational behavior. Feelings of worthlessness can result when one is unable to achieve impossible ideals or finds that others do not value what one does.

Persons with limitations of capacity often find that they are unable to live up to social values such as self-reliance and physical beauty. They may be faced with accepting such social values, thereby devaluating themselves. Or, they may have to reject these mainstream values and accept a marginal identity.

When people acquire limitations of capacity they may find themselves unable to perform in ways that were important to them. They may have to relinquish activities they valued and experienced as sources of personal meaning. When impairments prevent persons from living up to their own values, they risk losing a sense of self-worth and may find their lives devoid of meaning. Consequently, disability can challenge persons with conflicts between societal ideals, their own values, and their remaining capacities.

Interests. One of the most pervasive effects of disability on occupation is disruption of interests. The pleasures, comforts, and satisfactions that accrue from performance and enliven everyday existence can be decreased or eliminated by disability. Impairments that restrict behavior can limit the range of experiences for developing a sense of attraction to occupations. The fatigue, pain, and preoccupation with failure that can accompany a disability may also reduce or eliminate feelings of pleasure in occupations. Necessary adaptations of performance may alter the ambience and spirit of activities, thus reducing enjoyment or satisfaction in performance.

Impairment may altogether prevent persons from engaging in former interests, requiring that they rechannel or discover new interests.

Persons with emotional disabilities may experience a loss of attraction to occupations. For example, depression and reduced enjoyment in activities are related.[77] Persons with substance abuse problems are less likely to pursue their interests[89] and may replace enjoyment in performance with pleasure induced by substances.

Habituation. Habituation is related to disability in a variety of ways.[56] Disability can invalidate, restrict, and place extra demands on habits. Roles may be lost or altered dramatically by disability. On the other hand habits and roles can contribute to disability when they constitute maladaptive patterns of behavior.

Roles. Dysfunction in roles may be both a consequence and a cause of psychosocial dysfunction. Role failure may occur when one has not internalized appropriate role scripts and thereby cannot meet expectations of social groups. Cognitive or emotional impairments and restrictive environments may limit experiences to internalize roles.

Acquired impairments can disrupt or terminate role performance. One may be unable to discharge a role so as to meet one's own or others' expectations for the role, a situation leading to role strain and interpersonal conflict. Losing roles or having to take on less valued roles may alter one's sense of identity and worth.

Persons with disabilities find that they are often barred from certain roles by virtue of societal attitudes. Despite federal legislation to the contrary, persons with disabilities still face greater challenges in acquiring jobs.[51] Also, people with disabilities may find that they are relegated by others to sick or impaired roles, or that they are considered to be incapable of normal role behaviors. For example, just being in a wheelchair can change how a person is viewed by others. In this way, people with disabilities often find their roles socially restricted.

Habits. Habits can be a source of dysfunction when they constrain effective occupational performance. Disorganized or rigid habits may be a serious liability. People with dysfunctional habits may find that their routines are dissatisfying and prevent them from living up to their own and others' desires.

A disability can place important restrictions and demands on habits. For example, expanding the time necessary for self-care may place limits on the time available for other activities in the day. Special routines may be required to manage a chronic disease or disability (e.g., routines for bowel and bladder care, joint protection, or energy conversation).

Persons who acquire a disability may find that many of their previous routines are no longer possible or effective. The onset of disability can radically alter the spatial and temporal dimensions of routine performance.

What was once the familiar territory of everyday life may become foreign as one can no longer perceive and move about the world in the same way.

Mind-Brain-Body Performance Subsystem. Disabilities may involve disturbances to the neurological, musculoskeletal, and symbolic constituents of the mind-brain-body performance subsystem. The model of human occupation does not directly address these impairments as do many of the other models of practice discussed in this text. The model does, however, emphasize the importance of understanding the experience of mind-brain-body disability.[56] Hence the model calls attention to what it is like to have restrictions of motor capacity, sensation, perception, or cognition. It emphasizes that experience is the subjective framework within which a person must exist and perform. This model also calls attention to the actual performance skills that a person exhibits. Restrictions in motor, process, and communication or interaction skills can limit the effectiveness of a person with impairments.

Environment. The physical and social environment can have a wide range of effects on occupational dysfunction.[56] Physical spaces can pose natural and architectural barriers that interfere with the occupational performance of persons who have impairments. Most of the objects of everyday life are designed for able-bodied persons and may pose barriers or challenges to those with physical impairments. Also, disability may require one to use new objects that extend or substitute for restricted capacity. Consequently, wheelchairs, adapted equipment, catheterization supplies, grab bars, and other extraordinary objects may come to fill the world of a person with a disability. Persons in institutional environments may be deprived of access to normal everyday objects. In sum, persons with disabilities can be profoundly affected by the objects they encounter, must use, or lack.

Most social groups are deeply ambivalent toward persons with disabilities and group practices and attitudes often betray discomfort with the person who has a disability. Disability may remove persons from groups where they previously performed. Moreover, the person with a newly acquired disability may find that coworkers, friends, and others are uncertain, withdrawn, or undesirous of maintaining previous relationships.

Occupational forms are dramatically altered for the person with a disability. Impairments may make occupational forms impossible or alter how they must be done. Occupational forms that were once private and easy affairs may require the assistance of others and take a great deal of time and effort after the onset of a disability.

In sum, the environment is radically transformed when a person has a disability. Objects, spaces, occupational forms, and social groups can be sources of frustration and devaluation. They can pose social and physical barriers to occupational performance and satisfaction.

Therapeutic Intervention

The model of human occupation frames the process of adapting to a disability in the following ways. Maintaining a satisfying and productive life through positive choices is a major task for persons challenged by disability. Such persons often must learn to overcome and compensate for the volitional restrictions and dysfunction they may experience. When persons can draw upon a belief in their own efficacy, feelings of attraction and satisfaction from performance, and personal convictions, they are better equipped to deal with a disability. Habituation is also essential to how persons come to practical terms with a disability by organizing a life that allows them to routinely function to their own and others' satisfaction. Disability is a subjective experience within which persons must learn to live and perform. Moreover, persons must learn to employ their intact skills in ways that compensate for deficits and maximize success in necessary and desired occupational forms. Finally, the environment has the power to mitigate or exacerbate emotional, functional, and behavioral consequences of impairments. Indeed where impairments are immutable, environmental accommodations are important means of enhancing functions. This picture of how persons cope with and adapt to disability serves as a general framework for understanding what therapeutic intervention should seek to accomplish.

The most recent edition of *A Model of Human Occupation: Theory and Application* outlines a series of therapeutic principles.[52] These principles are organized into general, volitional, habituation, and performance categories and include the following general principles:

1. Therapy is an event that comes into a life in progress and must be understood and undertaken in that context.
2. The focus for change should be the action or process underlying the human system.
3. Change does not mean simply more or less; it means a different form of organization.
4. Changes can and should occur in many aspects of the human system simultaneously.
5. Change is often disorderly.
6. Therapy should involve experimentation to find the best solutions.
7. The only tool that therapists have at their disposal is to change the relevant environment to support or precipitate change in the human system.

These and the other principles are derived from theoretical arguments about order and disorder. They propose broad themes about how change may take place in highly complex human systems. While the principles are explained and supported with examples in the book, it is emphasized that the therapist's knowledge of each patient is necessary to know how to apply the principles.

For example, the model of human occupation suggests that improvement in a person's sense of efficacy requires positive experiences of undertaking and completing occupational forms that are valuable and interesting. Which occupational forms will work best depends on what a particular client enjoys and finds important. While some patients respond positively to modification of old interests so that they can be pursued, others find diminished performance in highly valued occupations too painful and must instead explore new occupations. Moreover, how many positive experiences it will take to shift a person's perception concerning efficacy cannot be specified ahead of time. As noted in the principle stated above, therapy requires experimentation to find out a client's reaction to a particular occupation. As therapy unfolds, the therapist gains important information about how an individual is changing. That emerging information is essential for anticipating what might come next and what strategy might help the patient continue to improve.

The principles provided by the model of human occupation provide a means for thinking about therapy. Therapy should be comprehended from a viewpoint that transcends any individual principles and reflects the attitude behind them all.

Technology for Application

Application of the model of human occupation in practice involves being able to use the theory as a guide to gathering and interpreting clinical data and as a guide to intervention.[64] When assessing, therapists should seek out data to answer questions they have generated from the theoretical perspective of the model. For example, therapists might ask questions such as the following: Is this person's habit pattern contributing to his poor role performance? How has chronic pain affected this person's enjoyment of previous interests? Is this person's sense of efficacy interfering with her ability to make an important occupational choice? Does this child hesitate to engage in social play because of the anxiety of failing in front of peers?

Assessments

Kielhofner et al.[66] note that therapists using the model of human occupation gather data through structured and situated means. Structured data gathering (typically referred to as assessments, evaluations, instruments, or scales) employs specified protocols. Situated methods are those devised by the therapist to match a specific situation. Structured methods have the advantage of using tested protocols, while situated methods capitalize on therapists' more intimate knowledge of patients and upon unique opportunities for getting useful information.

Structured Methods. The three most common structured data collection methods developed for and used in association with the model of human occupation are observational measures, self-report questionnaires or checklists, and structured interviews.

The Assessment of Motor and Process Skills (AMPS)[25] and the Assessment of Communication and Interaction Skills (ACIS)[28] have been developed to measure performance skills. The AMPS employs observation of patients performing occupational forms and consists of two scales that separately measure process and motor skills. The ACIS uses observations of persons involved in social groups to measure communication and interaction skills.

The Volitional Questionnaire[15,40] is an observational rating scale developed for obtaining information about volition from persons who cannot effectively self-report (e.g., persons with substantial cognitive limitations). Therapists observe and rate patients while they engage in work, leisure, or daily living tasks, indicating the amount of volitional spontaneity (versus passivity or need for support and encouragement) the individual demonstrates. This instrument is intended for examining the effect of different environments on volitional spontaneity and for tracking volition over time.

The Role Checklist[9,20,81] captures clients' role identification and determines the value a person attaches to roles. It can be filled out in a few minutes independently or with therapist assistance. The Role Checklist is interpreted by examining the pattern of responses; a summary sheet aids in the visual examination and interpretation of the response pattern.

The Interest Checklist was originally developed by Matsutsuyu[73] and later modified.[89] The current version of the Interest Checklist[66] includes opportunity for the respondent to indicate how interests have changed and to indicate whether the activity is one in which a person participates or wishes to participate in the future. Henry[38] has recently developed an adolescent interest checklist and is also developing child and adult versions.

The NIH Activity Record[30] and the Occupational Questionnaire[94] are self-report forms that ask the client to indicate what activity he or she engages in over the course of a weekday and a weekend day. The Occupational Questionnaire asks persons to report, for each half-hour period in which they are awake, what activity they are performing. Then each activity is rated as to (a) whether he or she considers the activity to be work, leisure, a daily living task, or rest; (b) how much he or she enjoys the activity; (c) how important the activity is; and (d) how well he or she does the activity. The latter three questions reveal the personal causation, interest, and value experienced in the activity. The questionnaire also provides data about habits (i.e., the typical use of time).

The Activity Record, developed for use with persons who have physical disabilities, includes the content from the Occupational Questionnaire and asks additional questions pertaining to pain, fatigue, difficulty, and rest during the activity. Consequently, it provides detailed information about how a disability influences performance of everyday activities.

The Self Assessment of Occupational Functioning (SAOF)[6] and the Children's Self Assessment of Occupational Functioning[17] are designed to assist collaborative treatment planning between the occupational therapist and the client. They provide data to the therapist concerning the client's perceptions of strengths and weakness.

Several interviews have been designed for use with the model. The Occupational Case Analysis Interview and Rating Scale[46] is based on a case analysis approach to using the model of human occupation.[16] This assessment was originally designed for short-term psychiatric treatment settings although it has been applied in other settings. The Assessment of Occupational Functioning was originally developed for use in long-term settings;[100] later revision of the scale resulted in a more generic version.[99] The Occupational Performance History Interview (OPHI)[61,62] can be used with a variety of populations. As a historical interview, the OPHI[61] seeks to gather information about a patient's or client's past and present occupational behavior. The Worker Role Interview[98] is designed for use with injured workers in work rehabilitation settings. More recently, the interview has been modified for use with psychiatric populations.[35] The interview allows the client to discuss various aspects of his or her life, work, and job setting that have an impact upon return to work.

One future challenge will be to develop better means of eliciting and analyzing narrative data in interviews. One step in this direction is a study by Mallinson et al.[72] that examined the narrative content of patient responses to the Occupational Performance History Interview. Kielhofner and Mallinson[65] also recently published guidelines for conducting more narratively oriented interviews. The Work Environment Impact Scale[74] is the first instrument designed for assessing the environment. It provides information about how objects, occupational forms, social groups, and spaces in the workplace affect work performance and satisfaction.

Therapists using the model of human occupation also use other structured methods of data collection, such as daily living assessments, standardized developmental assessments, standardized assessments of motor performance, standardized work evaluations, and so on. While such methods were not developed specifically for use with the model of human occupation, they are compatible with it.

Situated Methods. Situated data collection ordinarily involves observation or informal conversations. Situated methods are adapted to the unfolding circumstances in therapy. The therapist periodically obtains data relevant to conceptual questions that are still unanswered or that emerge in the course of intervention. Examples of situated data collection are having a conversation with a patient while beginning an activity, observing a client's performance in the classroom, listening to a patient's comments about the workplace where he was injured, noting the affect of a client during a group session, or listening to a client's occasional stories about what happened since she was last seen.

Reasoning with Data

Therapists collect data in order to create an explanation of the patient's circumstances.[64] This explanation emerges as the therapist integrates data on the client with concepts from the model of human occupation. What results is a particular theory of the circumstances of the individual patient. For example, no one's experience of value is exactly the same. One person may have a value system tightly organized around a set of fundamental religious beliefs. In such a person's value system, certain themes concerning morality, personal obligations, and ideals for conduct may predominate. Another's values will emphasize different issues. In either case, the important thing to discover in data collection is how the particular individual's way of experiencing and expressing value influences his or her occupational life and constitutes a strength or weakness for adapting in the face of disability.

In the same way, the model's theoretical arguments represent possible circumstances that may influence function or dysfunction. For example, one theoretical argument of this model is that volition influences the activity choices of individuals. Volition may be a source of strength, sustaining a level of occupational functioning because of the person's value commitments, satisfaction, and/or sense of being able to achieve desired outcomes. Conversely, volition may be impaired, leading to poor activity choices or preventing persons from making choices. In such cases, loss of important life goals, inability to experience pleasure in action, and a sense of helplessness may all contribute to the problem. The therapist collects data in order to figure out what particular set of conditions represent this patient's occupational dysfunction. By understanding the many factors that contribute to a patient's dysfunction, the therapist can decide upon and implement interventions.

Intervention Methods

The model of human occupation emphasizes that through therapy, persons are helped to engage in occupational behavior that maintains, restores, reorganizes, or develops their capacities, motives, and lifestyles.

Through participation in therapeutic occupations, persons transform themselves into more adaptive and healthy beings.

This model emphasizes that the occupations used in therapy are important and need to be carefully selected. Therapeutic occupations should relate to the life circumstances of the individual and the individual's desires and needs for future occupational behavior. Since this model emphasizes the process of individualizing therapy, case examples are very important. A wide range of case examples can be found in *A Model of Human Occupation: Theory and Application*, and in numerous other publications.

Programs

Because the model provides a comprehensive view of occupational function and dysfunction, it is often used as a framework for program development. Munoz and Kielhofner[75] have outlined a process of program development, describing how a practitioner can define and implement occupational therapy services using the model of human occupation. In addition, a wide range of programs based on the model are described in the literature. These include, for example, programs in child, adolescent, and adult psychiatry;[1,4,5,29,34,41,45,67,78,88,91,102] programs for persons with traumatic brain injury,[19,93] arthritis,[30] chronic pain,[33,83] learning disabilities,[86] dementia,[79,82] AIDS;[85,92] and programs in acute care,[2] home care,[69-71] early intervention,[90] and senior housing.[96]

Research

The model of human occupation has generated a range of research. Most research to date has focused on validating the theoretical arguments about order and disorder. One type of study asks whether relationships postulated by the model are found in specific study samples.[11,18,21,23,32,94] For example, research has asked whether personal causation is associated with adaptation. Other studies have inquired as to whether variables selected from the model discriminate between adaptive and maladaptive populations.[7,8,12,22,68,89,95,101] For example, studies have asked whether personal causation is different in those with and without psychiatric illness. Finally, some studies have examined whether variables from this model will predict future functioning.[3,39,80,87] Such studies have provided support for the theoretical arguments of the model. Nonetheless, much more research is required to test the theoretical arguments. Another, more recent effort, has been qualitative studies that have sought to expand understanding of volition, especially the concept of volitional narrative.[36,37,72]

A number of studies have been undertaken to investigate the properties of assessments being developed for the model. These studies have generally examined the reliability and validity of the assessments.[10,13,14,24,27,31,44,47,61,63,81,84,97,99,100] A few studies have examined the effectiveness of this model in practice.[58] The major task that remains is to examine the impact of therapy based on this model.

Discussion

Because of its broad focus, the model of human occupation is widely used, and many people have contributed to its development. Consequently, a substantial literature on this model exists and much technology for application has been developed. At the same time, this model's broad focus means that a great deal of developmental work is needed to validate and create a technology for applying it.

The technology for application is better in some areas than in others. For example, while the model has more assessments developed specifically for use with it than other models, it requires still more assessments if it is to be applied across the range of circumstances for which it has potential. Research on this model also needs to develop further. The situation for research is similar to that for technology. The model is applied in so many different circumstances that a great deal more research will be needed to test its relevance and usefulness.

The model of human occupation is unique in some of the issues it addresses. For example, it is the only model to directly address the motivation for occupation and the only one that emphasizes roles and habits. It also provides a unique view of the environment. Because of its broad focus the model is recognized as a holistic and comprehensive model for practice.[42]

Since the model was one of the first to develop a strong focus on occupation, many persons see it as a useful integrating framework for therapy and a useful explanation of the unique focus of occupational therapy. At the same time, the model does not directly address specific performance capacity and deficits, and must routinely be used in association with models that have such a focus.

TERMS OF THE MODEL

affords	Refers to the environmental opportunities for performance.
attraction	A proclivity to enjoy certain occupations or certain aspects of performance.
dispositions	Cognitive and emotive orientations toward occupations.
habits	Latent tendencies acquired from previous repetitions, mainly operating at a preconscious level, and influencing a wide range of behavioral patterns that correspond to familiar habitats.
habit map	An internalized appreciative capacity that guides the perception of familiar events and the related construction of action toward accomplishing some implicit outcome or process.
habituation subsystem	An internal organization of information that disposes the system to exhibit recurrent patterns of behavior.
interests	Dispositions to find pleasure and satisfaction in occupations, and the self-knowledge of our enjoyment of occupations; encompasses attraction and preference.
internalized roles	A broad awareness of a particular social identity and related obligations, which together provide a framework for appreciating relevant situations and constructing appropriate behavior.
knowledge of capacity	Awareness of present and potential abilities.
mind-brain-body performance subsystem	The organization of musculoskeletal, neurological, perceptual, and cognitive constituents that together make up the capacity for occupational performance.
objects	Natural and fabricated things with which persons may interact.
occupational forms	Rule-bound, coherent, sequences of action that are oriented to a purpose, sustained in

	collective knowledge, culturally recognizable, and named.
personal causation	A collection of dispositions and self-knowledge concerning one's capacities for and efficacy in occupations; encompasses knowledge of capacity and sense of efficacy.
personal convictions	A common-sense set of beliefs about what matters in life.
preference	The knowledge that one enjoys particular ways of performing or particular activities over others.
presses	Refers to the environment recruiting or requiring particular behavior.
self-knowledge	Commonsense awareness of ourselves as actors in the world.
sense of efficacy	The perception of control over one's own behavior (and underlying thoughts and emotions), as well as a sense of control in achieving desired outcomes of behavior.
sense of obligation	Strong emotional dispositions to follow what are perceived as right ways to behave.
social groups	Collections of persons that occur with regularity.
spaces	Physical contexts in which persons engage in occupational behavior.
values	A coherent set of convictions that assigns significance or standards to occupations and creates a strong disposition to perform accordingly. Values encompass personal convictions and a sense of commitment.
volition	A system of dispositions and self-knowledge that predisposes and enables persons to anticipate, choose, experience, and interpret occupational behavior.

SUMMARY

The Model Of Human Occupation

FOCUS

- Concerned with:
  - Motivation for occupation
  - Patterning of occupational behavior into routines and lifestyles
  - Nature of skilled performance
  - Influence of environment on occupational behavior.
- Intended for use with any person experiencing occupational dysfunction

INTERDISCIPLINARY BASE

- Builds on concepts from ego psychology, sociology, social psychology, anthropology, philosophy, and early occupational therapy literature

THEORETICAL ARGUMENTS

Order

- Humans are dynamic, self-organizing systems, unfolding and changing in time.
- Occupational behavior:
  - Involves cooperation of three subsystems (volition, habituation, and mind-brain-body performance)
  - Emerges from interaction of the human system with the environment
  - Affects subsequent organization of the human system
- Volition:
  - Arises from a need for action
  - Is a system of dispositions and self-knowledge comprising personal causation, values, and interests
  - Predisposes and enables persons to anticipate, choose, experience, and interpret occupational behavior
- Personal causation is:
  - A collection of dispositions and self-knowledge concerning one's capacities for and efficacy in occupations
- The composite of:
  - Knowledge of capacity (awareness of and attitude toward one's present and potential abilities)
  - Sense of efficacy (perception of control and sense of effectiveness in achieving outcomes)
- Values:
  - Are a coherent set of convictions that assign significance or standards to occupations and create a strong disposition to perform accordingly

- ○ Include:
  Personal convictions (ways of viewing life and the goals to be pursued in life)
  Commitments (strong emotional dispositions to follow what is perceived as the right ways to behave)
- Interests
  - ○ Are dispositions to find pleasure and satisfaction in occupations, and the self-knowledge of our enjoyment of occupations
  - ○ Include:
    Attraction (disposition to enjoy certain occupations or certain aspects of performance)
    Preference (knowledge that one enjoys particular ways of performing or particular activities over others)
- The process of choosing (activity choices and occupational choices), experiencing, and interpreting occupational behavior is an ongoing cycle that sustains and transforms volition.
- Habituation:
  - ○ Is an internal organization of information that disposes the system to exhibit recurrent patterns of behavior
  - ○ Allows people to behave efficiently and automatically in their environments
  - ○ Is composed of interwoven habits and internalized roles
  - ○ Habits:
    Are latent appreciative tendencies (i.e., habit maps) acquired from previous repetitions
    Allow one to recognize familiar events and contexts and to construct action
    Operate at a preconscious, automatic level
  - ○ Influence:
    How one performs routine activities
    How time is typically used
    Styles of behavior
  - ○ Internalized roles:
    Include a broad awareness of a social identity and related obligations (i.e., role script)
    Provide a framework for appreciating relevant situations and constructing appropriate behavior
  - ○ Influence:
    Manner and content of interactions with others
    Routine tasks
    Partitioning of daily and weekly cycles
- Occupational performance:
  - ○ Comprises motor, process, and communication/interaction skills

- ○ Involves musculoskeletal, neurological, cardiopulmonary, and symbolic constituents organized into a mind-brain-body performance subsystem
- ○ Emerges from interaction of the mind-brain-body performance subsystem with the environment
- The social environment (occupational forms and social groups) and the physical environment (objects and spaces):
  - ○ Affords (gives opportunities for performance)
  - ○ Presses (recruits or requires particular behavior)

Disorder

- Volition may lead to maladaptive activity and occupational dysfunction when persons:
  - ○ Feel inadequate
  - ○ Hold deviant, internally conflicted values
  - ○ Lack attraction to or pursuit of interest in occupations
- Volition may be restricted/affected by limitations of capacity, as when persons:
  - ○ Face painful knowledge of restricted or lost capacity
  - ○ Have difficulty assessing capacities in the face of progressive diseases or changing environments
  - ○ Fall short of social values
  - ○ Cannot perform in ways that are personally important
  - ○ Have to relinquish valuable or meaningful activities
  - ○ Have limited experiences to develop attraction and feel pleasure in occupations
  - ○ Need to rechannel or discover new interests to replace lost ones
- Roles:
  - ○ May be disrupted as a consequence of psychosocial dysfunction and may cause psychosocial dysfunction
  - ○ May be disrupted or terminated by acquired physical impairments
  - ○ May be unavailable to or restricted for persons with disabilities
- Habits:
  - ○ Can constrain effective occupational performance
  - ○ Can maintain dissatisfying routines
  - ○ May be restricted, altered, or invalidated by disability
- Restrictions in motor, process, and communication/interaction skills:
  - ○ Can limit the effectiveness
  - ○ May involve disturbances to the neurological, musculoskeletal, and symbolic constituents of the mind-brain-body performance subsystem
  - ○ Can emanate from the physical and social environment

Therapeutic Intervention

- Adapting to a disability involves:

- Maintaining a satisfying and productive life through (activity and occupational) choices
- Organizing life to routinely function to one's own and others' satisfaction
- Employing intact skills in ways that compensate for deficits and maximize success in necessary and desired occupational forms
- Environmental accommodations
- Principles derived from the theoretical arguments propose broad themes about how change may take place in highly complex human systems; the therapist's knowledge of each patient is necessary to know how to apply the principles.

TECHNOLOGY FOR APPLICATION

- Application involves using the theory as a guide to gather and interpret data and formulate intervention
- Therapists collect data to:
  - Answer questions generated from theoretical perspective of the model
  - Create an explanation of the patient's circumstances
- Therapists gather data through:
  - Structured methods that employ specified protocols (i.e., observation methods, self-report questionnaires or checklists, and interviews)
  - Situated methods devised by the therapist for a specific situation
- Engaging in occupational behavior:
  - Maintains, restores, reorganizes, or develops capacities, motives, and lifestyles
  - Transforms people into more adaptive and healthy beings
- Occupations used in therapy are important and need to be carefully selected to relate to:
  - The life circumstances of the individual
  - The individual's desires
  - Needs for future occupational behavior
- The model is often used as a framework for program development.

RESEARCH

- Types of studies:
  - Quantitative studies that ask whether relationships postulated by the model are found in study samples
  - Qualitative studies that have sought to expand understanding of volition
  - Investigations of the properties of assessments being developed for the model
  - Investigations of the effectiveness in practice

References

1. Adelstein, LA, Barnes, MA, Murray-Jensen, F, and Skaggs, CB: A broadening frontier: Occupational therapy in mental health programs for children and adolescents. Mental Health Special Interest Section Newsletter 12:2–4, 1989.
2. Affleck, A, Bianchi, E, Cleckley, M, Donaldson, K, McCormack, G, and Polon, J: Stress management as a component of occupational therapy in acute care settings. Occupational Therapy in Health Care 1:17–41, 1984.
3. Azhar, FT: The relevance of worker identity to return to work in clients treated for work related injuries. MS Thesis, Department of Occupational Therapy, University of Illinois at Chicago, 1996.
4. Baron, K: The model of human occupation: A newspaper treatment group for adolescents with a diagnosis of conduct disorder. Occupational Therapy in Mental Health 7:89–104, 1987.
5. Baron, K: Occupational therapy: A program for child psychiatry. Mental Health Special Interest Section Newsletter 12:6–7, 1989.
6. Baron, K, and Curtin, C: A manual for use with the self assessment of occupational functioning. Unpublished manuscript, Department of Occupational Therapy, University of Illinois at Chicago, 1990.
7. Barris, R, Dickie, V, and Baron, K: A comparison of psychiatric patients and normal subjects based on the model of human occupation. Occupational Therapy Journal of Research 8:3–37, 1988.
8. Barris, R, Kielhofner, G, Burch, RM, Gelinas, I, Klement, M, and Schultz, B: Occupational function and dysfunction in three groups of adolescents. Occupational Therapy Journal of Research 6:301–317, 1986.
9. Barris, R, Oakley, F, and Kielhofner, G: The role checklist. In Hemphill, B (ed), Mental Health Assessment in Occupational Therapy: An Integrated Approach to the Evaluative Process. Slack, Thorofare, NJ, 1988, pp 73–91.
10. Biernacki, SD: Reliability of the Worker Role Interview. Am J Occup Ther 47:797–803, 1993.
11. Bränholm, I, and Fugl-Meyer, AR: Occupational role preferences and life satisfaction. Occupational Therapy Journal of Research 12:159–171, 1992.
12. Bridle, MJ, Lynch, KB, and Quesenberry, CM: Long term function following the central cord syndrome. Paraplegia 28:178–185, 1990.
13. Brollier, C, Watts, JH, Bauer, D, and Schmidt, W: A content validity study of the Assessment of Occupational Functioning. Occupational Therapy in Mental Health 8:29–47, 1989.
14. Brollier, C, Watts, JH, Bauer, D, and Schmidt, W: A concurrent validity study of two occupational therapy evaluation instruments: The AOF and OCAIRS. Occupational Therapy in Mental Health 8:49–59, 1989.
15. Chern, JS, Kielhofner, G, de las Heras, CG, and Magalhaes, LC: The Volitional Questionnaire: Psychometric development and practical use. Am J Occup Ther (in press).
16. Cubie, S, and Kaplan, K: A case analysis method for the model of human occupation. Am J Occup Ther 36:645–656, 1982.
17. Curtin, C, and Baron, K: A manual for use with the children's self assessment of occupational functioning. Unpublished manuscript, Department of Occupational Therapy, University of Illinois at Chicago, 1990.
18. DeForest, D, Watts, JH, and Madigan, MJ: Resonation in the model of human occupation: A pilot study. Occupational Therapy in Mental Health 11:57–75, 1991.
19. Depoy, E: The TBIIM: An intervention for the treatment of individuals with traumatic brain injury. Occupational Therapy in Health Care 7:55–67, 1990.
20. Dickerson, AE, and Oakley, F: The role checklist. In Hemphill, B (ed), Mental Health Assessment in Occupational Therapy: An Integrated Approach to the Evaluative Process, Slack, Thorofare, NJ (in press).
21. Duellman, MK, Barris, R, and Kielhofner, G: Organized activity and the adaptive status of nursing home residents. Am J Occup Ther 40:618–622, 1986.
22. Ebb, EW, Coster, W, and Duncombe, L: Comparison of normal and psychosocially dysfunctional male adolescents. Occupational Therapy in Mental Health 9:53–74, 1989.

23. Elliott, M, and Barris, R: Occupational role performance and life satisfaction in elderly persons. Occupational Therapy Journal of Research 7:215–224, 1987.
24. Evans, J, and Salim, AA: A cross-cultural test of the validity of occupational therapy assessments with patients with schizophrenia. Am J Occup Ther 46:685–695, 1992.
25. Fisher, AG: The assessment of motor process skills (version 8.0). Unpublished test manual, Colorado State University, Occupational Therapy Department, Fort Collins, 1994.
26. Fisher, A, and Kielhofner, G: Mind-brain-body performance subsystem. In Kielhofner, G (ed): A Model of Human Occupation: Theory and Application, ed 2. Williams & Wilkins, Baltimore, 1995.
27. Fisher, A, Liu, Y, Velozo C, and Pan, A: Cross cultural assessment of process skills, Am J Occup Ther 46:876–884, 1992.
28. Forsyth, K, Salamy, M, Simon, S, and Kielhofner, G: A user's guide to the Assessment of Communication and Interaction Skills (ACIS), (Version 4.0). Unpublished manuscript, Department of Occupational Therapy, University of Illinois at Chicago, 1995.
29. Froehlich, J: Occupational therapy interventions with survivors of sexual abuse. Occupational Therapy in Health Care 8:1–25, 1992.
30. Furst, G, Gerber, L, Smith, C, Fisher, S, and Shulman, B: A program for improving energy conservation behaviors in adults with rheumatoid arthritis. Am J Occup Ther 41:102–111, 1987.
31. Gerber, L, and Furst, G: Validation of the NIH Activity Record: A quantitative measure of life activities. Arthritis Care and Research 5:81–86, 1992.
32. Gregory, M: Occupational behavior and life satisfaction among retirees. Am J Occup Ther 37:548–553, 1983.
33. Gusich, R: Occupational therapy for chronic pain: A clinical application of the model of human occupation. Occupational Therapy in Mental Health 4:59–73, 1984.
34. Gusich, RL, and Silverman, AL: Basava day clinic: The model of human occupation as applied to psychiatric day hospitalization. Occupational Therapy in Mental Health 11:113–134, 1991.
35. Handelsman, D: The construct validity of the Worker Role Interview for the chronic mentally ill. MS Thesis, Department of Occupational Therapy, University of Illinois at Chicago, 1994.
36. Helfrich, C, and Kielhofner, G: Volitional narratives and the meaning of occupational therapy. Am J Occup Ther 48:319–332, 1994.
37. Helfrich, C, Kielhofner, G, and Mattingly, C: Volition as narrative: An understanding of motivation in chronic illness. Am J Occup Ther 42:311–317, 1994.
38. Henry, AD: Adolescent Leisure Interest Profile. Center for Psychosocial and Forensic Services, Research, University of Massachusetts Medical Center, Worcester, MA, 1995.
39. Henry, AD, Tohen, M, Coster, WJ, and Tickle-Degnen, L: Predicting psychosocial functioning and symptomatic recovery of young adolescents and young adults following a first psychotic episode (unpublished paper). Boston Universtiy, Boston, MA, 1996.
40. De las Heras, C: A User's Guide to the Volitional Questionnaire, ed 2. The Model of Human Occupation Clearinghouse, Department of Occupational Therapy, University of Illinois at Chicago, 1993.
41. Hocking C: Anger management. Journal of the New Zealand Association of Occupational Therapists 40:12–17, 1989.
42. Hubbard, S: Towards a truly holistic approach to occupational therapy. British Journal of Occupational Therapy 54:415–418, 1991.
43. Jonsson, H, Kielhofner, G, and Borell, L: Anticipating retirement: The formation of attitudes and expectations concerning an occupational transition. American Journal of Occupation (in press).
44. Kaplan, K: Short-term assessment: The need and a response. Occupational Therapy in Mental Health 4:29–45, 1984.
45. Kaplan, K: The directive group: Short term treatment for psychiatric patients with a minimal level of functioning. Am J Occup Ther 40:474–481, 1986.
46. Kaplan, K, and Kielhofner, G: Occupational Case Analysis Interview and Rating Scale. Slack, Thorofare, NJ, 1989.
47. Katz, N, Giladi, N, and Peretz, C: Cross-cultural application of occupational therapy assessments: Human occupation with psychiatric inpatients and controls in Israel. Occupational Therapy in Mental Health 8:7–30, 1988.

48. Kielhofner, G: A model of human occupation, Part 2. Ontogenesis from the perspective of temporal adaptation. Am J Occup Ther 34:657–663, 1980.
49. Kielhofner, G: A model of human occupation, Part 3. Benign and vicious cycles. Am J Occup Ther 34:731–737, 1980.
50. Kielhofner, G: A Model of Human Occupation: Theory and Application. Williams & Wilkins, Baltimore, 1985.
51. Kielhofner, G: A Model of Human Occupation: Theory and Application, ed 2. Williams & Wilkins, Baltimore, 1995.
52. Kielhofner, G: Change making: Principles of therapeutic intervention: In Kielhofner, G (ed): A Model of Human Occupation: Theory and Application, ed 2. Williams & Wilkins, Baltimore, 1995.
53. Kielhofner, G: Environmental influences on occupational behavior. In Kielhofner, G (ed): A Model of Human Occupation: Theory and Application, ed 2. Williams & Wilkins, Baltimore, 1995.
54. Kielhofner, G: Habituation subsystem. In Kielhofner, G (ed): A Model of Human Occupation: Theory and Application, ed 2. Williams & Wilkins, Baltimore, 1995.
55. Kielhofner, G: Human system. In Kielhofner, G (ed): A Model of Human Occupation: Theory and Application, ed 2. Williams & Wilkins, Baltimore, 1995.
56. Kielhofner, G: Occupational dysfunction. In Kielhofner, G (ed): A Model of Human Occupation: Theory and Application, ed 2. Williams & Wilkins, Baltimore, 1995.
57. Kielhofner, G, Borell, L, Burke, J, Helfrich, C, and Nygard, L: Volition subsystem. In Kielhofner, G (ed): A Model of Human Occupation: Theory and Application, ed 2. Williams & Wilkins, Baltimore, 1995.
58. Kielhofner, G, and Brinson, M: Development and evaluation of an aftercare program for young and chronic psychiatrically disabled adults. Occupational Therapy in Mental Health 9:1–25, 1989.
59. Kielhofner, G, and Burke, J: A model of human occupation, Part 1. Conceptual framework and content. Am J Occup Ther 34:572–581, 1980.
60. Kielhofner, G, Burke, J, and Heard-Igi, C: A model of human occupation, Part 4. Assessment and intervention. Am J Occup Ther 34:777–788, 1980.
61. Kielhofner, G, and Henry, AD: Development and investigation of the Occupational Performance History Interview. Am J Occup Ther 42:489–498, 1988.
62. Kielhofner, G, Henry, A, and Walens, D: A user's guide to the Occupational Performance History Interview. American Occupational Therapy Association, Rockville, MD, 1989.
63. Kielhofner, G, Henry, A, Walens, D, and Rogers FS: Generalizability study of the Occupational Performance History Interview. Occupational Therapy Journal of Research 11:292–306, 1991.
64. Kielhofner, G, and Mallinson, T: Gathering and reasoning with data during intervention. In Kielhofner, G (ed): A Model of Human Occupation: Theory and Application, ed 2. Williams & Wilkins, Baltimore, 1995.
65. Kielhofner, G, and Mallinson, T: Gathering narrative data through interviews: Empirical observations and suggested guidelines. Scandinavian Journal of Occupational Therapy 2:63–68, 1995.
66. Kielhofner, G, Mallinson, T, and de las Heras, CG: Methods of data gathering. In Kielhofner, G (ed): A Model of Human Occupation: Theory and Application, ed 2. Williams & Wilkins, Baltimore, 1995.
67. Lancaster, J, and Mitchell, M: Occupational therapy treatment goals, objectives, and activities for improving low self-esteem in adolescents with behavioral disorders. Occupational Therapy in Mental Health 11:3–22, 1991.
68. Lederer, J, Kielhofner, G, and Watts, J: Values, personal causation and skills of delinquents and nondelinquents. Occupational Therapy in Mental Health 5:59–77, 1985.
69. Levine, R: The cultural aspects of home care delivery. Am J Occup Ther 38:734–738, 1984.
70. Levine, RE, and Gitlin, LN: Home adaptations for persons with chronic disabilities: An educational model. Am J Occup Ther 44:923–929, 1990.
71. Levine, RE, and Gitlin, LN: A model to promote activity competence in elders. Am J Occup Ther 47:147–153, 1993.
72. Mallinson, T, Kielhofner, G, and Mattingly, C: Like being stuck in flypaper: Metaphor and meaning in a clinical interview. Am J Occup Ther 50:338–346, 1996.

73. Matsutsuyu, J: The interest checklist. Am J Occup Ther 23:323–328, 1969.
74. Moore-Corner, R, and Kielhofner, G: The Work Environment Impact Scale. Unpublished manuscript, Department of Occupational Therapy, University of Illinois at Chicago, 1996.
75. Munoz, JP, and Kielhofner, G: Program development. In Kielhofner, G (ed): A Model of Human Occupation: Theory and Application, ed 2. Williams & Wilkins, Baltimore, 1995.
76. Nelson, D: Occupation: Form and performance. Am J Occup Ther 42:633–641, 1988.
77. Neville-Jan, A: The relationship of volition to adaptive occupational behavior among individuals with varying degrees of depression. Occupational Therapy in Mental Health 12:1–18, 1994.
78. Neville-Jan, A, Bradley, M, Bunn, C, and Gehri, B: The model of human occupation and individuals with co-dependency problems. Occupational Therapy in Mental Health 11:73–97, 1991.
79. Oakley, F: Clinical application of the model of human occupation in dementia of the Alzheimer's type. Occupational Therapy in Mental Health 7:37–50, 1987.
80. Oakley, F, Kielhofner, G, and Barris, R: An occupational therapy approach to assessing psychiatric patients' adaptive functioning. Am J Occup Ther 39:147–154, 1985.
81. Oakley, F, Kielhofner, G, Barris, R, and Reichler, RK: The Role Checklist: Development and empirical assessment of reliability. Occupational Therapy Journal of Research 6:157–170, 1986.
82. Olin, D: Assessing and assisting the person with dementia: An occupational behavior perspective. Physical and Occupational Therapy in Geriatrics 3:25–32, 1985.
83. Padilla, R, and Bianchi, EM: Occupational therapy for chronic pain: Applying the model of human occupation to clinical practice. Occupational Therapy Practice 1:47–52, 1990.
84. Pan, AW, and Fisher, A: The assessment of motor and process skills of persons with psychiatric disorders. Am J Occup Ther 48:775–780, 1994.
85. Pizzi, MA: The model of human occupation and adults with HIV infection and AIDS. Am J Occup Ther 44:257–264, 1990.
86. Platts, L: Social role valorisation and the model of human occupation: A comparative analysis for work with people with learning disability in the community. British Journal of Occupational Therapy 56:278–282, 1993.
87. Rust, K, Barris, R, and Hooper, F: Use of the model of human occupation to predict women's exercise behavior. Occupational Therapy Journal of Research 7:23–35, 1987.
88. Salz, C: A theoretical approach to the treatment of work difficulties in borderline personalities. Occupational Therapy in Mental Health 3:33–46, 1983.
89. Scaffa, M: Alcoholism: An occupational behavior perspective. Occupational Therapy in Mental Health 11:99–111, 1991.
90. Schaaf, RC, and Mulrooney, LL: Occupational therapy in early intervention: A family centered approach. Am J Occup Ther 43:745–754, 1989.
91. Scarth, PP: Services for chemically dependent adolescents. Mental Health Special Interest Section Newsletter 13:7–8, 1990.
92. Schindler, VJ: Psychosocial occupational therapy intervention with AIDS patients. Am J Occup Ther 42:507–512, 1988.
93. Series, C: The long-term needs of people with head injury: A role for the community occupational therapist? British Journal of Occupational Therapy 55:94–98, 1992.
94. Smith, N, Kielhofner, G, and Watts, J: The relationship between volition, activity pattern and life satisfaction in the elderly. Am J Occup Ther 40:278–283, 1986.
95. Smyntek, L, Barris, R, and Kielhofner, G: The model of human occupation applied to psychosocially functional and dysfunctional adolescents. Occupational Therapy in Mental Health 5:21–40, 1985.
96. Tatham, M: Leisure facilitator: The role of the occupational therapist in senior housing. Journal of Housing for the Elderly 10:125–138, 1992.
97. Viik, MK, Watts, JH, Madigan, MJ, and Bauer, D: Preliminary validation of the Assessment of Occupational Functioning with an alcoholic population. Occupational Therapy in Mental Health 10:19–33, 1990.
98. Velozo, C, Kielhofner, G, and Fisher, A: A user's guide to the worker role interview (research version). Department of Occupational Therapy, University of Illinois at Chicago, 1990.

99. Watts, JH, Brollier, C, Bauer, D, and Schmidt, W: A comparison of two evaluation instruments used with psychiatric patients in occupational therapy. Occupational Therapy in Mental Health 8:7–27, 1989.
100. Watts, JH, Kielhofner, G, Bauer, D, Gregory, M, and Valentine, D: The Assessment of Occupational Functioning: A screening tool for use in long-term care. Am J Occup Ther 40:231–240, 1986.
101. Weeder, T: Comparison of temporal patterns and meaningfulness of the daily activities of schizophrenic and normal adults. Occupational Therapy in Mental Health 6:27–45, 1986.
102. Weissenberg, R, and Giladi, W: Home economics day: A program for disturbed adolescents to promote acquisition of habits and skills. Occupational Therapy in Mental Health 9:89–103, 1989.

CHAPTER 11

THE MOTOR CONTROL MODEL

Four treatment approaches of similar origin, and with similar concepts and techniques, have traditionally been used in occupational therapy for persons with brain damage that results in difficulty controlling movement. These are:

1. The Rood approach
2. Bobath's neurodevelopmental therapy
3. Brunnstrom's movement therapy
4. Proprioceptive neuromuscular facilitation

These approaches are often thought of as interrelated concepts and techniques since they are "more similar than divergent."[14] They are referred to collectively as neurodevelopmental approaches because they are based on a view of the nervous system and emphasize its developmental nature. All four neurodevelopmental approaches share the goal of improving *motor control*—that is, the ability to use one's body effectively while performing an occupation. Motor control includes such diverse components as generating and coordinating movement patterns of the head, limbs, and trunk, and maintaining balance during occupational performance.

As a group these approaches have sought to explain motor dysfunction and to specify strategies of intervention aimed at improving motor control. These approaches are directed to motor dysfunction that occurs as a result of damage to the central nervous system (CNS). In CNS damage, neural communication to muscles is often preserved, but it becomes disordered because of the insult to central processing components of the brain.

These approaches are often taught and used together not only because they have similar goals and concepts, but also because they draw upon much the same interdisciplinary knowledge. More recently, interdisciplinary conceptualizations of how humans achieve motor control have changed dramatically.[5] As a consequence, occupational therapists have begun to articulate a new conceptualization of motor control that modifies and replaces many of the ideas of these four neurodevelopmental approaches. Importantly, this new approach also challenges some of the most basic assumptions of the previous approaches and replaces them with a new view of how persons control movement in the context of occupations.

While offering a distinctly different conceptualization of how humans control movement, the contemporary motor control model has nevertheless evolved from the traditional neurodevelopmental approaches. Hence, it is important to consider the concepts and techniques of these neurodevelopmental approaches and how they are being replaced or reconceptualized in occupational therapy's contemporary motor control model.

Interdisciplinary Base

The neurodevelopmental approaches as well as the contemporary motor control model are based on interdisciplinary concepts about how normal motor control is developed and learned. These concepts come from neurophysiology, neuropsychology, human development, psychology, and human movement science.[14] The neurodevelopmental approaches are based on older knowledge, whereas the motor control concepts represent contemporary concepts of motor control and motor development.

Traditional Interdisciplinary Concepts

Although the interdisciplinary base is complex, a few fundamental concepts are common to the neurodevelopmental approaches. Normal movement is presumed to emanate from "genetically wired configurations of neurons."[14] These biologically determined movement patterns, which occur in response to sensory stimuli, are referred to as *reflexes*. Different reflex patterns emerge as the nervous system matures in the course of normal development. Movement patterns associated with the spinal cord and lower brain centers appear first, followed by those associated with higher brain centers.

The emphasis on reflexes originates from the earliest interdisciplinary ideas about motor control dating back to the beginning of this century. This approach suggested that movement was achieved through collective action of multiple reflexes.[7,9]

Later research showed the reflex model to be insufficient to explain motor control. This led to the conceptualization of *hierarchical control*, which argued that movements are controlled from the top down. According to this argument, higher centers in the nervous system exert control over lower-level parts of the nervous system that organize reflexes.[7,9] The higher centers acquire and store motor programs that act as "instructions" for movement. So, for example, the theory holds that the pattern of movement required for reaching to grasp an object is stored in a CNS "generalized motor program" acquired from previous experiences of reaching and grasping. The program, an abstract representation of the sequence, duration, speed, and direction of movements, is required to effect the desired movements and necessary postural adjustments for reaching.

According to this hierarchical explanation, reflex patterns are integrated into voluntary movement and, therefore, come under higher level control. Both the emergence of reflexes and their eventual integration into hierarchically controlled patterns of voluntary movement are considered to be the result of ongoing development and reorganization in the CNS. Since the nervous system is considered the highest executive system involved in motor control, all abilities for and problems of motor control emanate from that system. Thus, the integrity of the CNS and its organization are considered the foundations for motor control.

Another important set of concepts taken from the earlier interdisciplinary literature was related to development.[7] Early neurodevelopmental concepts stress that there is an invariant sequence of development. Motor control develops from head to foot (*cephalocaudal*) and from the middle of the body to the distant limbs (*proximodistal*). This sequence of development is believed to be driven by maturation of the CNS and represents the gradual development of control of higher centers over lower centers. In this conceptualization, the environment does not have a direct role in influencing motor control. Rather, the organization of the CNS determines movement patterns, and changes in the CNS produce changes in motor performance.

A final concept common to all four approaches is *plasticity* of the nervous system. The neurodevelopmental approaches all assume that the CNS is a flexible system with potential for both organization and reorganization as the result of experience. Drawing upon the concept of neuroplasticity, the neurodevelopmental approaches argue that, since the experience of controlling movement is necessary to brain organization, such experience can be utilized in therapy to achieve organization or reorganization of the brain.

Contemporary Interdisciplinary Concepts

Newer interdisciplinary concepts have criticized and sought to replace the reflex-hierarchical concepts upon which the neurodevelopmental approaches are based.[5,7,9] The most important criticism directed at the idea of hierarchical control of movement is the observation that an almost infinite number of motor programs would be required to specify the necessary detail for even a simple task to be performed in variable contexts. As discussed in Chapter 4, this is known as the degrees of freedom problem. Briefly stated, the argument goes as follows: The various muscles and joints involved in motion can be used and combined in a very large number of ways (these possibilities are referred to as degrees of freedom). If each of these degrees of freedom were controlled directly by a central mechanism, the instructions it would have to store and give would be so complex as to be virtually impossible. Hence, hierarchical conceptualization of motor control has come to be considered implausible.

In its place, a new conceptualization based on dynamical systems concepts has been proposed.[5,7,9] This conceptualization focuses on the interaction of the human system with the environment. Moreover, the components of central nervous and musculoskeletal systems are considered to work together heterarchically—that is, cooperating together toward the production of movement, but without central executive control. Finally, the context and the task the person is performing are understood to have a major role in the organization of motor control (*heterarchical control*).

Within the dynamical system's framework, the degrees of freedom problem is addressed through the concept of *coordinative structures*, which are groups of muscles acting over many joints but constrained to behave together as a single functional unit to achieve a purposeful action. An example is natural tenodesis. Long flexor and extensor muscles acting over the wrist and finger joints coordinate together to produce wrist extension and finger flexion as a single functional pattern for grasping. Such coordinative structures compress the available degrees of freedom (e.g., all the possible planes of movement of the wrist and finger joints) into a single pattern, eliminating the need for detailed central instructions for all the muscles involved. The dynamics for this process are provided locally as an emergent feature of the joints and muscles in action. Hence, coordinative structures do not require hierarchical control of all the details of movement.

Of the many patterns that are possible for accomplishing that particular task, persons use certain preferred movement patterns when they perform routine tasks. These preferred patters of doing a task, such as reaching for an object, are conceptualized as *attractor states*. (The concept of attractor states was discussed in detail in Chapter 4.) These attractor states do not require centralized instructions (i.e., motor programs) that have precoded all the necessary movement patterns. Rather, the patterns of movement come together as a synergy during actual performance; that is, the movement pattern emerges from the dynamic interaction of the person with the environment and task.

The dynamical systems perspective argues, then, that motor control is distributed among many systems. The systems involved include parts of the CNS working together, the various components of the musculoskeletal system, the goal of the task, and relevant conditions in the environment (e.g., the size, shape, weight, and location of an object to be grasped and lifted). Dynamical systems theory views motor control as an emergent phenomenon, arising out of the dynamics of all these components as they interact. Hence, the systems explanation does not view the CNS as the central executor of movement and eliminates the need for precoded instructions that specify all the details of movement ahead of time. Rather than depending on a motor program that contains all the necessary information for movement, the control of movement depends on the dynamic conditions of interacting systems. Moreover, the dynamical systems view emphasizes that the parts of the CNS cooperate together to achieve performance, rather than being hierarchically organized with higher centers controlling lower centers. Consequently, dynamical systems theory envisions all parts of the human system coming together in a functionally related and context-dependent way, rather than in a fixed and centrally instructed way.[5,7,9]

The systems view also emphasizes that development is influenced not only by changes in the CNS, but also by changes in all the elements involved in motor control (e.g., environment, task, CNS, and musculoskeletal system). Rather than being a fixed sequence of motor changes, development is a variable process of learning to find individual optimal solutions to *motor problems* (i.e., motor challenges such as learning to reach out and grasp an object).[7,9]

From this discussion, it should be clear that there has been dramatic change in the interdisciplinary concepts upon which occupational therapy approaches to motor control have been founded. Hence, it is not surprising that the conceptual practice model of motor control is also in a process of dramatic flux. It appears most accurate to say, then, that a motor control model is currently being formulated in occupational therapy. I will first present an overview of occupational therapy's four neurodevelopmental approaches that are based in the earlier reflex-hierarchical concepts before going on to contrast these approaches with the contemporary approach based on dynamical systems.

Theoretical Arguments and Technology for Application of the Neurodevelopmental Approaches

This section highlights the main theoretical arguments and presents the technology for application of the four neurodevelopment treatment approaches. While these approaches are founded on much the same interdisciplinary base and overlap substantially, they are first treated separately since they have different emphases and somewhat different arguments about both disorder and recovery of function.

The Rood Approach

This approach is named for its originator, Margaret Rood, an occupational therapist and physical therapist. She originally developed this approach for the treatment of persons with cerebral palsy, but it has since been applied to a wide variety of motor control problems.

Order. According to Rood, normal motor control emerges from the use of reflex patterns present at birth. As these patterns are used and generate sensory stimuli in purposeful activities, they support voluntary control at a conscious (cortical) level. However, the patterns themselves are believed to be under unconscious (subcortical) control. Basic movement patterns do not require conscious attention, which instead can be directed to the goal or purpose of the task. This subconscious organization of motor control makes for efficiency in motor tasks. An additional observation of this approach is that different muscles have different responsibilities in the body—that is, they perform different kinds of work. Accordingly, Rood classified muscles into light work muscles (muscles whose function was primarily movement) and heavy work muscles (those whose function was primarily stabilization). These two types of muscles are under different types of nervous system control (i.e., control of heavy work muscles tends to be more reflexive and that of light work muscles more voluntary), and they respond differently to sensory stimulation.

Disorder. Rood[13] observed that, following CNS damage, the normal sequence of reflex development and learned voluntary motor control did not occur. Moreover, abnormal muscle tone was often present. *Muscle tone* refers to the state of stiffness or tension in muscle. Muscle tension is necessary to maintain postural states. A muscle that is sufficiently stiff is ready to be called on to contract appropriately when required. Muscle tone is maintained by the CNS in response to ongoing sensory information. When the CNS is impaired, muscles may not be adequately tense (hypotonic) or may be too tense (hypertonic).

Therapeutic Intervention. Underlying this approach is the hypothesis that appropriate sensory stimulation could elicit specific motor responses.[10] The therapeutic approach includes four goals:

1. To normalize muscle tone by using sensory stimuli to evoke an appropriate muscle response
2. To progress through the normal sequence of motor development, beginning with the person's current developmental level
3. To focus attention on the goal or purpose of an activity (because all movement is essentially purposeful)
4. To provide opportunities for repetition to reinforce learning

Much of Rood's technique centered on providing appropriate sensory inputs to evoke muscle response.[13] Sensory stimuli (e.g., applying ice, brushing, and stroking the area over muscles) and proprioceptive stimuli (e.g., manual joint compression, quick stretching, tapping, and pressure applied by the therapist, as well as resistance to movement) are used to facilitate muscles. Sensory stimuli such as slow rhythmic movement, neutral warmth, and maintained stretching are used by the therapist to inhibit muscles. Olfactory, gustatory, auditory, and visual stimuli are also used to facilitate or inhibit responses. These latter sensory stimuli are used when voluntary control is minimal and abnormal tone and reflexes are present.

Treatment progresses sequentially, from evoking muscle response with sensory stimuli, to using obtained responses in developmentally appropriate patterns of movement, to purposeful use of the movements in activities. Rood identified a normal developmental sequence of motor behavior to be followed in treatment. Ideally, the various techniques of sensory stimulation are used in occupational therapy to assist the patient to move voluntarily and to prepare the patient for active participation in purposeful activities.[10]

Technology for Application. Within the Rood approach, therapists identify the highest developmental motor pattern that the person can do with ease; treatment begins with the next level at which the person must struggle. Sensory stimulation and manual assistance may be used to help the person perform the movement until the person is able to achieve satisfactory voluntary control of the movement.

Within the field of occupational therapy, Rood's work initiated interest concerning the role of sensory stimulation in recovery of motor control. However, information from neuroscience suggests that how sensory stimulation affects motor responses is more complex than the Rood approach suggests.[2] For example, there is evidence that the physical response to sensory stimulation is mediated or modulated by psychological factors, such as the individual's emotional state and the perceived significance of sensory stimulation (e.g., touch). Hence, the relationship between sensory stimulation and motor response is not a simple linear one, as assumed in the traditional therapeutic use of sensory stimulation.

Bobath's Neurodevelopmental Treatment (NDT)

The Bobaths, a neurologist and physiotherapist team, originally developed the neurodevelopmental treatment approach for persons with cerebral palsy.[1] This approach is also believed to be effective for any person with abnormal movement due to a CNS deficit. For example, this approach is frequently included in the treatment of adult hemiplegia.[14]

Order. Neurodevelopmental treatment is based on the following premises:

1. Motor control involves learning the sensations of movement (not the movement per se).
2. Basic postural movements are learned first, later elaborated on, and integrated into, functional skills.
3. Every activity has postural control as its underlying foundation.

Disorder. Motor dysfunction following brain damage involves abnormal muscle tone (e.g., spasticity) and abnormal patterns of posture and movement that interfere with everyday functional activity. Moreover, when posture and movement are abnormal, the individual's sensation reflects these abnormal patterns and provides incorrect information to the CNS. Therefore, the person is unable to experience and learn or relearn normal movement.

Therapeutic Intervention. Treatment requires that abnormal patterns be inhibited and replaced with the normal movement patterns that will provide appropriate sensory information for motor learning. Abnormal patterns are inhibited and normal ones are elicited by providing appropriate sensory stimuli. When persons are enabled to perform correct patterns of movement, the sensory information about movement that they generate for themselves enables the learning of motor control. Thus, the basis of this approach is for the patient to learn how appropriate movement feels.

Technology for Application. Evaluation consists of determining the highest developmental level at which the person can consistently perform. Evaluation also aims to describe the distribution of muscle tone when the body is in various developmental positions and how tone changes in response to external stimulation or voluntary effort. The evaluation will identify, for example, whether a person is arrested at a particular developmental level of motor control or whether motor abilities are scattered across developmental levels with gaps in between. Thus, the evaluation provides an individualized picture of the person's development of motor control.

Treatment follows the developmental progression and emphasizes the correct *handling* of the person to inhibit abnormal distribution of tone or postures while stimulating and encouraging active motor performance at the next developmental level. Handling is based on the principle that there are key points of control for movement (usually, but not always, proximal areas, such as the shoulder girdle). The therapist handles these points to inhibit abnormal movement and facilitate normal movement.[14] Handling can take place in association with voluntary efforts of the patient and serves to facilitate more normal movement.

Other sensory stimulation, such as physically tapping muscles, may also be used. Once normal responses are elicited, they are repeated, and the person is given the opportunity to practice the movement in purposeful tasks. The thrust of therapy is to encourage voluntary control over normal responses.

The underlying belief of the NDT approach is that once a person is able to control a particular developmental motor pattern voluntarily, he or she will be able to integrate it into skilled activities. The goal of treatment is to prepare the person for functional performance. However, direct involvement in tasks that significantly challenge capacities is considered contraindicated since it may reinforce maladaptive muscle tone and motor patterns.

The NDT approach has been used in occupational therapy to support and facilitate normal movement in the context of purposeful activities.[14] Therapeutic activities can be adapted for patients with hemiplegia to follow the principles of this approach. Additionally, principles are incorporated into training adults with hemiplegia to perform daily living activities (e.g., teaching a person to inhibit abnormal muscle tone in his or her own body when the abnormal tone would otherwise interfere with dressing).[14]

Brunnstrom's Movement Therapy

Signe Brunnstrom, a physiotherapist, developed movement therapy as an approach to the treatment of motor control problems in persons with hemiplegia following cerebrovascular accident.[2]

Order. The view of order is based on the observation that normal development involves progression of reflex development. Reflexes are modified, and their components are rearranged into purposeful movement. This is accomplished as higher centers in the brain take over.

Disorder. Brunnstrom observed that persons who experienced cerebrovascular accidents regressed to lower levels of motor function (i.e., reflex behavior).[2] She identified and categorized stereotypical limb movement patterns that occur sequentially in recovery from hemiplegia. She referred to these patterns as limb synergies.* These synergies are patterned flexion or extension movements of the entire limb that are evoked by attempts to voluntarily move the limb, by efforts to move the unaffected limb, and/or by other sensory stimuli. Brunnstrom reasoned that since each of these reflex patterns was normal at some stage in the course of development, they could

---

*It should be noted that Brunnstrom's concept of synergies is quite different from the idea of synergies in the dynamical systems perspective. Brunnstrom saw synergies as resulting from the dominance of reflex patterns when higher cortical control was impaired. For example, she noted that persons with hemiplegia tended to flex the elbow when they flexed their shoulder in an attempt to reach. This flexion pattern was assumed to be present because of the dominance of reflexes. Dynamical systems offers a different explanation for this same phenomena that relies on the dynamics of the total situation. Because the shoulder flexors are weakened secondary to CNS damage it is easier to do shoulder flexion when the lever (i.e., the arm) being flexed is shorter. When the arm is flexed at the elbow it takes less force to flex the shoulder. Hence, elbow and shoulder flexion are coupled when shoulder flexors are weakened as a dynamic property of the musculoskeletal system attempting flexion of the shoulder against gravity.

be considered normal when they appeared in persons with hemiplegia resulting from brain damage. The occurrence of these patterns was simply evidence that the function of the damaged CNS had reverted to an earlier developmental stage.

Therapeutic Intervention. Brunnstrom's therapeutic approach begins with eliciting reflex synergies and using them as the basis for learning progressively more mature voluntary movement, much as it is learned in normal development. This approach stresses using the motor patterns that are available to the patient in order to progress through the recovery stages.[12]

Technology for Application. In this approach, evaluation involves determining the person's sensory status (since the ability to sense and recognize patterns of movement is important to treatment), which reflexes are present, and the current level of recovery. Brunnstrom[2] identified six levels of recovery from hemiplegia:

1. Flaccidity with no voluntary movement
2. Movement synergies beginning to appear
3. Voluntary control of synergies
4. Voluntary movements deviating from synergies
5. Voluntary independence from basic synergies
6. Voluntary isolated joint movements with near-normal coordination

Treatment is based on the following principles:

1. Using the developmental recovery sequence
2. Facilitating movement through sensory stimulation when no voluntary movement is present
3. Encouraging volitional control over stimulated movements
4. Reinforcing emerging synergies by asking the patient to hold positions and move voluntarily
5. Employing synergies that are under control in functional activities

The occupational therapy application of this approach centers on the use of controlled movements in purposeful activities. In stages 3 and 4 of recovery, when the patient has some voluntary control, activities can be

---

As this example points out, the same observed phenomena can be understood very differently from traditional neurodevelopmental approaches and from the dynamical systems perspective.

This example also points to the fallacy of NDT's assumption that engagement in real-life tasks is contraindicated on the grounds that such activity may reinforce abnormal patterns of movement. This assumption is predicated on the notion that a pattern of observed movement that deviates from what is considered normal is due entirely to "abnormal" messages from the CNS. As the example just shows, such movement patterns may instead be a feature of the total system attempting to cope with the dynamics of the situation, given the effects of CNS damage. From this perspective, engagement in occupational tasks would not be contraindicated. Rather, such occupational engagement would be the preferred method for achieving optimal solutions to overcoming and/or compensating for motor deficits.

adapted to make use of these motor behaviors. Sometimes this involves using the affected extremity to stabilize objects while the unaffected arm is used in the task.[12] Activities can be adapted to promote the use of existing synergies and to elicit motor behaviors that break out of, or combine, synergies and thus accomplish even greater volitional control of movement.[12]

Brunnstrom's approach differs from the Bobath approach. Bobath holds that motor patterns appearing after brain damage should not be used in retraining motor control. However, Brunnstrom argues that in the early stages of recovery, when only reflex activity is present, such activity must be used. Brunnstrom does agree, however, that reflex activity should be inhibited in the later stages of recovery.

Proprioceptive Neuromuscular Facilitation (PNF)

This approach was originally developed by a neurophysiologist and physician (Kabat) and later articulated and elaborated by two physical therapists (Knott and Voss) and an occupational therapist (Meyers). Proprioceptive neuromuscular facilitation (PNF) is defined as "a method of promoting or hastening the response of the neuromuscular mechanism through stimulation of the proprioceptor."[16] This approach is somewhat broader and more eclectic than the other three.

Order. Several principles define the view of order held by this approach.[11] According to this view, normal motor development proceeds cephalocaudally and proximodistally. Reflexes dominate early motor behavior and, with maturity, are integrated into voluntary motor behavior. Motor behavior is cyclic (alternating between flexion and extension phases). Normal goal-directed behavior is made up of reversing movements (e.g., flexing, then extending) and depends on a balance between "antagonistic" muscles (e.g., flexors and extensors). Motor behavior develops in an orderly sequence of total movement patterns. This development is not stepwise; instead, there is overlap between successive stages of motor development.

Increases in motor abilities require learning. This learning often involves acquiring a chain or series of steps and later integrating them into the task. Frequent stimulation and motor repetition support retention of learned motor abilities. A final, important principle is that motor learning requires multisensory information. Auditory, visual, and tactile systems provide sensory data along with proprioceptive information to program the learning of movement.

Disorder. In terms of this approach, disorder is any difficulty with motor control. PNF was originally developed for the treatment of persons with cerebral palsy and multiple sclerosis but has found application with a wide range of patients, including persons whose motor limitations are not of CNS origin.

Therapeutic Intervention. The therapeutic approach of PNF is multisensory. The kinds of sensory stimulation used include physical contact by the therapist, visual cues, and verbal commands. The central feature of treatment is the use of diagonal patterns of movement (i.e., moving extremities in a plane diagonal to the body midline) for recovery of motor function. Diagonal patterns are considered the treatment of choice because they involve natural movements that are part of normal development and require integration of both sides of the body.

Technology for Application. Evaluation is broad-based and may include determination of the developmental postures and movement patterns of which the individual is capable, as well as determination of the person's ability to use these capacities in functional activities. The goal of evaluation is to gather a comprehensive picture of the strengths and weaknesses of the patient in terms of capacity for movement and to identify these in sufficient detail so that appropriate techniques for intervention can be selected.

Several techniques are used to encourage the patient's engaging in natural diagonal patterns of movement. One method is irradiation, which seeks to facilitate specific muscle action by using stronger muscle groups to stimulate activity of weaker groups. Another technique, successive induction, aims to facilitate one voluntary motion by using another. A third technique, reciprocal innervation, uses voluntary motion to inhibit reflexes. Other techniques include appropriate positioning, the use of manual contact for positioning or stimulation, and verbal commands and instructions for movement. Other sensory stimulation, such as stretching muscles and providing resistance to movement, is also employed. Goal-directed movements combined with facilitation techniques are believed to be the most effective means of treatment.

Summary of Neurodevelopmental Approaches

While the previous discussions illustrated the different emphases of the four neurodevelopmental approaches, their commonalities will be discussed here. By summarizing the common views of these four approaches, they can be collectively compared with the contemporary motor control approach in occupational therapy.

Order. The neurodevelopmental approaches all share the following view of motor control.[7,9] They assert that the CNS is hierarchically organized (i.e., higher centers control lower centers) and that movement is controlled by sensory input to lower centers and through the encoded motor programs of higher centers. Development and learning occur because of maturational or experientially driven changes in the CNS. Essentially, motor control occurs because the human being learns to master movements and then use those movements to accomplish tasks. Fixed sequences of motor learning and development are viewed as necessary consequences of how the system hierarchically builds upon and modifies lower level movement patterns (e.g., voluntary movement builds upon reflex-driven postural control).

Disorder. According to the neurodevelopmental approaches, abnormal patterns of movement result directly from disorganization in the CNS. Damage to the CNS disrupts or interferes with sensory/perceptual inputs, motor programs, and the normal hierarchical organization of motor control. This, in turn, produces abnormal muscle tone, reflexes, and movement patterns.

Therapeutic Intervention. The neurodevelopmental approaches exclusively focus on understanding and remediating motor control deficits that are believed to result directly from the nature of damage to or disorganization in the CNS. The most basic concepts underlying the approach to intervention focus on:

1. Inhibiting abnormal muscle tone, reflexes, and movement patterns with sensory stimuli
2. Facilitating normal muscle tone and movement patterns with sensory stimuli

Underlying this focus is the assumption that all observed changes in the dynamics of muscle and movement are directly related to changes achieved in CNS organization.

The neurodevelopmental approaches emphasize learning through task repetition with constant assistance (e.g. handling, positioning, instructions) and feedback from the therapist. They also emphasize a developmental progression of learning parts of a task and proceeding to combine the parts into a whole.

Recovery and treatment are expected to follow normal developmental sequences from reflex to voluntary control, from gross to discrete movements, and from proximal to distal control. Consequently, these approaches emphasize using movements that are normal or that follow recovery sequences. The perceived importance of these sequences is based on the assumption that they are "hard-wired" in the CNS.

Technology for Application. In the neurodevelopmental approaches, evaluation focuses on:

1. Determining the status of muscle tone, sensation and perception, and postural control
2. Identifying abnormal reflexes and movement patterns
3. Ascertaining the developmental level of existing motor control patterns

The technology for treatment relies heavily on the use of external sensory stimulation and handling to elicit correct patterns of movement.

Moreover, these approaches emphasize practicing and mastering movement patterns with the assumption that, once normal movement patterns are mastered, they will generalize to functional motor control in occupational performance. Participation in occupational forms is not emphasized. When occupational forms are used, they are chosen because they are thought to elicit the appropriate movement patterns. Sometimes the use of occupational activities has been discouraged since they are seen as developing isolated splinter skills. Such splinter skills are viewed as specific to the task performed and, hence, not generalizable to other areas of performance. In general, occupation does not play a central role in the remediation of motor control deficits in the neurodevelopmental approaches.

Theoretical Arguments and Technology for Application of the Contemporary Motor Control Approach

The contemporary motor control approach is in the process of being more fully articulated in occupational therapy. While a number of authors have begun to refer to and make use of current motor control concepts, Mathiowetz and Haugen[4,7,9] and Trombly[15] have offered the most systematic articulation to date in the occupational therapy literature.

Theoretical Arguments

The theoretical arguments of this approach are strongly tied to the contemporary interdisciplinary conceptualization of motor control. While only recently elucidated in occupational therapy, they constitute a coherent explanation of order, disorder, and intervention as it concerns the control of movement in occupational performance.

Order. Motor control is viewed as emerging from the interaction of the human system (CNS and musculoskeletal components) with environmental and task variables. Movement is a self-organizing phenomenon that depends on this dynamic interaction; it is not solely dependent on the CNS. The CNS is viewed as a heterarchically organized system with higher and lower centers interacting cooperatively with each other and with the musculoskeletal system.

Movement patterns are not invariant sequences prewired into the CNS. Instead, they are stable (or preferred) ways to accomplish occupational performance, given the unique characteristics of the human being and certain environmental conditions. These preferred patterns of movement are attractor states that can be perturbed by changes in any of the participating systems or in the environment.

Motor control is learned through a process in which the person seeks optimal solutions for accomplishing an occupation. Hence, learning is dependent on the characteristics of the performer, the context, and the goal of the occupation being performed. Patterns of movement become attractor states when they are practiced. When they are practiced under a wider range of conditions, they are more stable than when learned under narrow conditions. Changes in the environmental conditions, the occupational form being performed, or the human system can result in a disintegration or a qualitative shift in the preferred pattern of movement.

A variable whose change can shift the motor behavior into another pattern is referred to as a *control parameter*. Control parameters may be changes in variables within the musculoskeletal system, the task or environment, or the CNS. So, for example, changes in strength, CNS maturation, size or weight of an object being handled, or the speed of action required for the task could all be control parameters that change motor behavior patterns.

The contemporary model of motor control in occupational therapy emphasizes the role of the occupation being performed and the occupational context in which it is performed. Occupational form, which refers to goals and procedures of the occupational activity being performed, is recognized as having an important influence on all motor control. Within this model, motor control is viewed as behavior that self-organizes specifically in the context of performing a given occupation.[15,17]

Finally the contemporary motor control model does not emphasize a fixed developmental sequence. Developmental pathways depend both on the unique characteristics of the individual and on variations in the environment in which motor control is learned.

Disorder. When persons have CNS damage, motor behavior results from the attempt to compensate for the damage while performing a specific occupational form in a given context. If the occupation or the environment in which the person is performing changes, the kind of motor behavior he or she exhibits may also change.[7,9,15] Hence, while disorders of movement are related to deficits in the CNS, they are not a direct consequence of those deficits. Rather, movement patterns are a consequence of the dynamics that occur between a person with specific abilities and limitations (as represented in both the CNS and the musculoskeletal system) and the occupational and environmental demands faced in performing. Thus, for example, an abnormal movement pattern may be jointly influenced by CNS impairment and muscle weakness and may be present only under certain occupational and environmental conditions.

Therapeutic Intervention. A central premise of this approach is that "functional tasks help organize motor behavior."[4] According to Haugen and Mathiowetz[9] therapy begins with identification of those tasks that are difficult to perform and by noting the preferred movement patterns the person uses for these tasks. The therapist then determines the personal and environmental systems that either support optimal performance or contribute to ineffective performance. This provides an identification of the supporting and limiting factors in motor control and serves as a basis for determining intervention. The therapist also seeks to determine the stability or instability of motor behaviors across occupational and environmental conditions. In this way, the range of conditions under which both functional and dysfunctional movement patterns are manifest can be determined. This reveals how strong an attractor state a particular (functional or dysfunctional) movement pattern is and, therefore, how easily it can be disturbed or shifted to another pattern.

Depending on what evaluation reveals, intervention can differ. For example, if a person's motor behavior is unstable, the therapist may help the client find the optimal motor solution and practice it so that it becomes more stable. If the patient is using a motor control strategy that accomplishes the goal of the task but is not the most efficient or safe, the therapist may help the client to find and stabilize different strategies of movement.

The contemporary motor control approach stresses learning the entire occupation rather than discrete parts. This approach also emphasizes allowing persons to find their own optimal solutions to motor problems rather than relying on instructions and constant feedback. Persons are allowed to experiment and problem-solve in the context of occupational performance. Feedback on the overall consequences of performance is considered more useful than discrete feedback about parts of the performance.

The goals of treatment in this approach focus on:

1. Accomplishment of necessary and desired occupational forms in the most efficient way, given the client's characteristics
2. Allowing the person to practice in varying and natural contexts so that the learned motor behaviors are more stable
3. Maximizing both personal and environmental characteristics that enhance performance
4. Enhancing the problem-solving abilities of clients so they will more readily find solutions to challenges encountered in new environments beyond the treatment setting

Overall this approach stresses a collaborative and client-centered approach that considers the client's role and motives.

Technology for Application. Since the contemporary motor control approach is in an early stage of development, its technology must be further developed and refined. The approach to evaluation is task-oriented, emphasizing the observation of a person's attempts to perform meaningful occupational tasks in context. Evaluation methods incorporate both quantitative and qualitative data gathering that examines how motor control varies in different occupational forms and contexts.[9,15] Evaluation begins with the observation of occupational performance and proceeds to examine underlying systems only when further understanding of how those systems are constraining performance is needed. For example, the therapist would not begin with evaluation of reflexes and muscle tone. Rather, the therapist would begin with examination of whether and how the person performed necessary occupational forms. Then, when difficulties are noted, the therapist might proceed to identify whether and how muscle tone and abnormal reflexes contribute (along with the environment and the occupational form) to difficulties in performance. Consequently, the focus of evaluation is on occupational performance, not on the underlying general motor abilities. This also means that the therapist begins by learning what occupational forms are necessary for the role performance of the patient or client. When therapists examine human systems to determine how they are contributing to difficulties in performance, the CNS is recognized as important, but as only one among several factors that codetermine performance. There are not yet validated standard methods of evaluation; however, principles of assessment and ways of incorporating existing assessments into the approach have been identified.[9] Since this model emphasizes the use of client-centered occupational forms, natural environments, and a process of active experimentation for optimal motor solutions, its techniques cannot be as readily specified as those of the neurodevelopmental approaches. These traditional approaches assumed that motor control was driven by a single system, the CNS. Hence, techniques were quite specific. The contemporary approach identifies multiple factors that influence motor control and argues that their relative importance and influence on a client's performance are situationally dependent. Hence, the actual techniques used in therapy require an individualized understanding of the client's situation across many dimensions. For those accustomed to the much more standardized approaches of the neurodevelopmental approaches, the motor control approach may, at first, appear much less prescriptive and specific. However, as more clearly defined principles and strategies of evaluation and intervention are articulated and accompanied by case examples, the technology of this model should become more readily accessible.

Summary and Comparison of the Neurodevelopmental and the Contemporary Motor Control Approaches

In the previous sections, I reviewed the traditional neurodevelopmental and the contemporary motor control approaches. In general, the contemporary motor control approach replaces the more mechanistic explanation of movement with a more dynamic and holistic viewpoint. In contrast to the neurodevelopmental approaches, which de-emphasized the role of the environment and of occupation in motor control and in the remediation of motor control deficits, the contemporary model places a great deal of emphasis on both these elements.

Research

Research on the Bobath approach is limited to some thesis projects that focus on isolated aspects of the approach.[14] Neurodevelopmental therapy is the most studied of the approaches, although the studies tend to be methodologically weak.[14] They do not clearly show that neurodevelopmental therapy is an effective treatment. One study suggested that nonspecific play activities were as effective in producing motor behavior gain. (Parenthetically, the findings of this study appear more compatible with the theoretical arguments of the contemporary motor control approach.) There are no published studies of the effectiveness of NDT with persons who have hemiplegia. Research concerning the PNF approach is limited and focuses primarily on normal populations.[11] Usually, each of these studies examined an isolated aspect of PNF, and the results from these studies are mixed. Overall, it can be seen that no systematic body of occupational therapy research has accumulated on the neurodevelopmental approaches.

At the same time, the contemporary motor control approach is too new to have been systematically subjected to research in occupational therapy. Preliminary studies[6,17] have begun to provide support for the theoretical arguments of this model.

Since both the traditional neurodevelopmental and contemporary motor control approaches are heavily based on interdisciplinary research, it is worth considering this research. Clearly, interdisciplinary researchers have strong evidence that contradicts many traditional concepts of motor control. Moreover, a robust research literature is developing that supports the dynamical systems approach. Hence, interdisciplinary studies suggest strongly that the traditional neurodevelopmental approaches need to be reconsidered, incorporated into, or replaced with the contemporary motor control approach.

Discussion

The transition from traditional neurodevelopmental approaches to a contemporary motor control approach raises a number of major challenges. Consideration will need to be given to which concepts and techniques from the traditional approach are still valid and useful in a contemporary framework. Moreover, further articulation of the theoretical arguments is needed, as well as a great deal of work to develop a technology for application of the contemporary motor control model.

The transition from traditional practice to practice based on the contemporary motor control model is likely to be somewhat uneven. The use of traditional neurodevelopmental approaches is widespread and characterized by strong allegiances of therapists to one or more approaches. Confusion about traditional versus new ideas is also a problem since some of the traditional approaches have attempted to incorporate new motor control ideas while implicitly retaining many of their original tenets.

These circumstances have already led to some disagreements between those who espouse traditional methods and those who are discussing the contemporary motor control approach and its explicit criticism of the traditional neurodevelopmental approaches. A good example of these disagreements is a letter to the editor of the American Journal of Occupational Therapy, in which a number of therapists strongly objected to a paper by Mathiowetz and Haugen that introduced new concepts of motor control that implicitly criticized the NDT approach.[3] These therapists argue that NDT has been updated to incorporate new concepts of motor control. However, in response to this letter, the authors of the original article point out that the new concepts of motor control require more than updating NDT.[8] They argue that the new concepts call for a paradigm shift and even question the appropriateness of the term neurodevelopmental, since it implies a view of motor control (i.e., a model of motor control driven by the CNS with a fixed developmental sequence) that is not in line with our current understanding of motor control.

Since the four neurodevelopmental approaches are long-standing occupational therapy approaches with significant following by practitioners, the change to a new model based on ideas that not only build upon but also criticize and call for replacement and reorganization of the older concepts and techniques will no doubt be controversial for some time. Also, until a new motor control model is more fully articulated and supported with technology for application, therapists will no doubt find it challenging to begin to alter their practices. As when any major transformation in a model of practice occurs, the change it calls for will occur unevenly in practice and will take place over a period of time.

Nonetheless, the kinds of changes in conceptualization and application that are called for by the contemporary motor control approach are very promising. First of all, they parallel a transformation in thinking about human performance that cuts across many disciplines. Secondly, they reaffirm many traditional occupational therapy ideas that emphasized the importance of occupation in learning motor skills and restoring motor capacity. The neurodevelopmental approaches were very much founded in the paradigm of inner mechanisms described in Chapter 3. The reorganization of these approaches into a more contemporary motor control model signals the transformation of practice that emanated from that older paradigm to practice consistent with the current paradigm of occupational therapy.

TERMS OF THE MODEL

attractor states	Preferred movement patterns that emerge from the dynamic interaction of the person with the environment, without centralized instructions.
cephalocaudal	Refers to sequence of motor development from the head downward.
control parameter	A variable whose change can shift a pattern of motor behavior into another pattern.
coordinative structures	Groups of muscles acting over many joints and constrained to behave together as a single functional unit to achieve a purposeful action.
handling	Therapist manipulation of the patient's body.
heterarchical control	Conceptualization that argues that movements are controlled by systems cooperating together toward the production of movement but without central executive control.
hierarchical control	Conceptualization that argued that movements are controlled from the top down (i.e., higher brain centers controlling lower ones).
motor control	The ability to use one's body effectively in interacting with the environment.
motor problems	Challenges for movement such as learning to reach out and grasp an object.
muscle tone	The state of stiffness or tension in muscle.
plasticity	The nervous system's potential for both organization and reorganization as the result of experience.
proximodistal	Refers to the sequence of motor development from the middle of the body to the distant limbs.
reflexes	Biologically determined movement patterns not under volitional control.

Motor Control Model

FOCUS

- Concerned with problems of movement following brain damage
- Consists of four traditional treatment approaches and a contemporary motor control model

INTERDISCIPLINARY BASE

- Concepts from neurophysiology, neuropsychology, cognitive psychology, and movement science

COMPARISON OF EACH OF THE TRADITIONAL MOTOR CONTROL APPROACHES

The Rood Approach	*Bobath's Neurodevelopmental Treatment*	*Brunnstrom's Movement Therapy*	*Proprioceptive Neuromuscular Facilitation*
Order			
• Normal motor control emerges from the use of subcortically controlled reflex patterns present at birth; they support voluntary control at a conscious (cortical) level. • Different muscles perform different work.	• Motor control involves learning the sensations of movement. • Basic postural movements are learned first and later elaborated on, and integrated into functional skills.	• Normal development involves a progression of reflexes that are modified; components are rearranged into purposeful movement as higher centers in the brain take over.	• Development of motor behavior is cyclic—i.e., made up of reversing movements (e.g., flexing, then extending) and depends on a balance between "antagonistic" muscles (e.g., flexors and extensors).

- ○ Light work muscles primarily provide movement and are more voluntarily controlled.
- ○ Heavy work muscles primarily stabilize and are more reflexively controlled.

- Motor behavior develops in an orderly sequence of total movement patterns with overlap between successive stages of motor development.
- Motor learning involves acquiring a chain or series of steps and later integrating them into the task through stimulation and motor repetition.
- Motor learning requires multisensory information (i.e., auditory, visual, tactile, and proprioceptive).

Disorder

- With CNS damage, the normal sequence of
- Brain damage results in spasticity and abnormal
- Cerebrovascular accident (and other brain damage)
- CNS damage and orthopedic problems

reflex development and learning of voluntary motor control is impaired and abnormal muscle tone is often present.

- patterns of posture and movement that interfere with everyday functional activity.
- When posture and movement are abnormal, sensation provides incorrect information to the CNS, preventing learning, or relearning, of normal movement.

Therapeutic Intervention

- Progress from appropriate sensory inputs to evoke muscle response when voluntary control is minimal and abnormal tone and reflexes are present, to using obtained responses in developmentally appropriate patterns of movement, to purposeful use of the movements in activities.

can interfere with normal patterns of movement, reducing capacity for functional activity.

leads to regression to lower levels of motor function (i.e., reflex behavior)

- Stereotypical limb flexion or extension movement patterns occur sequentially in recovery from hemiplegia (limb . synergies).

- Abnormal patterns are inhibited and normal ones elicited by sensory stimuli.
- When persons perform normal patterns of movement, sensory information about movement allows learning of motor control.

- Reflex patterns (normal at various stages in the course of development) elicited by brain damage can be built upon for relearning of motor control (thus, they should be initially facilitated and later inhibited).

- Use of multisensory stimulation (including physical contact, verbal commands, and visual cues)
- Employment of natural diagonal patterns of movement (i.e., moving extremities in a plane diagonal to the body midline)

TECHNOLOGY FOR APPLICATION

- Identify the highest developmental motor pattern that the person can do with ease
- Use sensory stimuli to normalize muscle tone
- Begin with current developmental level and progress through normal sequence of motor development
- Focus attention on the goal or purpose of an activity
- Provide opportunities for repetition to reinforce learning

- Determine the highest developmental level at which the person can consistently perform, distribution of muscle tone when the body is in various developmental positions, and how tone changes in response to external stimulation or voluntary effort
- Abnormal patterns stopped (inhibited through sensory stimuli) and replaced with normal movement patterns (elicited through sensory stimuli) to provide appropriate sensory information for motor learning in developmental sequence.
  ○ *Handling* of the person to inhibit abnormal distribution of tone or postures-while stimulating and encouraging active

- Identify person's sensory status (since sensation to recognize patterns of movement is important to treatment).
- Identify which reflexes are present and determine level of recovery as manifest in reflex synergies of movement.
- Elicit reflex synergies of movement and use them as the basis for learning progressively more mature voluntary movement
- Employ developmental recovery sequence:
  ○ Facilitate movement through sensory stimulation.
  ○ Encourage volitional control over stimulated-movements.
  ○ Reinforce emerging syner

- Determine available developmental postures and movement patterns and ability to use them in functional activities to generate a comprehensive picture of capacity for movement.
- Stimulate diagonal patterns for recovery of motor function through:
  ○ Facilitating specific muscle action by using stronger muscle group to stimulate activity of weaker groups (irradiation).
  ○ Facilitating one voluntary motion by using another

motor performance at the next developmental level.

- ○ Practice new abilities in purposeful tasks to encourage voluntary control over normal responses in purposeful activities.

gies through voluntarily use in functional activities.

- ○ Elicit motor behaviors in purposeful tasks that break out of, or combine, synergies for greater volitional control of movement.

(successive induction) and inhibiting reflexes by voluntary motion (reciprocal innervation).

- ○ Appropriate positioning, using manual contact to position or stimulate the individual
- ○ Giving verbal commands and instructions for movement
- ○ Sensory stimulation such as stretching muscles and providing resistance to movement
- ○ Goal-directed activities combined with facilitation techniques

COMPARISON OF TRADITIONAL NEURODEVELOPMENTAL APPROACHES (COMMON FEATURES) AND CONTEMPORARY MOTOR CONTROL APPROACH

Traditional Neurodevelopmental Approaches (Common Features)	Contemporary Motor Control Approach
Theoretical Arguments	
Order	
• CNS is hierarchically organized (i.e., higher centers control lower centers).	• Motor control is a self-organizing phenomenon that emerges from the interaction of the human system (CNS and musculoskeletal components) with environmental and occupational variables.
• Movement is controlled by sensory input to lower centers and through the encoded motor programs of higher centers.	• CNS is a heterarchically organized system with higher and lower centers interacting cooperatively with each other and with the musculoskeletal system.
• Development and learning result from changes in the CNS	
• Fixed sequences of motor learning and development	• Movement patterns are stable/preferred ways to accomplish occupational per-

formance (attractor states) given the unique characteristics of the human being and environmental conditions.

- Motor control is learned when the person seeks optimal solutions for accomplishing an occupation; it depends on the characteristics of the performer, the context, and the goal of the occupation being performed.

- Developmental pathways depend on unique characteristics of the individual and on variations in the environment.

- Motor dysfunction is a consequence of the dynamics that occur between a person with specific abilities and limitations (as represented in both the CNS and the musculo-

Disorder

- Abnormal muscle tone, reflexes and patterns of movement result directly from disorganization in the CNS

skeletal system) and the occupational and environmental demands faced in trying to perform.

Therapeutic Intervention

- Inhibition of abnormal muscle tone, reflexes, and movement patterns with sensory stimuli
- Facilitation of normal muscle tone and movement patterns with sensory stimuli
- Learning through task repetition with constant assistance (e.g., handling, positioning, instructions) and feedback from the therapist
- Progression from learning parts of a task to combining the parts into a whole
- Progression of recovery and treatment through

- Emphasis on person's attempts to perform meaningful occupational tasks in context
- Intervention dependent on:
  - Identification of those tasks that are difficult to perform, and noting the preferred movement patterns for these tasks and their degree of stability/instability
  - Determination of personal and environmental systems that either support optimal performance or contribute to ineffective performance
- Emphasizes:
  - Learning the entire occupation rather than discrete parts

developmental sequence (reflex to voluntary control, gross to discrete movements, and proximal to distal control)

- Using movements that are normal or which follow recovery sequences

Technology for Application

- Determines status of muscle tone, sensation and perception, and postural control
- Identifies abnormal reflexes and movement patterns
- Ascertains the developmental level of existing motor control patterns
- Uses external sensory stimulation and handling to elicit correct patterns of movement

○ Allowing persons to find their own optimal solutions to motor problems

- Examines occupational performance and proceeds to examine underlying systems when further understanding of how those systems are constraining performance is needed
- Emphasizes the use of client-centered occupational forms, natural environments, and a process of active experimentation for optimal motor solutions

- Requires practicing and mastering movement patterns

- Does not emphasize participation in occupational forms

- Requires an individualized understanding of the client's situation across many dimensions

RESEARCH

- Research on neurodevelopmental approaches is limited.
- Preliminary studies have begun to provide support for the theoretical arguments of contemporary motor control approach.

References

1. Bobath, B: Adult Hemiplegia: Evaluation and Treatment, ed 2. William Heinnemann, London, 1978.
2. Brunnstrom, S: Movement Therapy in Hemiplegia. Harper & Row, New York, 1970.
3. Cammisa, K, Calabrese, D, Meyers, M, Tupper, G, Moser, K, Crawford, K, Pope, L, Bostater, KA, Cooper, M, Wardill, J, Buelsing, D, Martin, L, Mitchell, S, Skoda, M, King, KM, Yuen, L, Fing, A, Hiraoka, K, Clevenger, VD, Gerard, N, Cornelissens, P, Lusk, T, Bierman, JC, Ocasio, S, Runyon, K, Shirey, T, Longsdon, M, and Cain, MA: NDT theory has been updated. Am J Occup Ther 49:176, 1995.
4. Haugen, JB, and Mathiowetz, V: Remediation of motor behavior through contemporary approaches—contemporary task-oriented approach. In Trombly, CA (ed): Occupational Therapy for Physical Dysfunction, ed 4. Williams & Wilkins, Baltimore, 1995.
5. Kamm, K, Thelen, E, and Jensen, JL: A dynamical systems approach to motor development. Physical Therapy 70:763–775, 1990.
6. Mathiowetz, V: Informational support and functional motor performance. Paper presented at the American Occupational Therapy Association National Conference, Boston, 1994.
7. Mathiowetz, V, and Haugen, JB: Motor behavior research: Implications for therapeutic approaches to central nervous system dysfunction. Am J Occup Ther 48:733–745, 1994.
8. Mathiowetz, V, and Haugen, JB: Authors' Response (to NDT Theory has been updated). Am J Occup Ther 49:176, 1995.
9. Mathiowetz, V, and Haugen, JB: (1995) Evaluation of motor behavior: Traditional and contemporary views. In Trombly, CA (ed): Occupational Therapy for Physical Dysfunction, ed 4. Williams & Wilkins, Baltimore, 1995.
10. McCormack, GL: Neurophysiology of sensorimotor approaches to treatment. In Pedretti, LW (ed): Occupational Therapy: Practice Skills for Physical Dysfunction. CV Mosby, St. Louis, 1990.
11. Meyers, BJ: Proprioceptive neuromuscular facilitation (PNF) approach. In Trombly, K (ed): Occupational Therapy for Physical Dysfunction. Williams & Wilkins, Baltimore, 1989.
12. Pedretti, LW: Movement therapy. In Pedretti, LW (ed): Occupational Therapy: Practice Skills for Physical Dysfunction. CV Mosby, St. Louis, 1990.
13. Rood, M: Neurophysiological mechanisms utilized in the treatment of neuromuscular dysfunction. Am J Occup Ther 10:4, 1956.
14. Trombly, C: Occupation Therapy for Physical Dysfunction, ed 3. Williams & Wilkins, Baltimore, 1989, pp 96, 78.
15. Trombly, CA: Occupation: Purposefulness and meaningfulness as therapeutic mechanisms, Am J Occup Ther 49:960, 1995.
16. Voss, DE, Ionta, MK, and Meyers, BJ: Proprioceptive Neuromuscular Facilitation: Patterns and Techniques, ed 3. Harper & Row, New York, 1985.
17. Wu, C-Y, Trombly, C, and Lin, K-C: The relationship between occupational form and occupational performance: A kinematic perspective. Am J Occup Ther 48:679–687, 1994.

CHAPTER 12

THE SENSORY INTEGRATION MODEL

The sensory integration model was originated by A. Jean Ayres as she studied the relationship between sensory processing in the brain and the behavior of children with learning disabilities. Ayres published two books, *Sensory Integration and Learning Disabilities*[2] and *Sensory Integration and the Child.*[3] Numerous publications by other authors have presented clinical application and research related to this model of practice. The most recent text concerning this model is *Sensory Integration: Theory and Practice;*[12] it reviews the concepts, research, and clinical applications of this model.

This model grew out of Ayres' observation that children with learning disabilities had difficulty interpreting *sensory information* from their bodies and the environment. She also observed that sensory processing problems were often related to deficits in motor and academic learning. Sensory integration is based on a conceptualization of how the brain functions as an organizer and interpreter of sensory information. It is concerned with failures of the brain to become properly organized for processing and integrating sensory information.

The sensory integration model is generally considered most relevant for persons who do not have frank neurological damage. The model addresses problems of sensory organization in the brain, but not outright physical damage to the central nervous system (CNS) such as occurs in stroke, cerebral palsy, and spina bifida. Accordingly, sensory integration disorder is recognized when the brain fails to organize properly in the absence of clear neurological damage to the CNS or peripheral sensory pathways.

Ayres believed that the problems of all children with learning disabilities were not homogeneous. Rather, she suspected that such children would manifest different types of sensory integrative problems. To pursue this line of reasoning, she constructed tests to study the behavioral manifestations of sensory processing problems. Findings from a series of studies comparing normal children and children with sensory integration problems were analyzed to identify patterns of sensory integration dysfunction. The identified patterns were interpreted in light of what was known about functional neurology and neuropsychology. Thus, the model provides empirical support for the existence of collections of problems and for the neurological explanations for those problems.

Interdisciplinary Base

The sensory integration model is based on experimental neuroscience literature,[11] on normal development studies, and on investigations with children who have learning disabilities.[8] In its early stages of development, the model was influenced by neurodevelopmental approaches (see Chapter 11). Since understanding of the brain is central to this model, new information from the neurosciences has constantly been incorporated into the model and used to revise its theoretical arguments. The most recent text introduced systems concepts into this model;[12] however, the model has not been reinterpreted in light of the most recent dynamical systems concepts.

Theoretical Arguments

Sensory integration theory is based in several assumptions. The first assumption is that of *neural plasticity*, "the ability of the brain structure to change or to be modified" as a result of ongoing experiences of sensory processing.[11] Another basic assumption is that there is a developmental sequence of sensory integrative capacities. This sequence unfolds as a result of the interaction between normal brain maturation and accumulating sensory experiences. While the brain's developmental sequence is considered to be biologically determined, it is also dependent on sensory processing to organize its biological potential in the course of development. A third assumption is that the brain functions as an integrated whole. The fourth assumption is that brain organization and adaptive behavior are interactive—that is, brain organization makes possible adaptive behavior, and adaptive behavior (which involves the processing of sensory information) influences brain organization. The final assumption is that persons have an inner drive to participate in sensorimotor activities. These assumptions are reflected in the theoretical arguments of the model.

The model proposes a number of constructs related to sensory processing and identifies and hypothesizes relationships between those constructs.

As Fisher and Murray[11] point out, the theory proposed by this model is tentative and thus constantly changing.

Order

The basic view of sensory integration concerning how persons normally come to organize and use sensory information is that:

> Learning is dependent on the ability of normal individuals to take in sensory information derived from the environment and from movement of their bodies, to process and integrate these sensory inputs within the central nervous system, and to use this sensory information to plan and organize behavior.[11]

The model proposes that this ability to organize sensory information and use it to learn and perform develops as the child interacts with normal environmental challenges. The processing of sensory information in the brain results in development of new neural interconnections that allow sensory information to flow through appropriate channels and be interrelated with other sensory data. Sensory integration results in formation of a meaningful picture of self and the world, which guides performance. For example, learning new motor skills, such as riding a bicycle, involves generation of an image of one's own body and a sense of the body's movements in relation to the bicycle, to the forces of gravity, and so forth. To be able to ride a bicycle is to have an appreciation of all these factors and to know how it feels to integrate them into the performance. Thus, the integration of sensory data also involves interpreting and making sense of that data.[11,18]

Sensory integration is a process in which sensory intake, sensory integration and organization, and adaptive occupational behavior result in a spiral of development.[11] The child's adaptive use of sensory information in the context of sensory motor activities further develops the sensory integrative capacity of the brain. This enhanced capacity provides the basis for further intake of sensory information in future sensory motor activities. Thus, the spiral continues, with the child building upon each new level of brain organization achieved as a result of previous adaptive behavior. According to the model, play is the major arena in which sensorimotor behavior takes place.

The sensory integration model was originally based on an evolutionary view of the brain, which emphasized that "as the brain evolved, higher and newer structures like the cerebral cortex remained dependent on adequate functioning of older structures."[18] More recently, the model stresses that the brain functions as a whole, with important connections between cortical and subcortical functions. The higher cortical processes require the sensory integration that occurs at lower subcortical levels. Moreover, lower subcortical levels depend on cortical functions for processing sensory information.[11] Nonetheless, the focus of sensory integration is on those sensory processes that are mostly subcortical and that profoundly affect higher cortical processes. Because these sensory integration processes are so fundamental, they are thought to affect a wide variety of emotional and behavioral aspects of the child's behavior, as well as the ability to learn academic skills.

Areas of Sensory Functioning. The sensory integration model is concerned with multimodal sensory processing (i.e., integrating at least two sources of sensory information). Most attention has been directed to tactile, vestibular, and proprioceptive sensory information, but auditory and visual sensory information have also been considered.[11] Ayres, in particular, emphasized *vestibular sensation* (sensory awareness of one's position in relation to gravity) as a basis for sensory organization in the brain. She indicated that the experience of gravity and the use of the body in relationship to gravity is a ubiquitous feature of human action.[2] For example, the pervasive challenge that infants face in movement is the struggle to rise against gravity.

Proprioception is the perception of joint and body movement and of the position of the body and its segments in space. Proprioception depends on sensory information from the muscles and joints. It also receives information via an important efferent feedback loop. This loop, associated with motor planning, allows sensory data about the position of body parts to be integrated with data about the motor effort exerted to effect placement or movement of the body parts. This feedback allows one to differentiate between active (voluntary) and passive (involuntary) movement and to form an image of the effects of one's efforts in placing and moving body parts.[9]

Together, vestibular and proprioceptive (vestibular-proprioceptive) sensation consists of "inputs derived from active movements of one's own body."[9] Vestibular receptors (located in the inner ear) detect movement of the head and elicit compensatory, head, trunk, and limb movements, which correct for any movement of the head, trunk, or limb. These receptors are also connected with eye muscles and enable the eyes to move to compensate for movement of the head.

The vestibular-proprioceptive system provides a consistent frame of reference from which other sensory data are interpreted; that is, the knowledge of one's position in space and the position of one's body parts provides a constant backdrop of awareness against which other sensory data can be understood. In particular, vestibular-proprioceptive sensory data serve as a reference point for monitoring and controlling movement. Tactile data provide information to the individual concerning physical contact with the external world. Visual and auditory data also provide information emanating from the external environment. Sensory integration is the process whereby all sensory data are organized and processed in the brain, converted to meaningful information, and used to plan and execute motor behavior.

Inner Drive, Play, and Mind-Brain-Body Relations. Ayres[3] argued that children had an inner drive to seek out organizing sensations. This drive is manifest in sensorimotor and play activities, and these activities are critical to the development of sensory integration in the child.[5] This drive begins with the self-organizing tendency of the brain, which requires the processing of sensory information, and is manifest in a subjective urge for exploration and mastery.[18]

The model further proposes that the mind and brain are interrelated.[13] Their interdependence requires that children have positive experience in using their bodies for the brain to be properly oriented to receive and organize sensory information and for the child to be motivated to seek out appropriate sensory experiences. Thus, experience and motivation are viewed as necessary elements of the process of sensory integration.

In the course of play, children fulfill their needs for action. As Bundy[5] points out, play is the primary medium of sensory integration experiences. In the occupation of play, the child is properly oriented to generate and process sensory information.

The Spiral Process of Self-Actualization. The various components of the view of order are combined into an overall schema, which the authors refer to as the spiral process of self-actualization.*[11] Figure 12–1 illustrates the process. As represented in the lower, gray band, the inner drive leads the individual to "seek out, and participate in the sensorimotor activities that provide the opportunities for *sensory intake.*"[11] Through a process of sensory integration, the CNS must process, organize, and modulate sensory intake from the body and the environment.[11] Further, the individual must organize and plan adaptive behaviors (which include both postural and motor skills). *Neuronal models* (i.e., neurologically encoded memories of "what to do" and "how to do it") can be used to plan new and more complex behaviors, and this is represented in the second loop (the dark line), which shows neuronal models being generated from sensory integrative experiences and leading to the organization and planning of new adaptive behaviors. Thus, neuronal models develop as the "result of sensory feedback derived from

---

*This conceptualization reflects an integration of many ideas developed over the years within the sensory integration model. It also reflects an attempt to synthesize sensory integration concepts with the conceptualization of motivation from the model of human occupation. Traditionally, sensory integration theory noted that the motivation of the child was important, but the main emphasis in concepts and arguments was on the neurological structures and processes involved in sensory processing and organization. This new conceptualization provides a clearer account of the nature and role of motivation in sensory integration. Moreover, it illustrates how concepts from different models can cross-fertilize each other.

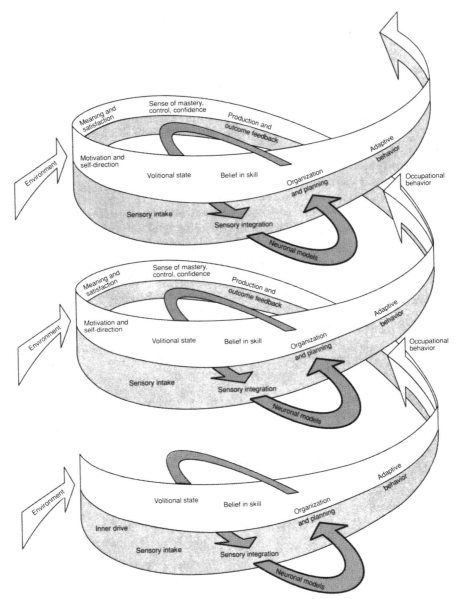

Figure 12–1. The spiral process of self-actualization. (From: Fisher, Murray, and Bundy,[11] p 19, with permission.)

the planning, the active performance (production), and the outcome of an adaptive behavior."[11]

The upper white band of the spiral shows how sensory integration is part of the occupational behavior of the child. Volitional state (the innate drive to participate in occupation and the belief in skill) also influences the selection of sensorimotor action. The child's occupational behavior generates feedback on the production and outcome of action. This feedback influences the child's sense of mastery, control, and confidence, as well as the experience of meaning and satisfaction in the behavior. This provides the basis for further motivation and self-direction, which in turn influences the ongoing processes of adaptive behavior, sensory integration, and occupational behavior.

Disorder

As noted, an important component of this model has been the identification, through research, of the types of sensory integration disorders and the explanation of these disorders in light of existing knowledge about nervous system function. The basic view of disorder in the sensory integration model is as follows: When individuals have deficits in processing and integrating sensory inputs, they also experience difficulty in planning and producing behavior—difficulties that, in turn, interfere with conceptual and motor learning.[11] The delineation of sensory integration dysfunctions has changed over time with new research findings. The patterns of disorder that are currently recognized are discussed in the following sections.

Vestibular-Proprioceptive Dysfunction. A first broad area of sensory integration dysfunction includes those problems that are vestibular-proprioceptive in nature. Vestibular and proprioceptive functions are linked together because current clinical assessment is unable to differentiate between these two functions. Problems associated with *vestibular-proprioceptive dysfunction* include hypotonicity of extension muscles, poor stability of proximal joints, poor postural adjustments, poor balance, lack of awareness of one's body, and disturbance of the body scheme.

Somatosensory Dysfunction. Included in the area of *somatosensory dysfunction* are problems with processing tactile and proprioceptive information together. Poor *tactile discrimination* is the specific inability to identify the location and timing of tactile stimuli. Problems associated with poor tactile discrimination include difficulty telling where and how many times one is touched, difficulty recognizing the shape of an object manipulated but not seen, and inefficiency in exploring the environment through touch. Proprioceptive difficulties are manifest in a poor sense of body position.

Sensory Modulation Disorders. A *sensory modulation disorder* exists when a child has difficulty maintaining normal limits of registering and responding to sensations. Such children tend to excessively overreact or underreact to sensory information or to shift between the two extremes.[19] *Sensory defensiveness* is one example of a sensory modulation disorder. It can be manifest by gravitational insecurity and aversive responses to vestibular stimulation (e.g., motion sickness). Sensory defensiveness may also include defensiveness toward tactile, auditory, olfactory, gustatory, and visual sensations.

The model proposes that *tactile defensiveness* is due to the inability to modulate or regulate tactile, sensory information. It is characterized by a tendency to avoid being touched, to avoid touching certain textures, and to avoid contact with other people. Other characteristics of a person with tactile defensiveness are an aversion to ordinarily non-noxious touch accompanied by an overreaction to touch by others (e.g., aggressiveness, withdrawal, negative responses). Tactile defensiveness is also associated with overactivity and is speculated to be related to such behaviors as emotional lability and isolation from others.

Gravitational insecurity is an overreaction (fear) to certain body positions, especially having one's feet off the ground or being out of the upright position. It is characterized by aversive responses to vestibular inputs, including nausea, vomiting, and other reactions associated with motion sickness.

Dyspraxia. Difficulty with volitional action directed to the environment is referred to as *dyspraxia*. All persons with dyspraxia have a difficulty with motor planning that is manifest as clumsiness.[7] Dyspraxia is not a problem of motor coordination (i.e., execution of motor behavior) but rather is related to difficulty in forming a plan of action. *Praxis* involves knowing how to do an action. Dyspraxia is mostly seen in difficulty with learning how to do a new task. Once the person with dyspraxia learns and practices a task, he or she can usually perform it adequately. However, for the person with dyspraxia, learning a particular skill does not seem to result in more basic learning that generalizes to other, similar types of performances. Dyspraxia often is manifest in childhood as clumsiness and through difficulty with ordinary tasks such as buttoning, tying shoelaces, and handwriting. While it is recognized that not all persons with dyspraxia have sensory integrative dysfunction, it is hypothesized that some forms of dyspraxia are related to deficits in sensory integration.

Problems with Bilateral Integration and Sequencing Praxis. The model proposes that disorders of *bilateral integration* (using the two sides of the body together) and sequencing praxis are related to vestibular-proprioceptive processing problems.[7] Disorders of bilateral integration and sequencing praxis include poor coordination of the two sides of the body, confusion of right and left, the tendency to avoid moving one's arms past the body's midline to the other side of the body, and difficulty in planning and sequencing movements, especially those involving both sides of the body.

Somatosensory Dyspraxia. It is hypothesized that *somatosensory dyspraxia* is related to deficits in somatosensory processing, the ability to process and integrate certain types of sensory information, particularly tactile and proprioceptive information. This is a more severe form of dyspraxia than bilateral integration and sequencing dyspraxia.

Problems with Praxis on Verbal Command and Visuopraxis. When evaluating persons for a possible sensory integration dysfunction, therapists may use assessments that provide a basis for hypothesizing about more complex cortical functions. The model suggests that difficulty with praxis in response to verbal commands is related to left-hemisphere dysfunction resulting from problems with auditory or language processing. Problems with *visuopraxis* can be more precisely analyzed as problems of:

1. Visuomotor coordination
2. Form and space perception
3. Construction abilities

Problems in these areas can be hemispheric (i.e., involving cortical versus subcortical functions). However, when fundamental sensory integrative functions do not develop, these dyspraxias can occur even when the hemispheres are intact. Hemispheric problems are not recognized as sensory integrative disorders, since they primarily involve cortical structures. Thus, they are not treated with sensory integrative approaches.

Therapeutic Intervention

As noted previously, Fisher and collaborators[9-12] view sensory integration as a systems process,* in which ongoing experiences of engaging in adaptive behavior result in further brain organization, which makes possible even more complex adaptive behaviors. When a person's brain fails to organize and process sensory information adequately, a disruption of this normal cycle of sensory integration is recognized.

Therapy based on the sensory integration model *always* aims at remediation of the sensory integration problem. Thus, the goal of sensory integration therapy is to improve the ability to integrate sensory information. This involves changes in the organization of the brain. Sensory integration approaches are based on the argument that:

> . . . provision of opportunities for enhanced sensory intake, provided within the context of a meaningful activity and the planning and organizing of an adaptive behavior, will improve the ability of the central nervous

---

*The most recent conceptualization of sensory integration uses older, open systems concepts rather than more current, dynamical systems concepts. One might expect that future conceptualizations of sensory integration would be modified somewhat to be in line with the most recent understanding of how persons learn to organize movement. One might contrast, for example, the systems-based conceptualizations (discussed in the chapters describing the cognitive-perceptual and motor control models, which employ a more contemporary systems view) with the theoretical arguments of this model.

system to process and integrate sensory inputs, and, through this process, enhance conceptual and motor learning.[11]

Therapy based on sensory integration emphasizes improving sensory processing at the subcortical level, because the subcortical processing of sensory information is believed to be the foundation for other, higher-level brain processes.[15]

Technology for Clinical Application

The sensory integration model has a well-developed technology for application. Assessment and intervention procedures have been thoroughly developed and clearly outlined.

Assessment

Assessment procedures in this model include the use of a formalized battery of tests, informal observation of performance, and data gathered from caregivers and other sources. Informal data along with the formal test battery results, are used to arrive at an assessment of whether a person has a sensory integration disorder and, if possible, to specify the nature of that disorder.

The Sensory Integration and Praxis Tests (SIPT) are a battery of tests designed to help the therapist identify and understand sensory integration disorders in children 4 through 8 years of age. The battery tests the relationships among "tactile processing, vestibular-proprioceptive processing, visual perception, and practice ability."[4] The tests are conceptualized as assessing the major behavioral manifestations of sensory integration deficits. The tests are grouped in four overlapping areas:

1. Tactile and vestibular-proprioceptive sensory processing
2. Form and space perception and visuomotor coordination
3. Practice ability
4. Bilateral integration and sequencing

The SIPT include 17 individually administered tests, which can be completed in about 90 minutes. All the tasks on the test are performance-oriented. They range from the Finger Identification Test, which asks the child to point to the finger(s) previously touched by an examiner, through the Standing and Walking Balance Test, to Design Copying, a test in which the child is asked to copy designs.

The tests are computer-scored. The company that does the scoring produces a report that includes statistical comparisons between the tested child and those observed in samples of normal and disabled children used to develop the tests. The SIPT were developed over nearly three decades, during which clinical experiences and research have been used to determine which testing procedures gave the most meaningful results. Statistical analysis of the items most useful in identifying dysfunction was used to develop and refine test items and testing procedures. Statistical studies, which have identified patterns of scores that indicate types of dysfunction, are the basis for interpretation of the test results.

Interpretation of the SIPT scores is based on meaningful clusters of scores. Research has shown that a particular pattern of low scores is indicative of a particular kind of problem. Thus, interpretation begins with examination of test scores to see if any such pattern exists.[10]

The SIPT are the mainstay of sensory integration assessment, but because of the restricted age range (4 to 9 years of age), other tests of motor, cognitive-perceptual, and sensory-processing capacity may be used. Observation and a history interview are also important. Careful observation of the person's neuromotor performance is used to identify subtle features. For example, a child with somatodyspraxia may not exhibit gross inability to perform purposeful tasks. Rather, such a child may tend to require more effort to perform tasks: the child may rely too much on trial and error, resulting in poor performance. The history interview is important in determining if the sensory integration problems result in functional problems in everyday life. Such information is important in determining the effect of the child's sensory integration status on occupational performance, which in turn influences decisions about treatment. Sensory integration treatment is meant to have a broad impact on behavior, so observations of neuromotor status and behavioral organization are also relevant to monitoring progress.[8]

Treatment Approach

Any discussion of the application of this model in practice must begin with a recognition that sensory integration procedures have been applied to a wide range of populations other than the children with learning disabilities for which the model was originally developed. For example, the model has been applied to adults, persons with frank brain damage, persons with schizophrenia, and individuals with mental retardation.[1,14] There has been considerable controversy over whether such individuals are appropriate candidates for sensory integration approaches. Additionally, many persons have been criticized for using techniques from sensory integration without a systematic application of its principles. While they may refer to the resulting therapy as sensory integration, it is, in fact, not. The text, *Sensory Integration: Theory and Practice*,[12] takes a conservative approach, arguing for a clear identification of the presence of sensory integration problems before the sensory integration approaches are used. The authors of the text believe that the model does have application with adults and may have potential for people with problems other than learning disability. The text outlines the authors' rationales for application of the model.

Treatment Guidelines. The sensory integration model provides specific guidelines for the kind of sensory integration experiences hypothesized to be of most benefit to a child. Treatment planning is based on identification of the child's deficits and the underlying reasons for those deficits, that is, the particular difficulty with processing sensory information. The vestibular-proprioceptive system provides a good example of the logic of intervention. Knowledge of the anatomy and physiology of the vestibular-proprioceptive system is used to determine what kind of sensory experience would most effectively stimulate vestibular organs and proprioceptors and elicit particular *postural reactions*. In this case, understanding neurological structures provides the logic for determining which therapeutic procedures should have particular impacts on the sensory system. The following quote from a discussion of treatment planning for a child (Steven) further illustrates the kind of specificity that can be achieved in choosing appropriate sensory integration therapy:

> Sensory integration theory suggests that Steven's difficulties with postural stability and bilateral integration and sequencing of projected limb movements should be addressed by activities that provide opportunities for him to take in enhanced vestibular-proprioceptive information. More specifically, the theory suggests that opportunities to take in linear vestibular-proprioceptive information in the context of activities that demand sustained postural control (in a variety of positions) and coordinated use of both sides of the body will be most appropriate. . . .[6]

Sensory integration theory does not yet present a complete picture of the various problems children manifest, nor does it explain all the underlying mechanisms. Thus, there are some gaps in information about how best to proceed in therapy. In such cases, the therapist should use all available information about the child to determine a prudent course of therapy.

Play as the Media. Bundy[5] has emphasized the importance of play as the vehicle for therapy based on the sensory integrative model. Creating a playful situation in which environmental demands are matched to the persons' capacity and challenging them to engage in new sensorimotor action creates the appropriate therapeutic context. The importance of play as the medium for therapy is underscored by the model's theory of mind-brain-body relations. This theoretical argument holds that appropriate organization of the brain for sensory processing is dependent on a positive mental and emotional orientation of the child during the activity.

The following description of a treatment session demonstrates how a therapist applies the understanding of the sensory integration disorder, achieves the needed sensory integration experiences, and maintains a playful context for the therapy:

[A]s Steven reached down and propelled himself, he tended to flex his entire body with the effort. Since [Colleen, the therapist] was looking for extension against gravity, and since Steven's flexion was becoming more and more pronounced, Colleen recognized that she must adapt the activity. Colleen grabbed a long dowel rod from the shelf behind her, held it at either end between her two outstretched arms, and entered into Steven's game. "Hey Superman!" she yelled, "Grab onto this branch and look in this window; I think there's someone who needs your help!" Stephen reached up and grabbed the bar with his arms outstretched. "Hold on," yelled Colleen. "Pull hard so you can come a little closer." As Steven began to flex his arms, Colleen watched closely to make sure that his body and head remained extended.[6]

This model emphasizes that the child must actively choose the actions that occur in therapy. In play, the child is given control and the enticement to choose appropriate sensory motor behaviors.

Equipment. Because of the special needs for sensory experiences (especially vestibular), sensory integration treatment has come to be associated with a variety of specially designed suspended equipment (trapezes, hammocks, and swings) and scooter boards. Such equipment, which is commercially available, provides the means of achieving desired sensory experiences in the context of play.

Research

The sensory integration model has been the subject of a great deal of research. Ongoing research has contributed to the development of the Sensory Integration and Praxis Tests[4] and, concurrently, to the validation of underlying sensory integration constructs. Pivotal studies in this area are the factor analytic studies, which identified meaningful clusters of test scores. These studies demonstrated that poor performance in a particular cluster of tests was typical of a child with a particular kind of sensory integration problem. Based on this research, it is thought that test score patterns can be indicative of the presence and type of a sensory integration problem.

A second area of research includes studies of the effectiveness of sensory integration therapy. According to Ottenbacher,[17] there have been enough studies of sensory integration treatment effectiveness to allow a meta-analysis. (Meta-analysis is a method of using data from several studies to determine whether there was a treatment effect across all the studies taken as a whole.) Ottenbacher[16] conducted such a meta-analysis and found evidence of treatment effectiveness, although he noted some limitations in the original studies used for the meta-analysis.

However, some controversy remains concerning the persons for whom sensory integration treatment is appropriate. One recent view of studies in the area of mental retardation concluded that sensory integration treatment was not warranted with that population.[1] A recent study of the efficacy of a sensory integration program on behaviors of inpatients with dementia also failed to show a significant effect on their behaviors.[20] Further research will be needed to clarify whether sensory integration treatment is effective and for whom it is appropriate.

Ottenbacher[17] writes that research is needed to assure the integrity of sensory integration intervention in studies. In the past, some studies that claimed to examine sensory integration-based therapy have defined the construct loosely and, therefore, did not provide true sensory integration therapy. He also notes that it is important to state clearly the intended outcomes of therapy and to select a meaningful and homogenous sample of subjects. Tickle-Degnen[21] notes that current studies have examined whether persons receiving sensory integration therapy have benefitted, but have not yet examined mediating factors. Such studies would help define what types of individuals benefit and under what conditions. Both Ottenbacher[17] and Tickle-Degnen[21] call for a series of ongoing studies to isolate and examine the effects of treatment based on the sensory integration model.

The sensory integration model and its underlying research base have been submitted to ongoing critiques. These critiques are all legitimate, but it is important to note that such criticisms are possible because there is a body of research upon which meaningful discussion and critique can be based.

Discussion

The sensory integration model is the most extensively researched and developed model of practice in occupational therapy. Nonetheless, the use of the model in practice has been subject to some criticism and controversy. Therapists have applied this model to populations that others deemed inappropriate for sensory integration treatment. Others have borrowed ideas and techniques from the model incompletely, resulting in clinical practices not justified by the theory.

This highly complex and well-developed model is both attractive to therapists and challenging to master. However, as noted, application of the model has not always been systematic. Clark, Mailloux, and Parham[8] note that "entry level therapists should not expect to be able to provide sensory integrative procedures upon graduation." They point out that considerable skill is required for use of this practice model. Therapists who wish to administer the Sensory Integration and Praxis Tests must become certified either through approved graduate or continuing education courses, and an examination process. The model represents an area of specialty practice in occupational therapy that requires training and experience beyond that of the generically trained therapist.

TERMS OF THE MODEL

bilateral integration	Using the two sides of the body together.
dyspraxia	Difficulty with volitional action directed to the environment.
gravitational insecurity	An unrealistic fear of certain body positions (especially positions in which the body leaves the ground).
neural plasticity	The ability of the brain to change or be modified.
neuronal models	Neurologically encoded memories of "what to do" and "how to do it."
praxis	The planning of motor action; involves knowing how to do an action.
postural reactions	Changes in one's body position to maintain equilibrium.
proprioception	The perception of joint and body movement and of the position of the body and its segments in space.
sensory defensiveness	Hypersensitivity to sensation resulting in a disorganized output.
sensory information	Sensations (e.g., from touch, movement).
sensory intake	Taking in of sensations from the environment or internally from the body.
sensory modulation disorder	Dysfunction in the ability to regulate sensory information (e.g., hyporesponsive or hyperresponsive).
somatosensory dyspraxia	Difficulty with voluntary action directed to the environment due to deficits in tactile processing.
somatosensory dysfunction	Deficits in processing tactile stimuli.
tactile defensiveness	Inability to modulate or regulate tactile sensory information.
tactile discrimination	Ability to identify tactile sensory information.
vestibular sensation	Sensory awareness of one's bodily position in relation to gravity.

visuopraxis	Problems of coordinating visual perception and movement including visuomotor coordination, form and space perception, and construction abilities.
vestibular-proprioceptive dysfunction	Deficits in processing vestibular and proprioceptive dysfunction manifest as hypotonicity of extensors; poor proximal stability, postural adjustments, and balance; lack of body awareness; and disturbed body scheme.

SUMMARY

The Sensory Integration Model

FOCUS

- Organization of sensory information in the CNS and its use in guiding adaptive motor behaviors that make up occupational performance

INTERDISCIPLINARY BASE

- Experimental neuroscience (brain structures and processes)
- Normal development studies
- Investigations with children who have learning disabilities
- Systems concepts
- Concepts of mind-brain-body relationships from neuroscience, philosophy, and psychology

THEORETICAL ARGUMENTS

Order

- Sensory integration is a systems process in which sensory intake, sensory integration and organization, and adaptive occupational behavior results in a spiral of development.
- The brain functions as a whole; higher cortical processes require the sensory integration that occurs at lower subcortical levels; lower subcortical levels depend on cortical functions for processing sensory information.
- Sensory integration is multimodal sensory processing (i.e., integrating at least two sources of sensory information) in which sensory data is organized and processed in the brain, converted to meaningful information, and used to plan and execute motor behavior.
- Children have an inner drive to seek out organizing sensations.
- Mind and brain are interrelated: subjective experience is a necessary part of the adaptive spiral of sensory integration.
- Play is the primary medium of sensory integration experiences; it provides the appropriate context for the child to be properly oriented to generate and process sensory information.

Disorder

- When individuals have deficits in processing and integrating sensory inputs, deficits in planning and producing behavior occur that interfere with conceptual and motor learning.
- Types of sensory integrative disorders:
  - Problems processing vestibular-proprioceptive sensations
  - Problems with processing tactile and proprioceptive information together (somatosensory problems)

○ Difficulty maintaining normal limits of registering and responding to sensations (sensory modulation disorder)
○ Difficulty with volitional action directed to the environment, a motor planning problem manifested in clumsiness (dyspraxia)

Therapeutic Intervention

- Aims at remediation (change) of the sensory integration problem
- Aims to improve the ability to integrate sensory information by changing the organization of the brain
- Improves the ability of the central nervous system to process and integrate sensory inputs by enhancing sensory intake, which occurs when a child plans and organizes adaptive behavior in a meaningful activity.

TECHNOLOGY FOR APPLICATION

- Assessment procedures include a formalized battery of tests (Sensory Integration and Praxis Tests), informal observation of performance, and data gathered from caretakers and other sources.
- Data are used to arrive at an assessment of whether a person has a sensory integration disorder and, if possible, to specify the nature of that disorder.
- Sensory integration experiences selected to benefit a child are derived from identification of the child's deficits, and the theory concerning the underlying reasons for those deficits—i.e., the particular difficulty processing sensory information.
- Play is a vehicle for therapy; environmental demands are matched to the persons' capacity and challenge them to engage in new sensori-motor action; in play the child is given control and enticement to choose appropriate sensorimotor behaviors.

RESEARCH

- Ongoing research has contributed to the development of the Sensory Integration and Praxis Tests and validation of underlying sensory integration constructs.
- Studies of the effectiveness of sensory integration therapy provide some evidence of treatment effectiveness.

References

1. Arendt, RE, MacLean, WE, and Baumeister, A: Critique of sensory integration therapy and its application in mental retardation. American Journal on Mental Retardation 92:401, 1988.
2. Ayres, AJ: Sensory Integration and Learning Disabilities. Western Psychological Services, Los Angeles, 1972.
3. Ayres, AJ: Sensory Integration and the Child. Western Psychological Services, Los Angeles, 1979.

4. Ayres, AJ, and Marr, DB: Sensory integration and praxis tests. In Fisher, AG, Murray, EA, and Bundy, AC (eds): Sensory Integration: Theory and Practice. FA Davis, Philadelphia, 1991. p 203.
5. Bundy, AC: Play theory and sensory integration. In Fisher, AG, Murray, EA, and Bundy, AC (eds): Sensory Integration: Theory and Practice. FA Davis, Philadelphia, 1991.
6. Bundy, AC: The process of planning and implementing intervention. In Fisher, AG, Murray, EA, and Bundy, AC (eds): Sensory Integration: Theory and Practice. FA Davis, Philadelphia, 1991, pp 341, 346.
7. Cermak, SA: Somatodyspraxia. In Fisher, AG, Murray, EA, and Bundy, AC (eds): Sensory Integration: Theory and Practice. FA Davis, Philadelphia, 1991.
8. Clark, F, Mailloux, Z, and Parham, D: Sensory integration and children with learning disabilities. In Clark PN, and Allen, AS (eds): Occupational Therapy for Children. CV Mosby, St. Louis, 1985, p 384.
9. Fisher, AG: Vestibular-proprioceptive processing and bilateral integration and sequencing deficits. In Fisher, AG, Murray, EA, and Bundy, AC (eds): Sensory Integration: Theory and Practice. FA Davis, Philadelphia, 1991, p 71.
10. Fisher, AG, and Bundy, AC: The interpretation process. In Fisher, AG, Murray, EA, and Bundy, AC (eds): Sensory Integration: Theory and Practice. Philadelphia: FA Davis, 1991.
11. Fisher, AG, and Murray, EA: Introduction to sensory integration theory. In Fisher, AG, Murray, EA, and Bundy, AC (eds): Sensory Integration: Theory and Practice. FA Davis, Philadelphia, 1991, pp 3, 4, 15, 19–21.
12. Fisher, AG, Murray, EA, and Bundy, AC (eds): Sensory Integration: Theory and Practice. FA Davis, Philadelphia, 1991.
13. Kielhofner, G, and Fisher, AG: Mind-brain-body relationships. In Fisher, AG, Murray, EA, and Bundy, AC (eds): Sensory Integration: Theory and Practice. FA Davis, Philadelphia, 1991.
14. King, LJ: A sensory-integrative approach to schizophrenia. Am J Occup Ther 28:529, 1974.
15. Murray, EA: Hemispheric specialization. In Fisher, AG, Murray, EA, and Bundy, AC (eds): Sensory Integration: Theory and Practice. FA Davis, Philadelphia, 1991.
16. Ottenbacher, K: Sensory integration therapy: Affect or effect? Am J Occup Ther 36:571, 1982.
17. Ottenbacher, K: Research in sensory integration: Empirical perceptions and progress. In Fisher, AG. Murray, EA, and Bundy, AC (eds): Sensory Integration: Theory and Practice. FA Davis, Philadelphia, 1991.
18. Pratt, PN, Florey, LA, and Clark, F: Developmental principles and theories. In Pratt, PN, and Allen, AS (eds): Occupational Therapy for Children. CV Mosby, St. Louis, 1989.
19. Royeen, CB, and Lane, SJ: Tactile processing and sensory defensiveness. In Fisher, AG, Murray, EA, and Bundy, AC (eds): Sensory Integration: Theory and Practice. FA Davis, Philadelphia, 1991.
20. Robichaud, L. Hebért, R, and Derosiers, J: Efficacy of a sensory integration program on behaviors of inpatients with dementia. Am J Occup Ther 48, 355–360, 1993.
21. Tickle-Degnen, L: Perspectives on the status of sensory integration theory. Am J Occup Ther 42:427, 1988.

CHAPTER 13

THE SPATIOTEMPORAL ADAPTATION MODEL

The spatiotemporal adaptation model, originally proposed by Gilfoyle, Grady, and Moore,[3] is based on the concept "that a person's developmental course is influenced by environmental experiences of movement and activity."[1] The model was introduced in a 1981 text and elaborated in a chapter in *Willard and Spackman's Occupational Therapy*.[1] A revised version was proposed in a recent second edition of the original text.[2] The authors indicate that the theory of spatiotemporal adaptation grew out of systematic observations of how normal children learn motor skills and how developmentally delayed or disabled children deviate from this process.[2]

The model stresses the importance of movement and movement-based abilities in the process of adaptation to the environment. The concept of spatiotemporal adaptation refers to the "process of adjusting basic posture and movement sequences to the gravitational demands of space and the temporal demands of timing movements."[3]

Interdisciplinary Base

The primary basis of this model is developmental theory, especially as it describes the emergence of motor behaviors. There is strong emphasis on the neurological underpinnings of development and on ecological factors in the development of motor behavior. The model also borrows concepts from theories of stress and its influence on adaptation. The most recent presentation of the model reflects influence from occupational therapy literature, especially that pertaining to childhood play.

Theoretical Arguments

The authors point out that movement provides the experiences from which the child comes to know objects in the environment and establish relationships with others. Movement is fundamental not only to physical maturation but also to psychological and social development. Play is recognized as the primary vehicle through which children engage in motor behavior and facilitate their own development.[1,2] The model emphasizes the developmental nature of motor skill acquisition. Further, it proposes that there is a dynamic relationship among central nervous system (CNS) maturation, the child's behavior, the environment, and the course of development.

This model views maturation of the CNS as a function of both innate programming for development and the child's purposeful behavior or play. Together, they are synergistic forces shaping development. Spatiotemporal adaptation is explained as an interactive and dynamic process, driven by both the maturing nervous system and the child's constant interaction with the environment. The emergence of new motor and play behaviors both depends upon and results in changes in the nervous system.

The environment provides challenges in the form of opportunities for purposeful behaviors. These challenges produce stress. When the child is able to respond to this stress with adaptive behaviors, the maturational process is facilitated. Play, the child's primary means of responding to the environment, exists and changes in concert with the developmental process: "the nature of play changes with the child and the child changes as result of play experiences."[1]

Order

The spatiotemporal adaptation model is explained in terms of systems concepts. The proposed relationship between biological structure and ongoing function embraces the systems emphasis on the importance of process over structure.

> Although life begins with certain neurological and anatomical structures, these structures do not determine functioning. The structures may inhibit or facilitate motor activity, but the child's interaction with the environment accounts for the development of the functional performance.[1]

The authors conceptualize development as an ever-widening spiral represented in the child's mastery of an ever-increasing range of skills and interaction, with a larger and larger orbit of environmental situations. The child's transitions from simple to increasingly complex and mature motor behavior is a central concern of the spatiotemporal adaptation model. In this regard the authors have observed of the developing child that:

> By attempting activities that appeared to be beyond their adaptive competence, children seemingly related components from previous behaviors to requirements of a new challenge, differentiated those components needed for the new activity, and adapted them to develop a more mature approach. Through this adaptation process, children used the challenging situations and adapted by "calling forth" their already developed capabilities to gain competence in movement patterns required for more difficult tasks.[2]

In elaborating how this process takes place, the authors have introduced four interrelated key variables:

1. Movement
2. Environment
3. Adaptation
4. Spiraling continuum

Movement. The authors note that the potentials for patterns of movement are provided by the structure of the musculoskeletal system. However, purpose provides the context for achieving movement; and which movement patterns are selected, used, and learned depends on the purposes to which children direct movement.[2] Over time, learned patterns of functional movement become automatic, allowing the child to direct conscious attention toward higher-level purposes. This process allows further shaping of other movement patterns toward accomplishing new objectives. The child's drive to be effective in the environment ensures that he or she will continuously employ new purposes, eliciting ever more complex movement patterns, which are adapted to the special objectives and demands of the environment in which the child is performing.

Environment. The child's development is facilitated through intense interaction with the environment. As the authors note, all aspects of development can be affected:

> Through movement and activity, a child acquires abilities to seek and obtain nutrition; to protect self; to perceive self and objects and their relationships; to pursue the world; and to acquire feelings of autonomy and competence. Movement puts the child in relationship with his/her surrounding, and through this relationship, a child can have an effect upon the environment, as well as be affected by the environment. Through this transactional relationship of child and environment, adaptation occurs.[1]

The various properties of the environment provide potentials and challenges for movement and thereby shape the direction of the child's acquisition of motor skills. The environment has four functions:

> The *holding function*, which serves to embed the infant and support the body; the *facilitating function*, which provides the source of stimula-

tion, arousal, intent and motivation to move; the *challenge function*, which helps the child reach higher levels of self's potential; and the *interactive function*, which promotes an interplay between self and the environment.[2]

Motor skill acquisition is ecologically driven, conforming not only to the child's inherent biological apparatus but also to the particular features of the environment toward which the motor behavior is directed.

Adaptation. Central in the framework of Gilfoyle, Grady, and Moore is the concept of *adaptation*. Adaptation is not a passive process of adjusting or coping with environmental demands, but rather an active process of engaging the environment according to one's intentions.[2] Adaptation is defined as "the continuous, ongoing state or act of adjusting those bodily processes required to function within a given space and time."[2] Adaptation includes a sensorimotor-sensory process by which the child links together sensation and motor behavior in the context of ongoing changes in motor abilities. It includes assimilation, accommodation, association, and differentiation processes.

Assimilation is the process of receiving sensory information both from outside (e.g., visual information) and from within (e.g., information about the position of one's body parts). *Accommodation* refers to the process of reacting to the stimulation with some motor action. *Association* occurs when the child relates sensory information to the motor action and when the child recalls previous motor actions for use in present situations. *Differentiation* is manifest when the child modifies behavior in an activity by distinguishing what motor behaviors are and are not required in a particular situation. Finally, *integration* refers to an organizational process wherein the child incorporates old motor action into new motor action and relates sensory input, motor output, and sensory feedback together. Thus, integration refers to the process of organizing together a range of information from past and present experience. The use of the term *sensorimotor-sensory* emphasizes the feedback process, whereby the child receives sensory information as a result of motor action.

The unfolding of adaptation is shaped by the predictable developmental sequence according to which children learn motor skills. While constrained by the developmental sequence, adaptation is still a purposeful process.* Children form their own intentions for action and experience their motor actions as personally meaningful in the context of their own background.

---

*One unique feature of this model is acknowledgment of the interrelated role of personality and motor development. Attention to factors such as personality is generally missing in explanations of motor development. Hence, it is a strength of this model to have acknowledged that personality and motor behavior codevelop. However, the concept of personality and how it develops and interrelates with motor development is not well developed. Hence, this is an area in which this model could expand significantly.

Spiraling Continuum. Spatiotemporal adaptation is conceptualized as a spiraling process (beginning with fetal adaptations and continuing throughout development) in which lower-level postures and movements become integrated into more developmentally mature, higher-level behaviors (Fig. 13–1). Thus, the model emphasizes the integration of old behaviors with new behaviors, which build upon the former. The spiral includes the four processes of assimilation, accommodation, association, and differentiation that lead to spatiotemporal adaptation. The spiral also involves the processes of sensory input, output, and feedback. Finally, the environment calls forth higher-level functions, thus shaping the spatiotemporal adaptation process.

Four principles characterize the *spiraling continuum.* First, the way in which a child adapts to new experiences depends on previously acquired motor behavior. Second, when previously acquired behaviors are inte-

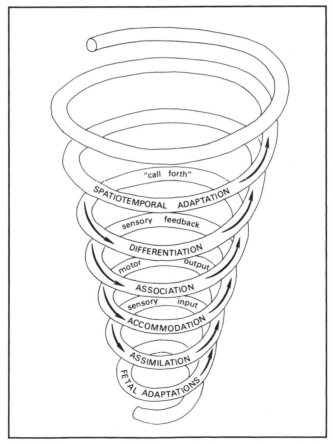

Figure 13–1. Spiraling continuum of spatiotemporal adaptation. (From Gilfoyle and Grady,[2] p 22, with permission.)

grated with present experiences, the former are modified, resulting in more complex behavior. Third, as the child integrates more mature behaviors, the maturity of behaviors acquired earlier is increased. Fourth, when environmental demands exceed the child's functional capacity, he or she will respond by reverting to lower-level functions. These, in turn, are modified to deal with the new challenge and result in new higher-level behaviors.[2]

Within the framework of the spiraling continuum, the authors provide an analysis of the development of:

1. Basic posture and movement strategies
2. Purposeful behaviors (creeping, sitting, rolling, and standing/walking)
3. Activities and skill, particularly as they involve the use of the hands

The spatiotemporal spiral is used as a framework for examining each of these developmental sequences. In each area of concern, the authors illustrate the sequential development by which more primitive motor behaviors become successively integrated into higher-level, more complex behaviors.

The authors also discuss the development of personality as a process in which more basic, primitive elements are successively integrated into higher levels. This development of the "self" begins with primitive awareness of one's body and extends up through the creation of a personal identity. The personality element provides a context, or a holistic viewpoint, from which to view motor behavior.[1]

Purposeful Sequences. The authors argue that adaptation depends on the child's attention to and active participation in purposeful events that provide meaningful experiences. Purposeful sequences are:

> directed toward goals outside the body or to events/occupations within the environment; thus, they are environment centered and motivated by the value to do something in relation to the environment.[2]

Only in the context of engaging in such self-directed, purposeful behavior will the child exhibit the higher-level adaptive responses that enable the maturational process. These higher-level responses become possible when the child builds upon and modifies previously acquired motor behaviors, adapting them to new purposes and challenges in the environment; that is, the child learns to adapt posture and movement strategies to other purposeful activities. Moreover, in so doing, the child is able to associate past and present sensory and motor experiences and to differentiate which motor behaviors work best in particular situations. Thus, the child's experience of purpose and meaning in motor action is central to the developmental process. Embedded in this view of purposeful activity is the thesis that lower-level, subcortical (unconscious) control of motor behavior is best organized when the higher-level, cortical (conscious) attention is directed to the purpose of an activity. In this way the lower-level, subcortical control is integrated and shaped toward the higher-level purposes being pursued.

In the current presentation of the model, occupation is proposed to be the "intervening variable for facilitating 'purpose' for adaptation of performance skills."[2] Occupation is recognized as the vehicle through which purpose is elicited. In children, the primary form of occupation is play. Thus, play is the context of purposeful action in childhood that facilitates the spatiotemporal adaptation process.

Phases of Development. The spiral process of spatiotemporal adaptation occurs in primitive, transitional, and mature phases of development. Each aspect of motor development goes through these stages of development. Since motor development occurs throughout body segments and in different domains of motor behavior, these phases are concurrent and overlapping.

The *primitive phase of development* constitutes the first several months of life. During this phase, movement patterns are undifferentiated and controlled by reflexes and external environmental conditions. The *transitional phase of development* begins a few months after birth and extends until the child has acquired mature movement patterns and skills. During the transitional phase, reflexes are being modified and strategies of movement are being differentiated. Transitional strategies allow the child to be in control of behavior, while not yet employing fully developed capacities. The performance of children during the transitional phase lacks the quality and efficiency of mature behavior and often requires children to work harder to accomplish the more complex tasks they are mastering.[2] The *mature phase of development* is characterized by the integration of automatic reactions into deliberate motor behavior. Behaviors have been differentiated so that appropriate and efficient movement occurs in the context of purposeful activity.

Stress. The environment presents situations that *stress* the child in positive ways. Environmental demands evoke the child's acquired strategies and behaviors as the child seeks to cope with the environment while pursuing purposes. However, when these learned ways of responding to the environment do not work, the child experiences stress. When such stress evokes higher-level functions, it is only temporary and results in further development. As such, stress is essential to development.

Disorder

The source of spatiotemporal dysfunction is damage to the CNS. However, the model focuses on what happens when this damage interferes with the spiral adaptation process. Nervous system damage disorganizes performance. Without the child's active performance in purposeful activities, the nervous system is deprived of the dynamic that facilitates development. Instead of making use of challenges in the environment, children may chronically employ primitive patterns of motor behavior as a way of interacting with the environment. This effectively shuts down the spatiotemporal adaptation process.[2]

Distress and Maladaptation. Damage to the CNS affects the spatiotemporal adaptation process. Due to impairments or limitations that such damage imposes, the child experiences distress in response to ordinary environmental challenges. *Distress* interferes with all aspects of adaptation. For example, the child may experience abnormal assimilation, such as sensory deprivation or overload. Distress also may affect accommodation and association. The child is then unable to use learned behavioral responses or to adapt those behavioral responses to sensory information and to environmental circumstances. Further, the child is unable to initiate new responses to environmental demands, negating the processes of differentiation and integration.

Normal children experiencing stress frequently resolve the problems encountered by trying to accomplish their goal in different ways. By modifying their approach to the problem, children expand their repertoire of solutions to particular types of problems. Ultimately, these children develop more mature, higher-level functions, which serve more challenging purposes.

Children with developmental problems are not so fortunate.[1] These children are often unable to move to higher levels of development because they do not adapt the old patterns of behavior to new stressful situations. Rather, these children may persist in the use of primitive functions or try to use lower-level functions to achieve higher-level activities. The persistence of nonadaptive strategies on the part of the child interferes with the spiral adaptation process. The child's persistence with purposeless lower-level performances leads to regression and ultimately produces developmental delay. So long as the child experiences distress, he or she will be unable to adapt lower-level behaviors to environmental demands, and higher-level behaviors will not emerge. Spatiotemporal distress affects all aspects of the child. It is manifest in a poverty, distortion, or absence of the sensorimotor and play behaviors ordinarily present at each developmental level.

Therapeutic Intervention

The view of therapeutic intervention is grounded in the concept of neuroplasticity. Plasticity refers to the nervous system's ability to undergo modification, particularly as a result of sensorimotor experiences. As the authors note, "The developing nervous system has capacity to compensate for impairments by forming new connections during the early periods of maturation."[3]

The normal process of maturation depends on the child's active participation in purposeful play in the environment. Therapy seeks to evoke this process by directing the child's attention and effort toward play activities that are purposeful for the child. To this end, the therapist structures both the environment and the child to provide opportunities in which the child can attend and participate without experiencing distress. This means that: (1) The child must be put in the optimal state (i.e., physically and emotionally prepared) to respond to the environment, and (2) The environmental challenges must be within the range of the child's abilities. When these conditions are created, the therapist elicits the spatiotemporal adaptation process, which the child enacts through purposeful behavior.

Purposeful activities are the core of the therapeutic process because they direct the child's attention toward the purpose or goal. This allows lower-level capacities to be integrated and adapted to higher-level functioning. Since play is the major purposeful activity of the child, "therapeutic use of purposeful play activities ordinarily sought by children is the occupational therapist's medium."[1]

The therapist supports the spatiotemporal adaptation process by making sure that the child receives appropriate sensory input and engages in adaptive motor output, thereby generating an adaptive sensory feedback. This process "enhances previously unresponsive brain cells, influences neural organization, establishes new engrams, thus facilitating maturation."[3]

The authors note that the expected therapeutic effect depends on what changes the child can bring forth. Unless the child is actively adapting action and activity, change will not occur. Thus it is critical that therapists guide the ongoing process vigilantly so that children generate meaningful experiences and create their own playful intentions for action.

The authors recognize that many children will have permanent limitations of capacity; in all cases, the aim of therapy is to help each child reach his or her highest potential. Therapy must consider the child's unique traits (both strengths and limitations) and should be based on realistic expectations for outcomes given the child's condition. The authors characterize the goals of intervention as prevention, remediation, or adjustment to dysfunction, as appropriate to each particular individual.[1]

Technology for Application

The model is not designed to provide a structured formula or "step-by-step" program of therapy.[2] The authors note that because each individual is unique, an individualized program of therapy is required. Further, they view the model as a system for organizing a variety of treatment techniques for application to an individual's needs.[2]

Assessment

While the authors offer no assessment tools that are particular to this model of practice, they do recommend appropriate assessment procedures. These include review of past data; interviews with the family, the child, and significant others; collecting a developmental and occupational performance history, using standardized and nonstandardized evaluations, and making clinical observations.

Treatment: Using the Spiral Process

The authors note that the spiral process provides principles to be followed in therapy. These principles are as follows:

1. The therapeutic environment should be organized to challenge the child to use existing and emerging capacities.
2. Environmental demands must complement the child's potential in order to allow success.
3. The child must be allowed and supported to guide and direct his or her own actions.
4. The child should be emotionally involved in the activity since the child's interest in activity influences his/her awareness of feedback.
5. Newly learned capacities should be repeated in order to assure their integration.

The authors point out that while the therapeutic process is developmental, it does not imply that in therapy a particular behavior or activity should be perfected before going to the next developmental behavior. Rather, overlap of learning performance is normal and should be allowed in therapy. They also point out that the therapy is not envisioned as recapitulating the normal developmental process. Rather, the special abilities and limitations of the child and the nature of his or her own progress through therapy should guide the sequence of learning, along with consideration of the normal developmental sequences.

Modes of Therapeutic Action. The authors identify three modes of therapeutic action. These are preparation, facilitation, and adaptation. *Preparation* includes preparing both the child and the external environment. Preparation of the child might include "enhancing neuronal and muscular functions for their readiness and use as posture and movement strategies."[2] It might also entail procedures done to the child, such as those that normalize postural tone or increase range of motion. External preparation involves readying the environment to elicit the appropriate purposeful behaviors from the child. *Facilitation* refers to "successive application of the necessary stimulus and/or assistance given to elicit an adaptive response."[2] It includes any of a multitude of ways in which an activity may be presented or changed (e.g., the position of the child or the presentation of tasks or objects). *Adaptation* refers to the process by which the child is challenged to organize his or her behaviors to environmental requirements, this involves the positive use of spatiotemporal stress.

Research

This model has not yet resulted in unique research to examine the theoretical arguments or the efficacy of intervention based on it.

Discussion

The strength of this model is the theoretical organization of information. The authors clearly present a framework for thinking about the normal process of spatiotemporal adaptation, how dysfunction in this process occurs, and how intervention can be done. This theoretical argument has been consistently developed and expanded to include relevant new information. While there is overlap between this model and the motor control and sensory integration models, the authors' different level of analysis makes this model potentially complementary to those others. On the other hand, the theoretical arguments of this model need to be updated in light of more recent concepts of motor control and related systems.

Another strength of this model is the way it delineates the role of occupational therapists in pediatric practice. Occupational therapy is recognized as "facilitating the adaptation of posture and movement strategies to purposeful activities through the active participation toward environmental-centered goals."[3] Specific goals include such behaviors as eating, coloring, and playing ball. The authors have articulated how occupational behavior is the dynamic medium through which children can be helped to achieve greater competence in their motor behavior.

Although the model is not intended as a recipe and should be used as a framework for deciding assessment and intervention, the utility of the model would be enhanced if more explicit applications were developed. In their most recent book, Gilfoyle, Grady, and Moore[3] refer to the use of technology (e.g., technologically adapted toys) that gives children with motor problems more access to environmental interactions. This brief section hints at one potential application of this model; that is, the spatiotemporal adaptation model could serve as a theoretical and practical framework for choosing and using rehabilitation technology to allow children with motor limitations to engage in play and thus support the spatiotemporal adaptation process. This is just one example of how more specific applications could be developed.

If this model gains support from a unique configuration of assessment and intervention strategies specifically derived from its theoretical arguments, it should develop into a robust treatment model. Conversely, if such technology is not developed, therapists may find it difficult to use this model in practice, and its value as a conceptual model of practice should be questioned. This is not to suggest that the model cannot prescribe the use of assessments and procedures indigenous to other models of practice or other theoretical approaches outside the field. However, if it continues to rely heavily on assessments and interventions based on other models and on related knowledge, it is less likely to be helpful for therapists as a separate treatment model. Moreover, since this model does provide a unique view of the process of developing motor skills through occupation, assessment procedures could be developed that reflect these unique tenets.

This model is not currently supported by a research base, except for the neurological, motor learning, and other interdisciplinary concepts that make up the interdisciplinary base of this model. Certainly, research could be developed to test the theoretical arguments of spatiotemporal adaptation, to develop assessment tools, and to test the efficacy of intervention based on the spatiotemporal model.

In conclusion, this model has some important strengths and weaknesses. While the theoretical arguments of this model are unique and relevant, neither research nor a technology for application have been pursued. These latter elements are critical to the utility and credibility of a conceptual model of practice and must be developed if this model is to remain in the mainstream of occupational therapy.

TERMS OF THE MODEL

accommodation	The process of reacting to stimulation with some motor action.
adaptation	The continuous, ongoing state or act of adjusting those bodily processes required to function within a given space and time; also refers to the therapeutic process by which the child is challenged to organize his or her behaviors to environmental requirements.
assimilation	The process of receiving sensory information both from outside and from within.
association	The process of relating sensory information to the motor action and recalling previous motor actions for use in present situations.
challenge function	One purpose of the environment: the promotion of self-growth.
differentiation	The process of modifying behavior in an activity by distinguishing those motor behaviors that are required in a particular situation.
distress	Excessive environmental demands that interfere with the child's adaptation.
facilitating function	One purpose of the environment: to stimulate, arouse, and provide motivation to move.
facilitation	Providing external stimulation to create a state of excitation in the nervous system.
holding function	One purpose of the environment: to provide support.
integration	An organizational process wherein a child incorporates old motor action into new motor action and relates sensory input, motor output, and sensory feedback to each other.
interactive function	One purpose of the environment: to promote interaction.
mature phase of development	Last phase of motor development in which automatic reactions are integrated into deliberate motor behavior.

preparation	Readying both the child and the external environment for movement.
primitive phase of development	Early phase of motor development (i.e., first months of life) in which movement patterns are undifferentiated and controlled by reflexes and the environment.
purposeful activities	Tasks that promote maturation of the nervous system.
purposeful behavior	Body-centered actions that promote maturation of the nervous system.
purposeful sequences	Integration of normal developmental sequences with events in the environment.
sensorimotor-sensory	Refers to sensory information that results from motor action.
spiraling continuum	Continual process involving the integration of primitive, lower-level skills into mature, complex skills.
stress	Refers to environmental demands that the child must cope with while pursuing purposes.
transitional phase of development	Second phase of motor development in which reflexes are modified and movement patterns start to become differentiated.

SUMMARY

Spatiotemporal Adaptation

FOCUS

- Developmental course as influenced by maturing nervous system and environmental experiences of movement and activity in play
- Purposeful movement as a foundation for knowing self and objects in the environment, and forming relationships with others

INTERDISCIPLINARY BASE

- Developmental and neurological theories pertaining to the emergence of motor behaviors
- Theories of stress

THEORETICAL ARGUMENTS

Order

- The child's interaction with environment shapes development.
- Adaptation:
  - Is a process of engaging the environment according to one's intentions
  - Involves a continuous, ongoing state or act of adjusting those bodily processes required to function within a given space and time
- Development is an ever-widening spiral corresponding to mastery of an increasing range of skills.
- Positive environmental stress evokes higher-level functions.
- Motor skill acquisition:
  - Follows a predictable developmental sequence, thus shaping the unfolding of adaptation
  - Develops through primitive, transitional, and mature phases
  - Conforms not only to the child's inherent biological apparatus, but also to the particular features of the environment
- Increasingly complex and mature motor behavior emerges by relating, differentiating, and adapting components from previous behaviors to requirements of a new challenge.
- Underlying motor skill acquisition is a sensorimotor-sensory process that links together sensation and motor behavior and includes assimilation, accommodation, association, and differentiation processes.
- Purpose provides the context for achieving movement and influences what movement patterns are selected, used, and learned.
- The child's drive to be effective results in the constant emergence of new purposes, eliciting ever more complex movement patterns.

- Occupation is the context in which purposes are formed and in which motor performance is shaped.
- As learned patterns of functional movement become automatic, the child can direct conscious intention toward higher-level purposes.

Disorder

- Damage to the nervous system may preclude active performance in purposeful activities and deprive the nervous system of the basic dynamic that facilitates development.
- In children who employ primitive patterns of motor behavior and engage in purposeless, lower-level performances, the spatiotemporal adaptation process shuts down: this produces developmental delay.
- When children are overstressed and unable to adapt lower-level behaviors to environmental demands, higher-level behaviors do not emerge.

Therapeutic Intervention

- The child's brain has the ability to undergo modification (i.e., neuroplasticity) as a result of sensorimotor experiences that enhance the response of previously unresponsive brain cells, influence neural organization, and establish motor engrams.
- The environment and the child can be structured to promote "purposefulness" so that the child attends to and actively participates in purposeful activity in the environment without distress.
- When a child receives appropriate sensory input, engages in adaptive motor output, and generates feedback, adaptive sensory feedback brain organization occurs and new motor skills can be acquired.
- Therapy must consider the child's unique traits (both strengths and limitations) and realistic expectations for outcomes given the child's condition.
- Intervention can be directed toward goals of prevention, (re)mediation, and/or adjustment to dysfunction.

TECHNOLOGY FOR APPLICATION

- No unique assessments have been developed.
- Interviews, developmental and performance histories, standardized and nonstandardized evaluations, and clinical observations are recommended.
- A structured formula is not proposed: but rather a system by which a variety of treatment techniques can be applied to meet individual needs.
- This approach recommends an individualized program of therapy geared to special abilities and limitations of the child and the nature of his/her own progress through therapy.
- Therapeutic principles include:
  - Environmental challenge complimentary to child's potential

- ○ Emotional involvement of child who must guide and direct action in therapy
  - ○ Opportunity to repeat and integrate newly learned capacities
- Three modes of therapeutic action include:
  - ○ Preparation of child and environment
  - ○ Facilitation (i.e., application of necessary stimuli)
  - ○ Adaptation (i.e., requiring the child to organize behaviors to environmental requirements)

RESEARCH

- No research unique to the model has been reported.

References

1. Gilfoyle, EM, and Grady, AP: Occupational therapy with children—Spatiotemporal adaptation. In Hopkins, HL, and Smith, ND (eds): Willard and Spackman's Occupational Therapy. Lippincott, Philadelphia, 1983, pp 459, 548, 550, 551, 562.
2. Gilfoyle, EM, and Grady, AP: Children Adapt, ed 2. Slack, Thorofare, NJ, 1990, pp 14, 19, 20, 193, 261.
3. Gilfoyle, EM, Grady, AP, and Moore, J: Children Adapt. Slack, Thorofare, NJ, 1981, pp 3, 211, 215, 216.

CHAPTER 14

CONCEPTUAL MODELS OF PRACTICE: THE STATE OF THE ART

I n the first part of this book I argued that the field's paradigm serves as a cultural and conceptual context within which models of practice are developed. The paradigm addresses universals in the field, while models deal with particular phenomena, elaborating the vision provided by the paradigm. The goal of this chapter is to make some observations concerning the state of the art of occupational therapy's conceptual models of practice and their relationship to the paradigm. These observations should serve as a starting point for further critical thought and analysis.

Influences of the Paradigm on the Theoretical Arguments of Models

In Chapter 4, I argued that the field's emerging paradigm includes three core constructs defining occupation as:

1. Part of human nature
2. An aspect of life that may become dysfunctional
3. A therapeutic agent

Moreover, the paradigm reflects a holistic and systemic viewpoint and embraces humanistic values that extoll the experiential and interpersonal dimensions of life. These elements are being articulated as part of a still-emerging paradigm. Moreover, this paradigm replaces a previous mechanistic paradigm, which articulated mechanistic concepts and a reductionist scientific viewpoint and values. Since the field's paradigm has undergone transformation, one expects that conceptual practice models will have shown changes that follow the direction of the new paradigm.

From a Mechanistic to a Systemic Viewpoint

Several conceptual practice models have their roots in the earlier, mechanistic paradigm described in Chapter 3. Examination of these models reveals that they have undergone transformation as the paradigms' viewpoint changed from mechanistic to systemic. The biomechanical model was first grounded in the mechanistic concern for the inner workings of the musculoskeletal system. Similarly, the cognitive-perceptual, sensory integration, and motor control models were originally based on a more mechanistic conceptualization of the central nervous system (CNS). Earlier articulations of these models achieved a view of the human musculoskeletal and neurological systems as fixed structures that determined or caused such functions as motion, cognition, and coordinated movement.

According to the mechanistic formulation, performance is a direct consequence of the inner arrangement and organization of the component parts of systems. This viewpoint was expressed, for example, in assertions that joint range of motion, muscle strength, and neural integration are both the necessary and sufficient causes of performance. Older, mechanistically based models assumed that performance would be satisfactory when there was order among the component parts of underlying structure. Concomitantly, disorder was understood to emanate *directly* from disruption and disorganization of the component parts of the musculoskeletal and neurological systems. Consequently, therapeutic intervention was conceptualized as repairing, enhancing, or compensating for deficits in the underlying structure in order to improve performance. The following are representative statements consistent with this perspective:

1. The ability to dress oneself requires a finite amount of strength and cognitive capacity.
2. Inability to dress oneself results when strength or cognition is reduced beyond a critical level.
3. Restoration of impaired strength or condition is both necessary and sufficient to restore dressing ability.

The systemic viewpoint of the emerging paradigm (described in Chapter 4) has lead to a different understanding of occupational performance. This viewpoint is reflected by changes in how models seek to explain movement, motor, and cognitive-perceptual phenomena. For example, the biomechanical, motor control, and cognitive perceptual models now emphasize that performance emanates from a dynamic relationship between the inner system, the environment, and the occupation being performed. These models now express a more complex and dynamic explanation of occupational performance. Similarly, they recognize that disruptions of components of the musculoskeletal and nervous systems are not direct causes of performance limitations. Rather, they recognize that the occupation being performed, the context, and the state of underlying systems interact in complex ways, with performance emerging out of the interaction.

To see more fully how this view differs form the previous mechanistic viewpoint, let us examine how the three statements concerning the relationship of strength and cognition to dressing might be formulated differently. Under the new paradigmatic viewpoint, they might appear as follows:

1. Strength and cognitive capacity contribute to the performance of dressing oneself; this performance is also a function of the occupational form of dressing and of the objects manipulated and other conditions in the environment.
2. When strength or cognition is reduced, the way in which factors come together in the dynamic process of performance may be altered if either of these variables changes sufficiently; this alternation may be manifest in changes and/or difficulties in the performance of dressing. Under different circumstances difficulty in dressing may be absent, present, or manifest to different degrees.
3. To the extent strength or condition can be repaired, the original pattern of dressing performance may be reinstated; alterations in the occupational form and or environment may be adequate to restore a functional dressing performance. Moreover, alterations in all these factors may, to some extent, be helpful or necessary to achieving functional dressing performance.

What should be obvious about this second set of statements is that they allow for a more complex and conditional view of what factors affect performance. They also offer a more open set of possibilities for how problems of performance can be addressed. Moreover, they conceptualize change (either change from a functional to a dysfunctional state or change from a dysfunctional to a functional state) as more than a simple linear relationship between two different factors (e.g., cognition and dressing). Both kinds of change involve a reordering of the total dynamics in which performance is embedded.*

---

*The importance of this way of understanding the complexity of factors involved in performance was brought home to me in a very personal way during the writing of this text. I suffered a herniation of the lumbar 3–4 disk with subsequent nerve compression, severe pain, and atrophy of the knee extensors. Surgery successfully relieved the pressure on the nerve, but my everyday routines were altered in a number of ways that were quite dynamic and context-dependent. Following surgery, I discovered that it was too painful for me to bend over to tie my shoes. On different days I achieved different solutions to the problem. One obvious solution was to substitute slip-on shoes (changing the objects used in dressing). However, when I dressed for work (a different

The systemic viewpoint is also found in newer models, such as the model of human occupation and the sensory integration model. While models differ in the extent to which systems concepts are incorporated and in the specific systems conceptualizations they employ, there is a clear trend across most models toward the systemic viewpoint expressed in the field's emerging paradigm. This transformation points out that authors of different models recognize the systemic viewpoint as something transcending the specific concerns and applications of a given model. When models give expression to the systemic viewpoint in their theoretical arguments, they affirm it as an generic paradigmatic viewpoint.* Hence the relationship between the paradigm and models of practice is one of mutual influence.

---

occupational form than dressing for home) I only had shoes that required tying. I discovered that it was possible for me to remain standing and raise one leg at a time to the top of the bed; this way I reduced the back flexion that occurred when I tied my shoes in my usual way, that is, bending over while sitting in a chair. This, of course, is a modification of the method of accomplishing the occupational form. I used this solution instead of kneeling down to tie my shoes (a solution that would also have kept my back straight) because the atrophy in my left knee extensors made it difficult to rise from a kneeling to standing position. Moreover, because we have a canopy bed, I could lean against one of the bedposts while raising my leg, which I also lifted with my arms. This assistance made it less likely that I would tilt my pelvis, an action that made me tend to extend my back (which also caused pain). On a couple of occasions when I was rushed to get to the train and my wife was nearby, I asked her to tie my shoes for me.

Hence, I generated different solutions to the task of getting my shoes on, depending on the dynamics of the circumstances. While painless flexion of my back was ordinarily a condition for getting my shoes on, my ability to get them on was in no way directly related to that capacity. As my capacity altered, it was one among many factors that ultimately determined how I achieved the necessary performance. A very interesting feature of all the solutions is that they emerged quite readily and automatically. It was only on reflection that I could say why it was more effective to stand and raise my legs than to kneel. Hence, these solutions were not the result a formal activity analysis and activity modification on my part. Most of the "logic" of my solutions was apparent only upon reflection after the fact.

This fairly automatic "emergence" of solutions was much like what I noted happening to my gait. Under ordinary conditions of walking or climbing stairs I did not have (as far as I was aware of) a limp. However, if I was trying to walk very fast or if I was carrying my briefcase (which is usually loaded with heavy papers, books, and a laptop computer) while climbing stairs, my ambulation/climbing became uneven. I tended to swing myself forward or up with my good leg to add momentum and, when climbing stairs, I would pull on any available rail to assist my weak leg. As the weak leg's remaining knee extensors hypertrophied (the body's solution to regaining the necessary strength to compensate for the atrophied muscle, which was not yet reinnervated), I noted that this tendency for an uneven gait was variable depending on just how fast I was trying to move and how steep was the grade or staircase on which I was walking/climbing. It was quite amazing to see how different solutions to walking and climbing just emerged in the dynamics of the situation.

*Over 20 years ago, in my master's thesis, I undertook an historical analysis of occupational therapy (an analysis that has evolved into Chapter 4 of this book). When I first examined the then-dominant biomechanical, neurological, and intrapsychic approaches of occupational therapy, it seemed that they had little or nothing in common. After struggling to understand how they stood in relation to each other, it eventually occurred to me that these approaches had in common an implicit way of explaining the phenomena they addressed and of thinking about therapy.

The Growing Centrality of Occupation in Models of Practice

Another influence of the paradigm on conceptual models of practice is the increasing centrality of occupation. This focus on occupation is found in two aspects of models. The first is the extent to which occupation is recognized as a factor in human performance. The second is the way in which occupation is viewed as a therapeutic agent.

Occupation as a Factor in Performance. The systemic viewpoint recognizes that order in human performance is not a direct function of a rigid and predetermined order in the underlying systems. Most importantly, occupation is recognized as having a significant role in recruiting the emergent order of performance. In this new perspective, occupation is part of the formula by which competent performance is possible. In the paradigm, this idea has been underscored by the concept of occupational form that was described in Chapter 4.

In a number of models there are examples of this focus on occupation as a factor in performance. The biomechanical and motor control models now argue that the purpose and the dynamic performance requirements of the occupation being performed (i.e., the occupational form) are just as important in determining which movements will be used as the underlying organization of the nervous system, muscles, and joints. The cognitive-perceptual model also includes discussion of the dynamic role that the occupational task plays in eliciting and organizing cognitive and perceptual processes.

The spatiotemporal adaptation model, which originally focused on the centrality of movement in adaptation, now focuses on how adaptation emerges in the context of occupational behavior. While the authors retain their original concern for movement, they now place this focus within the phenomena of occupation. The group work model focuses on the occupa-

---

The more I explored this insight, the more apparent it became that there were two levels of discourse going on in the field. At one level therapists were explaining how the musculoskeletal, nervous, and intrapsychic systems were related to function, as well as how to conduct therapy to address problems related to these systems. A second level of discourse (sometimes implicit, sometimes explicit) addressed more global questions concerning how the field looked upon its problems and methods and, ultimately, upon the nature of occupational therapy. Moreover, it also became apparent that these two discourses (one about the paradigm and the other about models) interwove and influenced each other. Although some of the terminology and ways of discussing the paradigm and models of practice have changed over the years, I am still struck by how this way of thinking about the conceptual foundations of occupational therapy describes a readily observable process of knowledge development.

Moreover, discussions with persons working on other models have reinforced my view that when therapists develop ideas while working on their specific models, they end up contributing ideas for the larger paradigmatic conversation in the field; that is, as authors look to the directions other models are taking for ideas about the directions they should perhaps consider, they end up incorporating paradigmatic constructs and viewpoints. This means that sometimes paradigmatic discourse actually takes place through models. This is why I say that paradigmatic discourse is sometimes implicit.

tional (or task-focused) nature of groups and on how group activities increase a person's occupational potential. This model emphasizes a view of task-oriented groups arguing for the central importance of the occupational behaviors in which group members engage.

The model of human occupation is somewhat unique in that it grew out of the occupational behavior tradition (which, as noted in Chapter 3, was the precursor to the emerging paradigm). Because of its origins, this model has always sought to articulate the centrality of occupation in the field. Nonetheless, it continues to be influenced by the articulation of new themes in core constructs. Examples of paradigmatic influence on this model include its incorporation of the concepts of narrative and occupational form to further articulate the model's explanation of motives and environmental influences.

Occupation as the Dynamic of Therapy. Most conceptual models of practice envision occupation as having the potential to generate change.* Evoking such diverse concepts as self-organization, neuroplasticity, learning, occupational choice, and adaptation, models have asserted that engaging in occupation has the potential to transform or change the human being. Such changes include reorganization of the brain, changes in attitudes, beliefs, and habits, and adoption of different strategies of solving problems.

The understanding of how occupation influences change is being elaborated into a more comprehensive set of arguments. From the mechanistic perspective, occupation was recognized as having therapeutic impact. However, the impact of occupation was understood in terms of narrow influences on discrete structures of the underlying system. For example, if occupation could be modified to elicit a desired movement, actively provide range of motion to a joint, or practice a particular skill, then it was thought to have a therapeutic impact. The goal of such use of occupation was precision in how the occupation was chosen, modified, and directed to have a specific therapeutic impact. Since the underlying structure was considered the sole determinant of how the human being functioned, the occupations needed to be appropriately modified to target the appropriate structure. Therapy changed performance by changing underlying structures. In this approach, whether the occupations were "natural" was not a primary concern. What was important was that they targeted specific underlying structures or provided exercise of specific capacities. This led to the use of "occupations" now considered to be of questionable value, such as stacking cones.[5] It also led to the devaluation of the many occupations previously used in occupational therapy. Such devaluation was manifest in arguments that using "real-life" occupations was too costly or time-consuming.

---

*One exception to this view of therapeutic change is the cognitive disabilities model, which argues that therapists should not make claims that participation in occupation can effect change.

Models have begun to argue that occupation influences the underlying order in human systems in a more complex way than previously thought. In the old view, therapy needed to alter or compensate for the underlying mechanism, which alone determined function. In the new view, occupation recruits, from among the musculoskeletal, neurological, and psychological components of the human being, configurations of action that strive toward the accomplishment of occupation's goals and purposes. Hence, order in the system's function is not solely a matter of the underlying structure of systems but also a function of the organizing influence of the occupational form. This is not to say that occupation does not directly alter underlying structures. However, the therapeutic impact of occupations is more extensive and complex than altering underlying structures.

Because occupation can evoke order among components of systems during performance, it has a more far-reaching capacity for organization or reorganization of function than previously recognized. Occupation serves as a context in which new order emerges among components of systems (even components that are permanently impaired).

This more complex view of the therapeutic potential of occupation can be found variously across the current formulations of models. One early example of the recognition that occupation provides a holistic context for reorganization is the application of the biomechanical model in work hardening. This approach recognized that therapy aimed at musculoskeletal conditioning for work was most effective when done in the context of the actual occupational forms one performed at work. Additionally, the biomechanical model has begun to articulate a more holistic view of occupational impact in its consideration of how occupational interest or meaning affect such factors as effort and fatigue.

The motor control model has begun to offer a sophisticated argument about the role of occupational forms in influencing the quality of movement and, by extension, the learning or relearning of functional movement patterns. The model of human occupation stresses that change involves achieving a new order among the subsystems that contribute to everyday occupational performance. It argues that occupations constitute a context in which this reorganization can be achieved. The model also offers a number of principles for change that underscore the complex way in which occupation evokes order and transformation.

This new vision of the therapeutic potential of occupation is only at a first stage of articulation in models of practice. Discourse about how occupation influences the human being and can achieve change has taken on a new direction, and is sure to be elaborated in the future.

Those models that offer new explanations of how occupation can be used as therapy are more complex. However, they offer more precision in understanding the nature of therapeutic change. Indeed, some of the disagreement about whether change is possible (see, e.g., the cognitive disabilities discussion in Chapter 7) is due to a misunderstanding of what is meant by change. Models espousing a more complex view of change recognize that the impairments that can exist in discrete structures and functions (e.g., damage to the musculoskeletal or nervous system, and deficits of motion, memory, and cognition) are not the sole determinants of occupational performance. Moreover, they also recognize that humans are complex self-organizing systems that can find and establish new orders among their (even dysfunctional) elements.

When models assume that changes in function require commensurate changes in underlying structures, they can only conceptualize therapeutic change in narrow terms. For example, if it is assumed that a neat linear relationship exists between brain status, cognition, and occupational performance, then it follows that cognition varies only as a function of brain change and performance as a function of cognitive change. The neatness of such a schema does not correspond with reality. As contributors to the cognitive-perceptual model point out, a particular cognitively related performance problem may be present in some occupational forms and contexts and not in others. Performance is an emergent phenomena that depends on the state of the brain, the occupational form, and the features of the environment. Performance is not a fixed and invariant function of cognition, nor is cognition a fixed and invariant function of the brain. Moreover the potential for change is embedded in the relation between all these elements. Both changes in discrete elements and in the relationship between elements are best achieved in an organizing context of occupation. Choosing the right therapeutic occupation means more than matching it to a presumed amount of cognitive or other deficit. It means, instead, finding out how performance varies across different circumstances and in different occupations and how optimal solutions for the reorganization of behavior can be achieved. Models that recognize humans as complex dynamical systems envision a much wider range of possibilities for the therapeutic use of occupation to achieve change.

Phenomena Addressed by Models

On the surface, conceptual models of practice are each about different things. After all, one model addresses the biomechanics of movement, while another addresses perception. Still others address motivation, lifestyle, and group dynamics. Hence, when all the models discussed in previous chapters are considered together, it becomes apparent that occupational therapy's theory and practice address a wide range of phenomena. To a significant degree this is why occupational therapists tend to think of their practice as holistic.

While the range of available models is an asset to therapists, the diversity of models presents a challenge. The therapist must determine which models to select and how to combine these models in practice. Toward this end, it is useful to consider the intellectual territory that is covered by the respective conceptual practice models. In Chapter 4, I noted that occupational therapy's paradigm called attention to biological, psychological, and sociocultural phenomena. The levels of phenomena addressed by each of the conceptual models of practice are shown in Figure 14–1. The biomechanical model is primarily focused at the biological level (i.e., concern for the musculoskeletal system). The cognitive disabilities model describes processes mainly at the psychological level. The cognitive-perceptual and motor control models describe those processes that span both psychological and the biological levels. The sensory integration model (which focuses primarily on lower brain functions) is aimed primarily at the biological level (i.e., how the brain processes sensory information). The spatiotemporal adaptation model is concerned with the biological level (i.e., development of motor capacity as influenced by the central nervous system) and the psychological level (as manifest in such themes as purpose and meaning). The group work model and model of human occupation are concerned with the personal and sociocultural levels, although the emphasis of each is different. The model of human occupation emphasizes the personal level, and the group work model emphasizes the sociocultural level.

From this simple mapping of conceptual models of practice, it is clear that each model addresses particular levels of phenomena and has a particular focus. Taken together, the models address the range of phenomena of concern to the field. However, no single model addresses the whole range of phenomena.

One readily concludes from this observation that, in practice, therapists must combine models in order to address the full range of phenomena with which the field is concerned. Models are rarely sufficient, of themselves, to provide a holistic approach to practice or a comprehensive understanding of the range of problems that should be addressed in therapy.

Technology for Application in Models

The models of practice discussed in the previous chapters vary in the degree to which they have developed a technology for application. Several models have assessment procedures and instruments, protocols for intervention, and useful case exemplars and program applications. Models that lack such technology are more difficult to apply. Moreover, such models are open to a loose or vague application. Hence, they may be employed without systematic reflection on the relationship between a model's theoretical arguments and how one puts them into practice.

Area of Focus	Phenomena of Concern	MODELS
Socio-cultural	Culture, Groups	Model of Human Occupation; Spatio-Temporal Adaption
Psychological	Motivation, Cognition, Perception	Group Work Model; Cognitive Disabilities Model; Cognitive Perceptual Model; Model of Human Occupation
Biological	Motion, Coordinated Movement	Biomechanical Model; Model of Human Occupation; Sensory Integration Model; Motor Control Model

Figure 14–1. Foci and phenomena addressed by conceptual models of practice.

Ideally, models of practice should provide technology that allows them to be applied in a disciplined way. This means that therapists should have understanding and confidence that they are employing methods and approaches that reflect the theoretical arguments of the model. Only when there is a systematic relationship between the theoretical arguments of a model and its application in practice can a useful dialogue between theory and practice occur. Such a dialogue requires two things. First, therapists must find meaningful guidance in the concepts and arguments of a model. Second, the application of concepts and arguments in practice must provide a forum for examination and critique of the models. When the connection is weak between the theory of a model and application in practice, then both the development of the model and the quality of practice suffer.

The connection between theory and application is not served unless therapists are challenged to actively think in the midst of practice. The most useful technology for application provides therapists with methods for actively engaging in the use of theory. Methods that can be carried out automatically, requiring little or no thought, add nothing to the dialogue between theory and application.

As conceptual models of practice become more systems-based and embrace more complex explanations of occupational behavior, therapists will be challenged to think more actively about their practice. Systemic thinking requires therapists to develop their intervention approaches from an theory-based understanding of the particular client. Such understanding must be actively generated by applying abstract theoretical concepts to a client's particular situation. Hence, dialectical thinking is required to move between abstract concepts and concrete situations, and to find meaningful connections and insights.

It is easier to use a model that gives specific instructions for treatment, requiring little or no judgment. In fact, not giving specific and detailed guidelines for intervention has been criticized as being simply ambiguous. However, therapists must seriously ask whether ready-made solutions for intervention emanate from oversimplified explanations of client function and dysfunction. I argue that therapists should distrust approaches that do not require active reflection on theory and attention to the unique circumstances of the client.

Further Directions for Model Development

In Chapter 5, I argued that a conceptual practice model should have theoretical arguments addressing order and disorder, a technology for application in practice, and research to examine its theory and application. The models discussed in the previous chapters vary in how fully each of these elements are developed. For example, the spatiotemporal adaptation model lacks a research base and a unique technology for application. Moreover, the theoretical arguments of the cognitive-perceptual and motor control models are much more loosely construed in the literature than other models. Nonetheless, models are always in flux. They do not come into existence overnight, and their impact on the field is best measured over time. The ultimate test of each model is the extent to which it is discussed in the profession's literature, reflected in therapists' viewpoints, and operationalized in practice. One must also take a long view on the impact of models in the field. By carefully considering these factors, readers of this text can and should draw their own conclusions about the relative merit of each model.

There are also indications that new models of practice will be recognized in the future. One good example is the occupational adaptation approach recently introduced into the literature.[3,4] The authors of this approach seek to explain the interaction between the person and the environment as a process of adaptation. For example, the authors use the concept of "relative mastery" to refer to how effectively a person meets environmental challenges. Like many models of practice discussed in this text, the occupational adaption approach emphasizes the process by which persons enhance their effectiveness and satisfaction though participation in occupations. Hence, it has begun to incorporate themes from the paradigm.

Occupational adaptation appears to be in a formative stage. Two articles have described some of the basic theoretical arguments and how they might be applied to the therapeutic context. Another article has used it as a framework for understanding professional development.[2] If the theoretical arguments are further articulated and a technology for application is developed, this approach will likely become a contemporary conceptual practice model.

The one thing that can be said with certainty is that new models will emerge and some existing models will not survive the test of time. Since models of practice represent the most dynamic arena of knowledge development in the field, constant change is always to be expected and valued.

Conclusion

The field's models constitute the current major theory building and research of occupational therapy. Moreover, they provide the corpus of knowledge unique to the field, and they are capable of guiding the everyday practice of occupational therapists. In the final analysis, occupational therapy practice will only be as valuable as the conceptual models upon which it is based.

The theoretical development of occupational therapy, as reflected in the models, shows a rich array of concepts and arguments. Nonetheless, on the whole, the models are still in early stages of development. Further theoretical clarification, development of technology for application, and research will be needed to augment these models. As current and future conceptual models of practice are refined and operationalized, both the field's conceptual foundations and practice should flourish.

References

1. Allen, CK, and Earhart, CA: Occupational Therapy Treatment Goals for the Physically and Cognitively Disabled. American Occupational Therapy Association, Rockville, MD, 1992.
2. Garret, SA, and Schkade, JK: Occupational adaptation model of professional development as applied to Level II Fieldwork. Am J Occup Ther 49:119–126, 1995.
3. Schkade, JK, and Schultz, S: Occupational adaptation: Toward a holistic approach for contemporary practice, Part 1. Am J Occup Ther 46:829–837, 1992.
4. Schultz, S, and Schkade, JK: Occupational adaptation: Toward a holistic approach for contemporary practice, Part 2. Am J Occup Ther 46:917–925, 1992.
5. Trombly, C: Occupation: Purposefulness and meaningfulness as therapeutic mechanisms. Am J Occup Ther 46:960–975, 1995.

CHAPTER 15

PROFESSIONAL IDENTITY AND COMPETENCE

T his text began with the argument that the field's conceptual foundations provide occupational therapists with identity and competence. The intervening chapters considered the nature of knowledge in the field, the development of the field's paradigm, and the status of its current models of practice. In this chapter, I consider how these conceptual foundations translate into identity and competence.

Professional Identity

Professional identity is founded on the paradigmatic constructs, viewpoint, and values that bind members of a profession together and give the profession a public identity. While each occupational therapist's identity comes from a unique set of personal experiences, it is ultimately shaped by the profession's paradigm.

Historical Challenges to Professional Identity in Occupational Therapy

As we saw in Chapter 3, occupational therapy has struggled with professional identity, especially in association with its second, mechanistic paradigm. Commenting on the lack of clear professional role delineation in occupational therapy two decades ago, O'Shea[12] noted that "instead of assuming a proactive stance in determining the focus of practice, occupational therapists have tended to accept the professional image fashioned by others." Supporting such an assertion, Barris[2] found that occupational therapists who lacked a clear sense of their own identity allowed their work to be defined by their work setting rather than by their profession. Hence, it was not uncommon that therapists developed identities more closely parallel to those of their colleagues from other professions (e.g., physical therapists and psychologists) than those of their counterparts within occupational therapy. Many therapists working with persons who had physical dysfunction adopted pure exercise and physical agents (therapeutic media traditionally used by physical therapists) as prominent features of their practice. Therapists in psychiatric practice often adopted the psychotherapeutic emphasis on talk as a therapeutic medium and stressed the interpersonal relationship over the activity performed (if activity was performed at all). As Barris[2] observed, the process of identity diffusion was further exacerbated in new areas of practice where occupational therapists were:

> discarding their own more familiar and traditional forms of treatment and replacing them with techniques borrowed from physical therapy, gestalt psychology, and social work among others.

Practice across different occupational therapy specialties has been so divergent as to obscure the "common ground" that made all practitioners *occupational* therapists. The gap between specialties was not the only dichotomy associated with the lack of a clear paradigm in the field. Therapists also tended to separate the physical from the psychosocial dimensions of their patients' problems. Occupational therapists found it difficult to bridge concerns with the objective, biomechanical aspects of patients' dysfunction with the issues that inevitably arose from the patients' subjective experiences of disability.[9,15] Along the same lines, therapists working in psychosocial practice tended to ignore the biological dimensions of their patients' problems.[5]

Perhaps the most pervasive impact of this paradigmatic uncertainty is the difficulty therapists have had with their own identity. Over the years, many students and colleagues have shared with me their frustrations in not being able to explain (to themselves, much less others) what their profession was.* Members of a profession without a clear paradigm bear an undue burden in attempting to make sense of their life work.

To be sure, the problem of professional identity is not nearly as acute for occupational therapists today as it was a decade ago. There is an increasing level of discourse concerning what constructs, viewpoint, and values are

---

*In fact, it is fair to say that much of my own work for the past two decades, and particularly the arguments in this book, are the product of a personal search for the identity of occupational therapy, born out of the same kinds of frustration.

central to occupational therapy. As the ideas represented in the paradigm enjoy more universal consensus, there should be increasing clarity about the profession's identity.

Emerging Identity

In Chapter 4, I attempted to characterize the emerging paradigm in occupational therapy. This paradigm, as it is accepted and further articulated by others, will influence individual occupational therapists' understanding of their profession and its role and mission within society. Even more importantly, the paradigm will provide members of the profession with a perspective on the nature of their work (i.e., the aspect of human well-being addressed, the kinds of problems to be solved, and the approach to problem solving). Based on the characterization of the emerging paradigm of the field offered in Chapter 4, I would argue that the emerging identity of occupational therapists might sound something like the following:

The concern of occupational therapy is with the well-being of persons in everyday occupation (i.e., work, play, and daily living tasks). Occupation is a necessary aspect of life, contributing to physical, emotional, and cognitive well-being. Through occupation, individuals achieve a productive relationship to their social environments.

Occupational therapists solve problems that prevent persons from having a satisfying and productive engagement in occupation. These occupational dysfunctions are serious problems that distress and compromise individuals' health and result in lost potential for society. Occupational therapists understand and address the complex biological, psychosocial, and environmental factors that contribute to occupational dysfunction. They are experts in the use of guided participation in occupations to enable people to change, develop, and adapt and thereby enhance their health. Occupational therapists recognize the rights of persons to choose and engage in those occupations that are meaningful for themselves and functional for their environments.

Of course, the preceding is only one expression of occupational therapy's professional identity. Each therapist must formulate a sense of professional identity in personally meaningful terms. This means active and ongoing reflection not only on one's unique experience, but also on the ongoing discourse in one's field. As Fidler[6] notes, "A reexamination of one's frame of reference, one's treatment model or paradigm, and how it is being operationalized should be undertaken periodically."

There is, then, an important balance that must be maintained between the individual as a professional and the profession as a whole. All occupational therapists must envision and enact their own professional identities in personal and unique ways. At the same time there should be universally recognizable features in every occupational therapist's identity.

According to the emerging paradigm discussed in Chapter 4, some essential features of this shared identity are:

1. The concern with occupation in human life
2. The focus on occupational dysfunction as the problem area for practice
3. The use of occupation as a therapeutic agent
4. A holistic viewpoint that encompasses the biopsychosocial aspects of occupation and their systemic interrelationship
5. A humanistic value orientation that recognizes the right of persons to experience themselves as meaningfully occupied and extolls both the intra- and interpersonal dimensions of the therapeutic process

The following example should illustrate the impact on professional identity of these elements of the emerging paradigm. When physicians view a person with arthritis, the professional identity of medicine orients them to the disease process and possibilities for altering its course and immediate physical effects. Thus, physicians recognize in the joint inflammation or deterioration a physiological process with a generally known course, which is sometimes responsive to medication (at least for symptom reduction) and which in advanced cases may require surgical repair or replacement of affected joints. In the end, the anatomical integrity of joints as affected by the physiology of the arthritic disease process is the primary concern of the physician. Physicians seek to limit the effects of the disease on the body and to reduce or eliminate pain. To a large extent, physicians do not need to consider the patient as an individual or be concerned with the patient's subjective experience. Rather, accurate diagnosis depends on recognizing those features of the disease that transcend the individual manifestation of a single case.

Occupational therapists will be primarily concerned with:

1. How movement limitations and pain resulting from the arthritis affect the ability to perform in everyday occupations
2. How performance itself can affect the status of arthritic joints
3. How the impairment affects the ability of the person to engage in those occupations that are necessary and/or meaningful components of everyday life

The occupational therapy focus will be on preserving as much of the patient's occupational life as possible within the constraints and risks imposed by the disease. The occupational therapist will consider how biological, psychosocial, and environmental factors influence adaptation in occupational behavior. Consequently, therapists recognize the need for physical strategies (e.g., splints to protect joints during activity and modification of how activities are done). Together, these strategies reduce biomechanical stress, pain, and fatigue, and maximize the amount and quality of activity possible. Additionally, therapists acknowledge the importance of psychosocial strategies to enable the patient to make lifestyle decisions, set priorities, negotiate roles with others, and pursue the kind of life story he or she wants. Finally, the therapist will use strategies of changing and adapting the physical and sociocultural environment surrounding the individual to enhance occupational functioning. These are all relevant therapeutic strategies for supporting optimally productive and satisfying occupational behavior. They require that therapists come to understand their patients as persons with subjective desires, concerns, and experiences.

In the occupational therapist's perspective, health implies a functional and satisfying occupational life pattern. Identifying and eliminating or mitigating the disease is the primary challenge for a physician. The challenge for the occupational therapist is to detect, understand, and eliminate or reduce occupational dysfunction. The physician will use interventions aimed primarily at altering the course and consequences of the disease. The occupational therapist will employ methods that aim to minimize the impact of disease-related factors on occupational behavior. These methods may seek to alter disease-related states in the individual, but they will also include making adjustments in lifestyle, altering how occupational forms are completed, and modifying the environment.

In contrast to physicians, who rely on their understanding of the universal features of the disease and how it can best be addressed, the occupational therapist will look to the patient's life for the indications of what needs to be addressed. While the physician concentrates on what is similar about this patient's disease course and symptoms, and that of others with the same disease, the occupational therapist focuses on what is unique to this patient's experience of arthritis and its impact on this patient's particular lifestyle. While the physician will employ generically known therapeutics to address the symptoms and disease course, the occupational therapist will need to identify strategies that fit how this patient needs and wants to live. The physician will rely on the patient's respect for medical authority, compliance with prescribed medication, and submission to the advice and recommendations for a course of medical therapy. The occupational therapist must build an alliance based on mutual respect and trust in which the patient has both a right and obligation to collaborate in defining what should be achieved and how it can be accomplished in therapy.

As the example illustrates, differences in professional identity specify different roles and activities of professionals. Such differences are important to persons with disabilities, because they ensure that their complex problems will be addressed from multiple perspectives.

Professional Competence

While a professional identity derived from the paradigm provides the necessary definition of the nature of occupational therapy, practitioners need more to be able to *do* occupational therapy—that is, to think and act as competent therapists. This *competence* is influenced by the field's paradigm, but it also requires the active use of the field's conceptual models of practice.

Thinking with Models

Competence requires that therapists bring the knowledge from models to bear on the problems of their patients or clients. Whatever else occupational therapists do, they must *think with* the conceptual practice models of their field.

But how do therapists employ models? Schon[16] argues that all professional decision making and action begins with a process he calls naming and framing the problem; he explains:

> Problem setting [is] the process by which we define the decision to be made, the ends to be achieved, the means which may be chosen. In real-world practice, problems do not present themselves to the practitioner as givens. They must be constructed from the materials of problematic situations which are puzzling, troubling, and uncertain. In order to convert a problematic situation to a problem, a practitioner must do a certain kind of work. He must make sense of an uncertain situation that initially makes no sense. . . . When we set the problem, we select what we will treat as the "things" of the situation, we set the boundaries of our attention to it, and we impose upon it a coherence which allows us to say what is wrong and in what directions the situation needs to be changed. Problem setting is a process in which, interactively, we *name* the things to which we will attend and *frame* the context in which we will attend to them.

Parham[13] argues that theory is central to occupational therapists' ability to name and frame problems:

> Theory is a key element in problem setting and in problem solving. It is a tool that enables the therapist to "name it and frame it." Both language and logic are needed to identify a problem (name it) and to plan a means for altering the situation (frame it). Theory provides these by giving us words or concepts for naming what we observe, and by spelling out logical relationships between concepts. This allows us to explain what we see and to figure out how to manipulate a situation to cause change.

When professionals name and frame a problem by applying a conceptual practice model, they must know how to map the theoretical arguments onto the actual features of the situation that requires professional action. Mapping theory onto the real world and transforming theoretical knowledge into practical action are complex processes. As Schon[17] points out, the problems of practice present themselves as "messy, indeterminate situations." Consequently, therapists must first make a judgment about which among alternative theories is most appropriate to formulate the nature of the problem and its action implications. In addition, therapists must close the inevitable gap between the generalities of the theoretical arguments of models and the problems contained in each unique situation. While the theoretical arguments of models deal with common features shared by people, "clinical problems deal with the uniqueness of patients rather than with their similarities."[14] Bridging theoretical concepts to practice means negotiating between "a form of knowledge that is general and a form of knowledge that is specific to a context."[10] Consequently, it is important to recognize that theories are not simple instructions for getting to a destination. Rather, theories provide "maps" of reality, providing a way of seeing the terrain of practice and thereby choosing the destination and a route for getting there.

Using theory is a complex business and there is no way around it. Occupational therapists must actively employ the knowledge of the profession as a way of seeing, understanding, and acting on the problems they solve in their practice. This places a great deal of responsibility on the therapist. We need also to ask: What is the responsibility of the profession to provide conceptual foundations that support therapists in discharging this responsibility?

The answer to this question is that the profession must develop and organize its knowledge into a format that supports the competence of therapists. The field does this through the creation and development of conceptual practice models.

The inherent organization of models of practice facilitates the application of theory in practice. There are several reasons for this. First of all, by virtue of providing a set of theoretical arguments that interweave logically the ideas of order, disorder, and therapeutic intervention, models organize theory in a way that lends itself to being mapped onto practice problems. Hence, the way theory is organized within the conceptual practice model facilitates naming and framing problems. Secondly, within their technology for application, models contain tools that assist and facilitate their application to problem solving in practice. For instance, assessments based on the theoretical arguments of a model provide a concrete means of translating concepts to the real world. The goniometer (which measures the degrees of available motion about the axis of a joint) gives expression to the biomechanical concept, range of motion, an interest checklist gives expression to the concept, volition, from the model of human occupation. In the same way, case examples, protocols of intervention, and other kinds of technology also provide means and exemplars for translating theory into action.

These features of conceptual practice models facilitate the therapist's work of relating theory to practice. Conceptual practice models are so valuable to the field because they organize knowledge in ways that nurture and sustain the process of application.

The Necessary Dialectic between Models and Practice. An intense dialogue should exist between models and the work of applying them. The inherent openness of the process by which theory is transformed into practical action means that using theory should be not only challenging but also empowering. The practical dimensions of minute-by-minute professional work require that the therapists creatively recognize events and objects in the real world as instances of the theoretical concepts and facts from models. Practice also requires that therapists connect the gaps between what theory explains and what the world presents. Conceptual practice models, by providing ways of looking, seeing, and formulating action, serve as springboards for the artistic wisdom that practitioners accumulate through experience.

The same wisdom that comes from applying theory should direct how theoretical arguments are developed and improved. Hence, articulating, applying, and researching models requires an active dialogue in which theory informs practice, and practice informs theory.

While conceptual practice models can be talked about in texts like this one, they come alive in the discourse between theory and practice. One hopes that clear presentation and critical analysis of models in the literature contributes to better understanding, and helps to shape further development, of models. However, unless the conceptual practice models of the field are part of the dynamic conversation of the profession, they become so many wasted pages in a text. Models must find their expression in the work of practice, in the ways therapists think about and articulate their decisions and actions. Those who develop conceptual practice models must assure the accountability of these models to interdisciplinary thought, to the scrutiny of research and, most importantly, to what the model enables therapists to accomplish in their practice. A lively and articulate professional conversation is needed if information is to flow through and influence the process of developing models. What can be discovered in the dialectic between models and practice is more important than what models have to say in the first place.

Using Models to Name and Frame Problems

By conceptualizing order and disorder and therapeutic intervention related to the phenomena it addresses, each conceptual practice model enables therapists to name, frame, and solve a unique set of problems. Moreover, the methods of problem solving (i.e., technology for application) flow logically from the view of order and disorder. Table 15–1 briefly summarizes how each model conceptualizes order, disorder, and therapeutic intervention.

Therapists must carefully select from the models a variety of ways of seeing and explaining the problems of their patients or clients. For example, consider a patient who has suffered a spinal cord injury, is currently in rehabilitation, and appears depressed and unmotivated. Conceptual practice models provide ways of achieving more in-depth understanding of such a patient's condition (the process of naming and framing the problem).* For example, from the perspective of the biomechanical model, the patient would be viewed in terms of the specific effects of the spinal lesion on muscle enervation and the consequent loss of active and passive range of motion, strength, and endurance. This model provides a basis for "insight" into the features of musculoskeletal functioning, patterns of innervation disrupted by a lesion, and the consequent disorganization in the total biomechanical system. The model also provides a way to consider such factors in light of their impact on the movement capacity of the individual in occupational tasks. That is, the problem of lost motion is framed as an interruption of the ability of a person to interact with the world of physical objects and force. Thus, movement limitations are framed as problems of not being able to move about in and to manipulate the physical terrain of daily life. This perspective is reflected, for example, in a description of a patient with spinal cord injury in an occupational therapy text:

> Although physical endurance is low as observed in frequent rest periods during a 60-minute treatment session, the patient's wheelchair tolerance is 8 hours per day. . . . Although finger function is absent bilaterally, Mr H is able to pick up light objects of varied sizes and textures utilizing natural tenodesis grasp in both his dominant right and non-dominant left hands.[1]

This partial description of the problem is guided by the biomechanical model's concept of movement (as reflected in range of motion, strength, and endurance) and by the model's concern for how movement limitations affect performance in occupational tasks. Thus, one aspect of the patient's situation is made more understandable and is framed as a particular kind of problem when seen through a model of practice.

It is important to note that the biomechanical model allows naming only a particular kind of problem (movement limitations) and is silent on the emotional or motivational dimension of the patient's situation. Hence, there is a need for more than one model if one wishes to acknowledge (name) and understand (frame) other problems experienced by the patient.

---

*Not all patient circumstances will be addressed by the current conceptual models of practice. For example, a child with cerebral palsy seems to have normal intelligence but is so impeded with motor problems that it is difficult for her to communicate with others. Information concerning technological adaptations developed in rehabilitation engineering may enable the child with cerebral palsy to communicate with a communication device. Similarly, a patient who recently underwent plastic surgery to reconstruct parts of his hand after a serious traumatic injury needs to begin to use the hand to prevent adhesions, but with consideration for the nature of the surgery and the process of wound healing. Knowledge from the medical model concerning the physiological process of postsurgical healing and scarring can assist the therapist to proceed judiciously in a program of hand rehabilitation. As these instances show, therapists will always require related knowledge from outside the field to augment application of conceptual practice models.

Table 15–1. *Theoretical Arguments and Therapeutic Applications of Conceptual Models of Practice*

Model	Biomechanical	Cognitive Disabilities	Cognitive-Perceptual	Group Work	Human Occupation	Motor Control	Sensory Integration	Spatiotemporal Adaptation
Order	Motion based on joint integrity, strength, and endurance	Cognitive processes that guide behavior	Perceptual and cognitive capacities underlying performance	Group process influencing individual performance	Choices in organization and performance of occupations in environment	Development of skilled motor action based on CNS organization	Organization of sensory information in brain for adaptive movement	Purposeful movements as foundation for knowledge of self, environment, and others
Disorder	Limited range of motion, strength, endurance	Cognitive limitation restricting behavior	Perceptual and cognitive disorganization	Individual occupational performance deficits	Personal and environmental problems influencing choice, organization, and performance	Problems of motor action based on CNS damage	Brain disorganization in which integrative sensory processing and adaptive movement is impaired	Disturbance of purposeful movement and related developmental processes
Assessment	Extent of reason for limitation of motion	Level of cognitive function	Extent and nature of cognitive/perceptual deficits	Group process and individual participation and change	State of personal and environmental factors influencing choice, organization, and performance	Nature of motor impairment	Presence and nature of sensory integrative dysfunction	Description of movement, and personal and environmental factors influencing development

Remedial Therapy	Positioning, exercise, and conditioning to prevent deformity and improve capacity	Training in cognitive and perceptual capacities	Use of group process to influence individual change	Directed experiences to change personal and environmental factors influencing choice, organization, and performance	Use of sensory input and goal-directed action to elicit and organize movement patterns	Specialized opportunities for adaptive movements to elicit sensory information and organize brain	Environmental challenge for purposeful movement to develop motor capacities
Compensatory Therapy	Orthoses/prostheses, adapted equipment/activity	Alter task/environment to match level of cognitive capacity	Teaching patient ways to make allowances for limitations, adapting environment	Environmental and personal adaptations to permanent limitations			

From the perspective of the model of human occupation, one could explain this same patient's motivational status. This model would be concerned with how the spinal cord injury has affected the patient's personal causation (sense of competence), interests, and values. This model orients the therapist to construct a picture of the patient's intense feelings of loss of capacity and control, fears about the future, disruption of his ability to participate in and enjoy old interests, and the disintegration of long-term goals. These factors, viewed together, provide a way to name the patient's unmotivated status as disruption of the volitional narrative (i.e., an inability to see the future as it once was imagined, coupled with the lack of an alternative future story). This view at the same time enables the therapist to frame the problem as requiring the construction of a new volitional narrative in order to achieve a more positive motivational status.

The two models, together, provide ways of conceptualizing the impact of spinal cord injury more holistically, and they allow the therapist to "see" in more depth the nature of two very different aspects of the patient's circumstances. The biomechanical and human occupation models provide a way to "name" the musculoskeletal and motivational problems and to "frame" their meaning for function (e.g., limited movement affecting functional tasks and disrupted volitional narrative, affecting motivation). Moreover, the problem is set as one in which the patient needs to be *motivated* and *moving* in ways that are still possible within the limitations imposed by the disability. This naming and framing provides a logical context for intervention.

For example, the therapist recognizes from the biomechanical model that a functional (tenodesis) grasp can be achieved when the pattern of muscle innervation resulting from the cord injury leaves finger flexors paralyzed, but wrist extensors are still intact. The therapist knows that when flexors have been allowed to contract and become tight, wrist extension produces a passive grip. That is, when the wrist is actively extended, the flexor tendons passively pull against the fingers, closing the hand. A treatment plan for increasing tenodesis potential includes allowing flexor tendons to tighten while building strength in the wrist extensors, followed by practice, using the resulting movement pattern to perform functional tasks (e.g., picking up an object). The therapeutic plan is based on an understanding of both what functions a tenodesis grasp can afford and the biomechanical means to achieve it. The therapist's concern—that the patient be able to move in a way that will allow him to do some things he may wish to do—is supported by an understanding of how that goal might be possible, given his biomechanical status.

Similarly, using the model of human occupation, naming the problem (disruption of volitional narrative and its elements of personal causation, values, and interests) and framing the problem (volitional disruption leading to depression and difficulty making adaptive choices for occupational behavior) sets the logical context for treatment of the volitional aspects of a person with spinal cord injury (i.e., rebuilding his confidence in his ability to perform valued roles, establishing goals based on a sense of values, and integrating these goals into an acceptable future story). The following description of treatment of a young man with spinal cord injury illustrates this:[7]

> His occupational therapist carefully selected occupational forms which appealed both to his role as a father and to his male-oriented interest pattern. For example, with therapist guidance, Alex chose to make a toy wooden truck for his new son. . . . To assist Alex in thinking about his future life, his therapist spent time with him to discuss where he saw his life headed and what was important to him. These ideas were translated into short-term goals for each week and into long-term goals which were reviewed periodically. This process was important since it gave Alex a concrete opportunity to tell his future story to his occupational therapist while receiving help in figuring out how to begin living that story in small steps. This gave a stronger sense of reality to Alex's volitional narrative.

As illustrated in the previous discussion, the selection of models of practice to name and frame the problem was an important first step. A competent therapist is one who knows how to select and use a model of practice to make sense of a situation. The therapist must know that the problem of disrupted motion due to innervation of muscles is addressed by the biomechanical model. The therapist must also know that the motor control, sensory integrative, cognitive-perceptual, and cognitive disabilities models would not be appropriate in this case, because they address problems unrelated to traumatic insult to the spinal cord. The therapist could select the model of human occupation because it addresses motivational problems that are present. Moreover, if the therapist identified a need for socialization with role models who have adapted to spinal cord injury, the group work model might be appropriately chosen.

Other circumstances may call for different models. The sensory integration model may be used to make sense of the clumsiness of a schoolchild. The spatiotemporal adaptation model may provide a way of conceptualizing the developmental process of a child with cerebral palsy. The cognitive-perceptual model may shed light on the memory and problem-solving difficulties of the victim of a stroke. In each case, a problem is named and framed by the model of practice.

Each model of practice frames a problem of occupational dysfunction and provides the therapist with a perspective for enhancing the occupational functioning of the individual. The models provide rationales for how occupation can be used as a therapeutic agent. Thus, they serve as a means by which the therapist operationalizes the professional identity provided by the field's paradigm.

Table 15–1 provides a basic map of the kinds of problems that can be named and framed with current models in occupational therapy. In brief, they are problems of motion, cognition, perception, motivation (choice), lifestyle organization, skilled motor action, sensory integration, purposeful movement, and group participation.

Therapists should select and use those models that together provide a holistic picture of the biological, psychosocial, and environmental circumstances that influence a person's occupational functioning. It is usually not possible to create an adequate picture with a single model of practice; therefore, the therapist will often use models in tandem.

The effectiveness of strategies suggested by one model can be enhanced through insights provided by another model. If we consider the earlier example of combining the biomechanical model and the model of human occupation, we see that intervention goals derived from both models may be met together. For example, if a person with spinal cord injury participates in a therapeutic occupation that has meaning because of a connection to a former life role, biomechanical goals may be enhanced (since a patient may feel less fatigue and exert more effort in a meaningful activity). Volitional goals may be realized simultaneously (a sense of possibilities for competence and a regeneration of interest and meaning may emerge from the activity). By combining models, therapists can achieve a more holistic and efficacious approach.

The Art of Using the Field's Conceptual Foundations

I noted earlier that the use of theory is a complex, indeterminate process. In the end, the use of the field's conceptual foundations is an art. In this final section, I will consider the nature of this art.

Traditional thinking asserts that practical or applied reasoning is a localized version of scientific thought.[9,16] This viewpoint assumes that the rational professional uses the same formal logic that characterizes science to apply the theory to practical problem solving. However, this is often not the case. As Mattingly and Fleming[11] have illustrated, clinical reasoning in occupational therapy is much more complex and multifaceted.

The occupational therapist, by virtue of concern for the occupational dysfunction, is drawn into the personal drama of unique individuals and must help them discover what kind of acceptable life is possible within the constraints and possibilities for change posed by their current condition. Hence, narrative reasoning (thinking with stories) becomes particularly important for considering how the person's disrupted life story can be constituted or reconstructed.[11]

The following is one way to describe the relationship between models and narrative reasoning. Conceptual practice models serve as means for constructing the "scripts" for the therapists' narrative accounts of their work.

That is, while the story the therapist generates provides the structure for emplotting events, models provide the themes that allow incidents to be interpreted, motives to be attributed, characters to be constructed, outcomes to be anticipated, and so on. For example, the biomechanical model provides a way of seeing what a partially paralyzed upper extremity means for pursuing a given story line, and the model of human occupation provides a way of seeing how an avoidance of action is a manifestation of the patient's volitional belief that he has lost all his major areas of competence and is unable to do what he likes to do. Models inform the therapist about what kind of story can be told.

The following example illustrates this point. I was working with an adolescent psychiatric patient whose life was ruled by anxiety. It was clear that his anxiety had been learned over many years, as his impulsiveness, clumsiness, and poor judgment resulted in many failures noticed and labeled by his parents, teachers, and others in control. In various ways, these people sought to circumvent his potential for failure and disruption by attaching all manner of rules and consequences to his behavior. By the time this young man reached his 13th year (when I worked with him), he saw himself as an incompetent person and saw his world as a potential disaster zone.

My primary goal was to alter his volition (i.e., to increase his belief in skill, to reduce his expectation of failure, to increase his interest in doing things, and to enable him to value his own actions). These objectives for volitional transformation represented both my theoretical understanding of him and narrative about who he had become (i.e., what his life story had been), and who he could be (i.e., how his life story could unfold). The latter included my view that, if he could come to improve his volition, he would chose to be active instead of passive and would be less anxious and more involved in life. Further, I imagined that these kinds of changes would give him a better chance at succeeding in school and eventually getting a job, as well as achieving satisfaction in his life. In constructing a narrative about his circumstances and a direction for his life to unfold, I had actively drawn upon a conceptual model of practice.

Thinking in terms of stories also allows one to create therapeutic episodes that have meaning for patients.[8] Having in mind a story for the patient allows the therapist to organize and improvise therapy as an episode relevant to that story. Another example illustrates this point.

I was working with an elderly patient who had suffered a cerebrovascular accident that had rendered her wheelchair-bound and robbed her of effective use of one upper extremity. When I interviewed this woman about her life, I ascertained that she had worked, raised children, and had a successful marriage that culminated in years of caring for an ailing husband. With her newly acquired disability and advanced years, however, she was convinced that her lot was to be a "helpless cripple" until she died. Her younger sister, a woman with deep religious feelings, also had accepted that it was God's will that she should care for her sister in her remaining life. Her well-intentioned but deadly plan was to wait on her sister and require nothing of her in return.

As an individual and as a therapist, I found this an intolerable future story, and I told her that I saw a large reservoir of remaining capacity that she not only could, but should, exercise. Furthermore, our mutual exploration of her past revealed an activity that had meant more to her in everyday life than anything else: baking cookies and breads. The story context in which this activity had meaning involved her loving relationship with her husband and the nurturing of her children. Each afternoon she carefully planned and baked goods that would be fresh and waiting as her children and husband returned from school and work. The sequence of her careful execution of the activity, her growing excitement and hurried preparation as the time of arrival of husband and children neared, and the warm and satisfying episodes that ensued were clearly very meaningful for her. That she should lose every remnant of this activity seemed an intolerable condition for her remaining years. Her sister's household, to which she would return, was populated with children and adults who could enjoy and value her baking. When I shared this idea with her, she protested that her ravaged body and failing health prevented her from engaging in such activities. After some exhortation, she agreed to try a cooking session (in which she adamantly predicted failure) only because I was "such a nice young man."

In preparation for the event, I prepared the clinic kitchen, fabricated a piece of needed adaptive equipment, and borrowed a recipe of her favorite baking project (chocolate chip cookies). On the appointed day, amid mild protests, she began the activity. With adaptive devices, some ad hoc instruction, and a bit of help, she completed the task, noting (inaccurately) that I had "done it for her." Finally, she crumpled the recipe and tossed it in the wastebasket.

According to my plan, ward and therapeutic staff appeared at the door and set about to greedily eat the cookies, showering compliments and gratitude. During this sequence, her affect slowly changed as she proudly announced that she had "done it all alone." When everyone left, we washed the dishes and put the kitchen in order. As we were about to leave the room, she stopped to ask if she could retrieve the recipe from the wastebasket.

As with the above instance, there is something about a "good" therapy session that is not unlike a "good" story. As Bruner[4] points out, a good story can never be the object of the question, "So what?" A good story moves us; we are intrigued by its significance and interested to know how it will unfold. It stands alone as something worth paying attention to in order to see what will happen. A good therapy session matters because it has bearing on how the larger story of the patient's life might unfold.

Bateson[3] observed the necessity of drama and suspense in the occupational therapy session 40 years ago, when he noted:

[E]very incident in occupational therapy is unique. An unrepeatable message is created by unforeseeable and unrepeatable events. In this respect, the modality resembles art. . . . After all, it is inevitable that every act of creation is, *ipso facto*, an act of discovery and the message which you are trying to communicate is a discovery. In the nature of the case, neither you nor the patient can know what is to be discovered. If the patient already knows, no change has been achieved. . . .

Occupational therapy is a deeply human process in which we seek to bring persons into encounters with life occupations—encounters that we hope will transform the course of their lives. There is high art in creating these dramas. This art both surpasses and relies upon the conceptual foundations that allow us to see the complexities of problems faced by our patients and clients.

References

1. Adler, C, and Pedretti, LW: Spinal cord injury. In Pedretti, LW, and Zoltan, B (eds): Occupational Therapy: Practice Skills for Physical Dysfunction. CV Mosby, St. Louis, 1990, p 598.
2. Barris, R: Toward an image of one's own: Sources of variation in the role of occupational therapists in psychosocial practice. The Occupational Therapy Journal of Research 4:1, 1984.
3. Bateson, G: Communication in occupational therapy. Am J Occup Ther 4:188, 1956.
4. Bruner, J: Acts of Meaning. Harvard University Press, Cambridge, 1990.
5. DiJoseph, LM: Independence through activity: Mind, body, and environment interaction in therapy. Am J Occup Ther 11:740, 1984.
6. Fidler, G: The challenge of change to occupational therapy practice. Occupational Therapy in Mental Health 11:1, 1991.
7. Kielhofner, G, and Mallinson, T: Application of the model in practice: Case illustrations. In Kielhofner, G: A Model of Human Occupation: Theory and Application. Williams & Wilkins, Baltimore, 1995, p 272.
8. Mattingly, C: Thinking with stories: Story and experience in a clinical practice. Unpublished doctoral dissertation. Massachusetts Institute of Technology, Cambridge, MA, 1989.
9. Mattingly, C: The narrative nature of clinical reasoning. Am J Occup Ther 45:998, 1991.
10. Mattingly, C: Perspectives on clinical reasoning for occupational therapy. In Roberson, S (ed): In Focus: Skills for Assessment and Treatment. American Occupational Therapy Association, Rockville, MD, 1988, pp 81–88.
11. Mattingly, C, and Flemming, M: Clinical Reasoning: Forms of Inquiry in a Therapeutic Practice. Philadelphia: FA Davis, 1994, p 40.
12. O'Shea, BJ: Pawn or protagonist: Interactional perspective of professional identity. Canadian Journal of Occupational Therapy 44:101, 1977.
13. Parham, D: Nationally Speaking: Toward professionalism: The reflective therapist. Am J Occup Ther 41:557, 1987.
14. Rogers, JC: Eleanor Clarke Slagle Lectureship—1983; Clinical reasoning: The ethics, science, and art. Am J Occup Ther 9:601, 1983.
15. Rogers, JC, and Masagatani, G: Clinical reasoning of occupational therapists during the initial assessment of physically disabled patients. Occupational Therapy Journal of Research 2:195, 1982.
16. Schon, D: The Reflective Practitioner: How Professionals Think in Action. Basic Books, New York, 1983, pp 4, 41.
17. Schon, D: Educating the Reflective Practitioner. Jossey-Bass, San Francisco, 1987.

CHAPTER 16

THE FUTURE OF OCCUPATIONAL THERAPY'S CONCEPTUAL FOUNDATIONS

I have had two aims in writing this text. The first has been to survey the conceptual foundations of occupational therapy, portraying the range of theory, research, and practical knowledge and tools that have been developed. The second, and equally important, aim has been to argue for a particular way of thinking about the development of occupational therapy's conceptual foundations. Hence the following three arguments run as threads throughout the preceding chapters.

First, there is not an obvious or universally accepted answer to the question of how a profession does and should develop its conceptual foundations. Consequently, I argued for a particular view that begins with the observation that the conceptual foundations of a profession provide identity and competence to its members. I further argue that the conceptual foundations can be distinguished into:

1. A paradigm that reflects the most basic constructs, viewpoint, and values of a profession
2. Conceptual practice models that articulate and apply the theory underlying practice
3. A collection of related knowledge employed in practice but not unique to the field

The paradigm supplies identity to the profession, and the conceptual practice models (supported by related knowledge) provide the foundation for practitioners' competence.

Second, occupational therapy's history of paradigm development is marked by radical transformation. These paradigm changes have created problems for the public identity of the profession as a whole and for individual members of the profession seeking to define their life's work. Currently, occupational therapy is taking the important step of articulating its unique focus on occupation and thereby creating an identity for itself. I assert that this focus on occupation needs to be reflected throughout the conceptual foundations and applied in the practice of occupational therapy.

Third, conceptual practice models are unique bodies of knowledge that reflect the pragmatic realities of an applied field. By integrating theory, methods of application, and applied and basic research, these models bring together the basic tasks of a profession. I argue that models emerge and develop toward a particular organization so as to lend themselves to these necessary tasks of the profession. Models meet the field's most basic requirement for knowledge to give substance to its practice.

These three arguments have been brewing for some time. Reilly[28] first recognized that occupational therapy had been severed from its original grounding in concern for occupation in human life, and she initiated the move to return the field's attention to occupation. She also led the way in arguing that occupational therapy should develop its own knowledge base independent of medicine. Her most seminal article,[28] published over 30 years ago, proposed that the proper scholarly focus in occupational therapy is the nature of occupation and its relationship to human adaptation.

Reilly sought to operationalize her vision in collaboration with colleagues and graduate students at the University of Southern California. She referred to the tradition of concepts subsequently developed as "occupational behavior." In nearly two decades, the occupational behavior tradition accumulated a wide range of concepts relevant to the study of occupational behavior and its relationship to health and adaptation. These concepts were reflected in masters theses, published articles, and Reilly's book, *Play as Exploratory Learning.*[30] The topics of these works included the nature of motivation for work and play, the evolution of tool use, the nature of skilled behavior, temporal adaptation, achievement, competence, interests, values, and role behavior. In Reilly's words, occupational behavior was intended to be a "general theory of occupational therapy."[29]

As Reilly's student, I took up and sought to elaborate the occupational behavior argument that the field's scholarly focus should be on occupation. In 1975[10] and in an account (with Janice Burke[17]) of the field's first 60 years, I introduced the concept of *paradigm* to the field's literature, using it as a framework for analyzing the history of knowledge development in occupational therapy. In that first article, we adapted the concept of paradigm from

Kuhn[19] who first introduced it in an analysis of the development of the physical sciences. Our historical account of occupational therapy and the concept of paradigm have undergone transformation in subsequent publications. My current understanding of occupational therapy's paradigm has evolved from many years of thinking and writing, and from helpful collaboration, criticism, and reflection by others.

Following Reilly's lead, I have always asserted that the field needed to embrace occupation as the core of its paradigm. In the early 1980s, I made the following argument:

> A universal first premise to which occupational therapy can attach its theories is the concept of occupation. That premise acknowledges that body and mind are intimately interrelated and that the person is organized and balanced through interaction with the social environment. As a synthesis of body, mind, and society, occupation is a naturally integrating concept for biological, psychological, and social knowledge.
>
> The concept of occupation also provides a useful filter for occupational therapy knowledge. It delineates which human needs or facets are served. Further, it directs us to select as our unique configuration of theories, those that explain occupation and its health-giving potential.[12]

I further argued that it would be important to study occupation, reasoning that "since an occupational therapist's unique and powerful tool is occupation, it behooves the field and the individual therapist to achieve a deep and penetrating understanding of it."[14] Along with others, I sought to develop a stronger focus on occupation in the book, *Health Through Occupation*.[13] These efforts, along with other contemporary arguments, appear to have nudged the field toward adopting the paradigm that is currently emerging.

At the same time I and others were urging the field to find its center in the concept of occupation, another problem concerning the field's conceptual foundations was becoming apparent. Over the years, many papers were published that discussed concepts of occupational behavior and how they might influence practice. Mosey[22] observed that the occupational behavior tradition contained no less than 28 papers that met her criteria for frames of reference and wondered if the body of knowledge was too disparate. Even more to the point, I, along with others trained in the occupational behavior tradition, found that its concepts, themes, and frameworks were not readily moved into practice.

While occupational behavior succeeded as a scholarly tradition calling occupational therapy's attention to its core constructs of occupation, it did not resonate optimally with the demands of practice. I became increasingly convinced that this had to do with how knowledge was being organized. That is, while the occupational behavior tradition generated many seminal papers introducing important concepts, it did not consistently organize its concepts and arguments in ways that facilitated using them in therapy.

To make this point as fairly as possible, I will use as an example a paper I published in 1977. Titled "Temporal adaptation: A conceptual framework for occupational therapy," the paper dealt with the theme of time use and time perspective in occupation.[11] The paper is still cited occasionally, which would seem to indicate that it offers some useful concepts. At the time the paper was written, I was working in an inpatient psychiatric unit. While the ideas in the paper had some influence on how I practiced, there was no formal connection between what I had written and how I practiced. At best, I was loosely guided by some of the ideas represented in the temporal adaptation framework. Hence, I knew firsthand that there was a real problem of connecting concepts to practice and that the problem was not simply with the content. It had to do with how knowledge was articulated and organized.

At that time, a small group of us began to work on the problem of how we could relate to our own practice the concepts we believed were important. We were searching for a more formal and consistent connection between concepts and practice. Janice Burke, Cynthia Heard, and I engaged in an effort to develop what we called a "model" (i.e., the model of human occupation). Over the next few years, we sought to articulate this model and to identify how it could be used to guide practice. Importantly, as we experimented with using this model in practice, it changed. From our efforts, I gained an initial understanding of how a model should be organized to facilitate its connection to practice.

After the model was first published, I began to collaborate with colleagues in my new academic setting (Roanne Barris, Anne Neville, and Janet Hawkins Watts) to implement studies for examining and refining the model. At this time, I was very influenced by examining how the research program for the sensory integration model had developed.

These and other experiences served to point out the differences and the relative importance of the paradigm and models. For example, my exposure to the occupational behavior tradition during my graduate studies taught me the importance of the work of building consensus about occupational therapy's identity and its universal themes, viewpoint, and values. However, as I attempted to put my occupational behavior background into practice, it became apparent that having an identity backed by a collection of concepts was not enough. It was also necessary that concepts be systematically coupled with practical application. This led to the efforts and experiences of creating a model.

Later, as I began to survey the field, it was apparent that the work of linking concepts to practice was being taken up by a number of others. While they were not explicitly calling their efforts models, they were, nevertheless, organizing knowledge in ways that resembled what I now call conceptual practice models.

Along the way, it became apparent that the *process* of knowledge development was worth reflecting on and talking about. This insight brought forth a first set of arguments concerning occupational therapy's conceptual foundations (i.e., that they consist of both a paradigm and models) introduced a decade ago in an article that I coauthored with Roanne Barris[16] and reiterated in the book, *A Model of Human Occupation*.[15] Following that, a more detailed description of the conceptual foundations was offered in the first edition of this text.[18]

This brief chronology should provide some perspective on how the current arguments have evolved over the past 20 years. However, it would be a serious omission to leave out two other important arguments about occupational therapy's conceptual foundations that have arisen simultaneously and have shaped my own views—sometimes because I agreed and sometimes because I disagreed. These are Mosey's view on applied scientific inquiry and the occupation science movement at the University of Southern California. I will first discuss each of these arguments and then return to a consideration of how they agree with and differ from the arguments in this book.

Applied Scientific Inquiry

No other theorist in occupational therapy has so thoroughly and consistently addressed the theme of knowledge organization in occupational therapy as Anne Mosey. In *Occupational Therapy: Configuration of a Profession*,[32] and more recently in *Applied Scientific Inquiry in the Health Professions: An Epistemological Orientation*,[24] Mosey has proposed that the most global construct in a profession was a *model* supported by *frames of reference*:

> The model defines and delineates the broad outlines of a profession as it is understood by the profession and by society. Frames of reference further delineate a particular area or aspect of a profession and, as such, are the link between the profession's model and practice.

The Professional Model

Mosey[20] defined the model as follows:

> A profession's model is the typical way in which a profession perceives itself, its relationship to other professions, and its association with the society to which it is responsible. The model of a profession is characterized by a description of the profession's philosophical assumptions, ethical code, theoretical foundation, domain of concern, legitimate tools, and the nature of and principles for sequencing the various aspects of practice.

Philosophical assumptions concern the nature of humans and their relationship to others and to the nonhuman environment. These assumptions also form the basis for the field's ethical code, its domain of concern, and legitimate tools for practice. Mosey[20] characterizes occupational therapy's philosophical assumptions as the right to meaningful existence, the developmental nature of humans, the right to seek potential through choice and to reach it through interaction with the environment, and the inherent need for a balance among work, play, and rest.

The theoretical foundation of a profession consists of theories selected from academic disciplines, other professions, and the profession's own scholarship. These include biological sciences, psychology, sociology, the arts, medicine, and traditional occupational therapy concepts. Mosey's thesis is that the primary role of a profession is to *apply theory*, rather than to generate theory.

The domain of concern identifies the areas of human welfare that the field serves. It thereby defines the profession's areas of expertise. Mosey[24] identifies occupational therapy's domain of concern as consisting of three elements: occupational performance areas, performance components, and context. She notes that occupational performance areas are "organized patterns of behavior that are characteristic and expected of an individual in a given position within a social system."[24] These areas include: (a) family interaction, (b) activities of daily living, and (c) play, leisure, recreation, and friendships. Performance components are "the basic skills that enable the individual to participate in the various occupational performance areas."[24] Mosey categorizes these components into biological, cognitive, psychological, and social areas. The context refers to the developmental stage of the person, and the physical, social, and cultural environments in which he or she performs.

Mosey uses the phrase "the nature of and principles for sequencing the various aspects of practice" in referring to how the profession defines the problems it solves and how it goes about solving them. She defines the legitimate tools of occupational therapy as the conscious use of self, purposeful activity, groups, the teaching-learning process, and the process of analyzing and adapting activities.

Frames of Reference

According to Mosey,[20] the purpose of a frame of reference is to organize theoretical knowledge for application. She defined a frame of reference as[20]:

> . . . a set of interrelated internally consistent concepts, definitions, and postulates that provide a systematic description of and prescription for a practitioner's interaction with a particular aspect of a profession's domain of concern.

As Mosey describes them, frames of reference consist of a theoretical base, a delineation of function–dysfunction continua related to the phenomena explained by the theory, a list of behaviors indicative of function and dysfunction, and postulates regarding intervention.

Mosey is clear that "a frame of reference is not a theory."[20] She differentiates theory from a frame of reference by noting that, although frames of reference are based on theories, their functions are different. The function of theory is to predict; the function of a frame of reference is to guide action. In this regard, she notes[20]:

> Theory cannot be directly applied. A *theory* is an abstract description of a circumscribed set of physical phenomena that delineates the characteristics of the phenomena constrained therein and their relationship to each other. . . . In occupational therapy, the structure used to transform theory into applicable information—to link theory to practice—is called a *frame of reference.* . . . Frames of reference used by occupational therapists comprise the concepts, definitions, and postulates derived from one or more theories that have been reformulated in such a way as to provide guidelines for evaluation and intervention relative to an element in the profession's domain of concern.

Thus, Mosey argues that theories are fundamentally disinterested in issues of application, and that the frame of reference "borrows" concepts from theories in order to apply them. She views theory and the knowledge for application of theory as requiring different organizational structures.

Occupational Science

In the 1980s, faculty members at the University of Southern California under the leadership of Elizabeth Yerxa developed a doctoral program organized around a new concept they called "occupational science." It was defined as "the scientific discipline that provides explanations of the human as an occupational being."[3] More recently, it was noted that the purpose of occupational science is to "generate knowledge about the form, the function, and the meaning of human occupation."[32]

The occupational science movement clearly has its roots in Reilly's occupational behavior tradition, though it articulates a particular vision of knowledge development that was not part of occupational behavior. Reilly[29] saw occupational behavior as a professional body of knowledge, organized to reclaim occupational therapy's historical concerns with occupational well-being and the use of occupation as a therapeutic agent. Reilly expressed an "obligation to generate ideas in research relevant to our field and to develop them as soon as possible within a clinic."[29] Proponents of occupational science distinguish between the profession of occupational therapy and occupational science. The latter is proposed as new discipline, separate from but supporting the applied science of occupational therapy. As a discipline, occupational science would be more like sociology or biology, which are not directly concerned with matters of practical application. Indeed, such traditional disciplines have held firmly to the ideal of a disinterested stance toward inquiry, going wherever new insights and empirical findings led, without the encumbrance of concerns for the practicality of such knowledge.

By distinguishing itself from the profession of occupational therapy and announcing itself as an academic discipline, occupational science took a brand new position about knowledge development. This position did not address the issue of how the profession of occupational therapy should develop its knowledge. Rather, it asserted that a field of inquiry that directly addressed the phenomena of occupation was needed.[32] Proponents of occupational science further asserted that this new academic discipline would naturally benefit occupational therapy, since it would generate knowledge especially useful for the field.[32] As Zemke and Clark[32] note, "Occupational science is apt to create changes in the way that therapists perceive and approach their work because of what they will have learned about occupation from occupational scientists."

The Heuristic Model of Occupational Science

Since the efforts of occupational science to become a discipline are recent, it is not yet clear what its focus, theoretical directions, and research will be. Occupational science authors have argued that "as occupational science evolves, numerous systems models will be constructed to give a sense of coherence and unity to the complexity of knowledge that is generated."[3]

One paper on occupational science describes a heuristic model that "circumscribes the discipline's major theoretical constructs as well as its conceptual boundaries."[3] This model is grounded in general systems theory, and aims to portray the human as an occupational being. According to this model, the individual is an open system composed of a hierarchically arranged set of subsystems that influence the system's output—and that output is occupational behavior. Moreover, the model portrays the individual in interaction with the environment over the life span. Finally, the model emphasizes that one's pattern of engagement in occupations may facilitate or limit one's adaptation to the environment.

This occupational science model (Fig. 16–1) includes six subsystems, which together make up the individual and influence occupation from within. The physical subsystem includes physiochemical processes (e.g., neuromuscular anatomy and physiology) that support occupational performance. The biological subsystem, made up of those characteristics of living systems related to biological adaptation acquired through evolution, includes such elements as the biological drive for competence and the process of sensory integration. The information processing subsystem is composed of the cognitive processes underlying organized behavior. It includes perception, conceptual appreciations, learning, memory, and planning. The sociocultural subsystem includes the individual's perceptions of

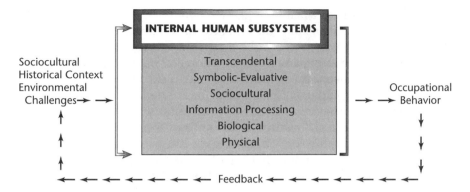

Figure 16–1. The occupational science model. (From Clark et al.,[3] with permission.)

society and culture and the expectations that arise from them. An example of a concept related to this subsystem is role enactment. The symbolic-evaluative subsystem includes symbolic processes that influence the individual's valuation of occupation and encompass symbolic processes such as language, art, moral judgment, and emotion. The transcendental subsystem is concerned with meaning that a person ascribes to life experiences. Transcendence connotes the influence on behavior of such factors as ideas, emotions, hope, and goals.

Clark and coauthors[3] characterize the assumptions of this model as follows:

> . . . (a) that occupation cannot be explained through the focus on a single level (subsystem) of the human system; (b) that occupation must be studied within the context of both the immediate environment and the person's history; (c) that occupation is fired by the human system's drive for efficacy and competency; (d) that although it may be observed as behavior, occupation cannot be fully understood without consideration of its significance to the individual (for example, eating for survival vs. eating as a respite from work); and (e) that the most productive study of occupation requires a synthesis of knowledge from the biological and social sciences.

The occupational science model appears to be intended less as an explanatory or theoretical framework than as a tool to describe themes relevant to the kind of inquiry occupational science will pursue. Hence the term model, as used in the occupational science movement has a very different meaning from the concept of conceptual practice models used in this text and from Mosey's concept of a professional model.

Inquiry in Occupational Science

In the short period that occupational science has existed, its proposal for what kind of inquiry and knowledge development it will pursue has changed. The earliest writings suggested that occupational science was clearly committed to pursuing the road toward being a traditional academic discipline.[3,31] Following these early arguments, Mosey[25] proposed that it would be best to clearly partition occupational science from occupational therapy. She reasoned that by clearly dividing the discipline and the profession, the former would be freed to pursue basic science and establish itself as a discipline in the eyes of its peer disciplines. At the same time, the profession of occupational therapy would be freed to pursue its purpose of applied scientific inquiry.

Mosey[25] makes the point that establishing a new discipline is a bold and risky venture requiring concentrated effort and significant achievement. Any new discipline will come under severe scrutiny by existing disciplines and must prove itself as a legitimate science before being taken seriously. For example, Csikszentmihalyi[6] expressed some skepticism about the emergence of a separate domain of occupational science, arguing that before occupational science can be recognized as a legitimate discipline, "a set of laws specific to occupations will need to be discovered, laws that are not reducible to the symbolic systems of already existing disciplines."

In response to Mosey's recommendation for a partitioning of occupational science and occupational therapy, proponents of occupational science[4] argued for a more symbiotic relationship between the discipline and the profession. They note that:

> in contrast to other disciplines, most occupational science researchers are (and are in the future expected to be) either occupational therapists or persons who are sympathetic to the values and needs of the occupational therapy profession; therefore, their research on occupation will be more directly targeted toward practice considerations than, for example, sociologically based research that touches on occupation.[4]

Hence, the authors appear to be an arguing for a less clear distinction between occupational science and occupational therapy than initially proposed.

Mosey[26] charges that this blurring of distinctions would be detrimental to both occupational science and occupational therapy. She argues that "disciplines are interested in describing the fundamental nature of phenomena within their sphere of inquiry, and ultimately in developing relatively inclusive, valid theories about that phenomena." Hence, she criticized the claim of occupational science to be in service to the profession as "not a great beginning for a discipline" and as making it unlikely that occupational science will be "accepted as a peer by the established disciplines."[26]

At the same time, Mosey argued that occupational therapy should not concern itself and devote its resources to support of occupational science because it was in critical need of developing its applied science. She noted:

> No science-based profession can survive and thrive without engaging in applied scientific inquiry focused on developing theoretically based, safe, effective, and efficient sets of guidelines for action.[26]

Mosey further argued that society demands that occupational therapy—along with other health professions—demonstrate the efficacy of its practice. Occupational therapy must, she reasoned, focus its energies and resources on accomplishing this task if it is to continue to be valued by society.

At this point, occupational science has not delineated how it plans to achieve legitimacy as an academic discipline. In this regard, Mosey's caveats are certainly worth pondering. In the meantime, proponents of occupational science seem to be concerned with shoring up relationships with occupational therapy. For example, Clark's Slagle lecture emphasized how "occupational science research speaks to practice."[5]

Since occupational science is emphasizing how the knowledge it generates will affect occupational therapy[2,4,5] it is worth asking how such knowledge from occupational science is likely to be organized for use in occupational therapy practice. In a special issue of *Occupational Therapy in Health Care* devoted to elucidating the occupational science movement, Jackson[9] discusses an application of occupational science to a high school program for disabled adolescents. In this paper she discusses several themes and concepts that she identifies as belonging to occupational science. These concepts provide the underlying logic for the proposed program. This paper resembles kinds of papers generated in the occupational behavior tradition (e.g., papers on temporal adaptation,[11] role acquisition,[7] and personal causation[1]) about which I wrote earlier in this chapter. Hence, I would raise concern about whether the occupational science movement might re-create some of the same dilemmas I faced two decades ago concerning the difficulty of moving concepts into practice. If occupational science is to contribute meaningfully to occupational therapy practice, it will need to pay careful attention to the issue of what kinds of conceptual structures are needed to guide practice.

Agreements and Disagreements Concerning Conceptual Foundations

At this point I will consider some important commonalities and differences between the view of occupational therapy's conceptual foundations provided in this book, Mosey's view of applied scientific inquiry, and occupational science.

The Focus on Occupation

I have argued that occupational therapy's scholarship and science should converge on the study of occupation, proposing that this study of occupation is influenced by the vision provided by the field's paradigm. I further have argued that the theme of occupation should be and is influencing how conceptual practice models articulate their theoretical concerns.

Originally, Mosey[21] argued against organizing occupational therapy knowledge around occupation (which she referred to as a monistic approach), preferring a pluralistic collection of diverse themes. Because Mosey sees occupational therapy as drawing its theory from multiple interdisciplinary sources, she was suspicious of any effort to organize occupational therapy knowledge around a single construct such as occupation. However, in her more recent work,[24] she defines occupational therapy's domain of concern as occupational performance areas and their underlying components and surrounding contexts. Hence, it appears that Mosey is now more willing to accept the importance of the theme of occupation to the field.

The occupational science movement calls for a focus on occupation. For example, Yerxa and coauthors[31] state that occupational science will study "the human as an occupational being including the need for and capacity to engage in and orchestrate daily occupations in the environment over the lifespan." They further note that occupational science will:

> . . . study individuals in interaction with their environments, not as decontextualized beings. It will focus on the person, not on a cell or reflex. The science of occupation will retain the complexity of occupation, recognizing that it can be understood by using models, specifically open systems models. These will be concerned with the processes by which all levels of the human system contribute to the output of occupation. It will be developmental in scope encompassing the entire lifespan.
>
> Occupational science will study the person's experience of engagement in occupation recognizing that observing behavior is not sufficient for understanding occupation. The organization and balance of occupations in daily life and how these relate to adaptation, life satisfaction, and social expectations will be central issues as will timing, planning and anticipation. Occupational science will seek to learn more about intrinsic motivation and the drive for effectance. Finally it will need to be true to its humanistic roots by preserving human complexity, diversity, and dignity.[31]

This vision of occupational science clearly parallels the core constructs that I characterized as underlying the field of occupational therapy in Chapter 4.

Knowledge Organization

Concerning the issue of how knowledge should be organized, Mosey's applied scientific inquiry, occupational science, and the view I have proposed in this book share important similarities and differences. These are summarized in Table 16–1.

Both Mosey's arguments and those in this book are concerned with how occupational therapy should organize its knowledge. Both perspectives share the view that there are two basic levels of knowledge: (1) the global

Table 16–1. **Proposals for Knowledge Organization**

	Occupational Science	**Mosey**	**Present Argument**
View of Knowledge Organization	Occupational science is a discipline separate from, but supporting, the profession of occupational therapy. Occupational science includes both basic and applied research.	Occupational therapy is a profession that only applies scientific knowledge.	Occupational therapy is a profession that engages in integrated basic and applied science (within conceptual practice models) as part of the necessary work of generating knowledge for practice.
Profession-Wide Knowledge Organization	No discussion of how knowledge should be organized within occupational therapy. Argues that occupational science is a separate discipline that has a special interest in providing knowledge useful for occupational therapy. Within occupational science a *model* is proposed as a heuristic tool that identifies the discipline's major theoretical constructs and conceptual boundaries.	*Model*: Describes structure and content of profession; consists of philosophical assumptions, ethical code, theoretical foundation, domain of concern, legitimate tools, and the nature of and principles for sequencing the various aspects of practice	*Paradigm*: Shared professional culture that shapes theory development and practice; consists of core constructs, focal viewpoint, and values.

Organization of Knowledge for Practice	No proposed structure. Existing literature suggests that each new application would generate a unique conceptual framework.	*Frames of Reference*:
		• Apply theory
		• Consist of:
		  ○ Theoretical base
		  ○ Function–dysfunction continuums
		  ○ Behaviors indicative of function and dysfunction
		  ○ Postulates regarding intervention
			Conceptual Practice Models:
			• Articulate theory and guide practical application
			• Consist of
			  ○ Interdisciplinary base
			  ○ Theoretical arguments
			  ○ Technology for application
			  ○ Empirical base

knowledge that describes the field as a whole (i.e., the model or the paradigm, depending on whose concepts are used), and (2) the structures for clinical application (i.e., the frame of reference or the conceptual practice model).

One can easily draw parallels between Mosey's arguments and mine. For instance, Mosey's concept of the model as a global structure that defines the profession parallels the concept of paradigm expressed in this book. In the same way, the idea that frames of reference organize knowledge for application is similar to the way in which models are defined in this book. However, important differences characterize the two schemes of knowledge organization. Mosey sees the model as a collection of themes, the configuration of which reflect occupational therapy's nature. She disagrees with the use of the concept of paradigm, which, she argues, belongs to pure sciences, whose purpose it is to develop new knowledge.[23]

The concept of paradigm as used in this book, serves to define the profession, but it also serves as an important shared intellectual perspective that shapes necessary theorizing within occupational therapy. Mosey sees no such role for the model, nor does she consider the creation and testing of theory to be an obligation of the field. Moreover, since frames of reference only *use* theory and create a means of applying it, they need not be concerned with problems of organizing or empirically validating theoretical arguments. I use the concept of paradigm to stress the fact that occupational therapy, like other basic disciplines, has a mission to develop knowledge. That is, the paradigm shapes the way models will organize their theoretical arguments.

I stress that conceptual models of practice make theoretical arguments; Mosey notes that frames of reference only create applications of existing theory. Conceptual practice models address a particular component of occupational behavior or performance (e.g., motivation, movement, perception, sensory integration) and seek to explain how this aspect of occupation is organized. They also seek to explain states of disorder or dysfunction and to describe the potential impact of occupation to preserve or change the organizational status, thereby maintaining or improving performance. In addition, conceptual models result in a technology for application (e.g., assessments and procedures for intervention). Finally, they generate a research base.

Proponents of occupational science have not concerned themselves with how occupational therapy should organize its knowledge. Rather, they have asserted that the study of occupational science demands formation of a new discipline. They have identified a heuristic model to guide the development of occupational science. However, this model is a framework for scientific inquiry, not for defining occupational therapy. When articulating knowledge intended to influence occupational therapy, occupational science writers appear to be following the lead of the occupational behavior tradition (i.e., creating multiple frameworks for application).

Applied Science versus Basic Science

Mosey[23] and writers in the occupational science movement have engaged in debate over the legitimate role of basic science versus applied science in occupational therapy. Occupational science was originally described as a basic science. In discussing the role of occupational science, Primeau, Clark, and Pierce[27] noted that basic science aims at describing, explaining, and predicting events as part of the search for knowledge and truth. They contrasted it with applied science, of which occupational therapy is an example.

Mosey argued for the partitioning of occupational science from occupational therapy because she sees the proper focus for inquiry in occupational therapy as applied science. According to Mosey[23]:

> Basic scientific inquiry is concerned with the development of valid theory through exploration of unknown or inadequately known phenomena. In contrast, applied scientific inquiry is concerned with the development of effective technology and techniques through extrapolation from previously articulated theories or empirical data.

In response to Mosey's call for a partitioning of occupational science from occupational therapy, authors of occupational science have emphasized the intent of occupational science to engage in applied work.[2,4,32] Moreover, they have argued that applied and basic science are not dichotomous, but instead form a continuum.

By focusing their arguments on the issue of applied versus basic science and their appropriateness for an academic discipline and for a profession, both Mosey and the proponents of occupational science have partly skirted a much more crucial set of issues that I will take up in the next section. These issues have to do with how to best develop the necessary knowledge for the practice of occupational therapy.

Developing Knowledge for Practice

Mosey makes an observation that is certainly valid for many theories: that is, if one examines theories in many traditional disciplines (e.g., sociology, philosophy, physics), these theories do not entertain within their logical structure guidelines for applying their concepts to practical problems. To the extent this is true, Mosey is correct in arguing that a structure for application is needed before theories translate into practice.

What I disagree with, however, is the implicit conclusion that creating theory and developing its application are, de facto, different enterprises that cannot be coupled into a single effort. One of the most influential efforts to understand the human psyche in modern history linked practical problem solving and theorizing. The work of Sigmund Freud clearly coupled efforts to develop a method for dealing with psychiatric disorders with efforts to decipher the organization of the psyche. A less well-known effort by the

German philosopher, Jürgen Habermas, has sought to understand how social theory can be transformative—that is, transcend the traditional discussions of methodological differences in social science and create better ways of knowing and being.

Indeed, if one looks seriously across efforts of knowledge development, there are ample examples of knowledge generated from or closely linked to solving practical problems. I would argue that much of the separation of theory and application of basic and applied work is simply a matter of institutionalized convention. Universities, funding agencies, disciplines, and professions have perpetuated the separation of understanding and action. *

The view of paradigm and conceptual practice models that I have espoused in this book proposes a way of building the conceptual foundations of the field without artificially separating theory and practice. I argued in Chapter 2 that conceptual practice models reflect the particular theoretical, practical, and scientific concerns of occupational therapy. Models are organized to simultaneously theorize about occupational behavior, to explain occupational dysfunction, and to elucidate both the dynamics of the therapeutic process and the practical means for achieving therapeutic goals. Finally, each model yields empirical support for the theoretical arguments and for the efficacy of applications that emanate from them.

Models integrate theoretical, practical, and scientific concerns in the field, creating cohesion and dialogue between these activities. Thus, models hold a central place in the development of knowledge in the field. Moreover, models demonstrate that the division of theory and application, of which Mosey speaks, is not a necessary condition. In fact, in occupational therapy, where theorizing is primarily in the service of practice, theoretical and practical concerns must be synergistic.

I argue that it is most efficient and effective that the field develop and use a finite number of conceptual practice models. This allows for cumulative refinement and for development of technologies for application. The argument between Mosey and proponents of occupational science has focused on whether basic and applied science are dichotomous or continuous. However, this argument skirts the more important issues of whether and how basic and applied inquiry might be able to be profitably integrated.

---

*The distinction between theory and practice is not entirely without foundation. There is a legitimate distinction to be made between tacit or practical knowledge and understanding. For example, we can move our bodies and converse without understanding how movement is made possible by the body or how language is learned and governed. However, understanding can improve upon or correct what we tacitly know how to do. For example, biomechanics can teach us better ways to do a variety of physical tasks so as to maximize our efficiency and avoid injury. Similarly, organization theories can help us become more effective communicators and better at dealing with social conflict. The whole enterprise of professional knowledge is aimed at creating knowledge that improves upon, corrects, or augments much of what we as ordinary persons know how to do.

In my view, basic and applied inquiry are synthesized within conceptual practice models. The theory of each model focuses on different aspects of occupation. For example, the sensory integration model focuses on sensory processing for performance; the model of human occupation theorizes about motivation influencing the choice of occupation; the biomechanical model theorizes about the musculoskeletal structures and processes and their use in moving in the context of occupations; and the group work model theorizes about the influence of collective behavior on occupational performance. The theoretical arguments of these models cover basic science concerns for how systems are organized and how they may be disrupted by disease, trauma, and other factors. However, these theoretical arguments also address questions of application—that is, they consider how occupations can be used to maintain or change organization and function within the phenomena of concern. Thus, occupational therapy develops both basic and applied knowledge within frameworks that are specifically organized to address practice. Research may be directed to *basic scientific questions* that emanate from the models. For example, "How are volitional images formed, and how do they shape choices for occupational behavior?" "How is the body used in the performance of occupations?" "How do cognitive processes influence performance?" Such questions can be asked about both adaptive and maladaptive states. The answers to these basic science questions have immediate relevance for clinical application. The more we know about the organization and disorganization of factors that influence occupational behavior, the more effectively we can design clinical methods for assessment and intervention. In addition, basic research will identify natural strategies for change that can be incorporated into clinical application. Finally, methods of data collection developed for basic research activities often result in the development of clinical assessment procedures.

Research emanating from conceptual models of practice can also address questions of application, such as how therapeutic occupation can be used to compensate for, preserve, or change the structures underlying occupational performance and adaptation. When practical applications of theory are shown to work, they provide further evidence of the viability of the theoretical system. In other words, if the theory can be used to predict, understand, and control processes in the clinical context, then we can be more confident that the explanations it provides have truth value—the goal of basic science.

Separation of basic and applied science and quarrels over the relative merit of each miss the larger possibilities that can arise from their integration within conceptual practice models. Occupational therapy requires such integration, because it needs both basic explanations of the phenomena with which it is concerned and proven, useful clinical strategies of assessment and intervention. The structure of models of practice that I have proposed is a framework intended to tie together the central concerns of the field: generating unique occupational therapy disciplinary knowledge, conducting basic and applied research, and developing means for practical application.

Figure 16–2 illustrates how basic and applied research serve as feedback loops within a model of practice. Both basic and applied research questions derive their logic from the theoretical arguments and test the truth of the theoretical arguments. Applied research examines the usefulness of the technology for clinical application that proceeds from those arguments. Applied research also provides indirect evidence of the validity of the theoretical arguments; if the technology works, then the explanations on which it is based have greater credibility. The diagram also illustrates ways in which the basic and applied research within occupational therapy generate information relevant to interdisciplinary fields.

In the end, the issue is not the relative merit of basic versus applied science. Rather, the pressing issue for occupational therapy concerns how to best articulate and test knowledge so as to guide and validate the practice of the field. Conceptual practice models place the processes of applied and basic inquiry into a framework that addresses that issue.

Conclusion

This chapter is an attempt to place the arguments in this book in the context of other important perspectives and to consider the implications of each for the future of occupational therapy. I identified a number of issues concerning the organization of knowledge, the focus of scholarship on occupation, and the nature and appropriateness of applied and basic research. In doing so, I have tried to illustrate the merits of the particular organization of knowledge proposed in this text. I proposed that the field's generic nature can be understood as contained in a paradigm that identifies

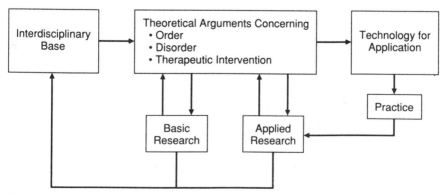

Figure 16–2. Applied and basic research emanating from conceptual models of practice.

the occupational nature of humans, occupational dysfunction, and the therapeutic use of occupation as the themes to which future knowledge development should be directed.

I also argued that conceptual practice models should be the focus for knowledge development, since they articulate, test, and apply occupational therapy theory. Moreover, I hold that research (both basic and applied) should be tied to these models. There will always be the need for exploratory research, to identify new themes and concepts to be integrated into models or to generate new models. But in the interest of developing a cumulative science of occupational therapy, the models of practice should provide the primary focus of research.

I described commonalities with and differences between both the occupational science movement and Mosey's applied scientific inquiry. In contrast to Mosey, I assert that, to be a viable profession, occupational therapy must actively develop its own theories. While occupational therapy may benefit from having occupation science share the concerns of the field for occupation and its application, it cannot afford to ignore the urgency of developing a strong conceptual foundation for the profession. The health care system increasingly clamors for health professions to articulate the nature and to demonstrate the worth of their services. Professions that lack a clear definition of what they do and that lack evidence of the efficacy of their service will not fare well in the next century. In this regard, I agree with Mosey that occupational therapy needs to focus its energies and resources on defining, refining, and demonstrating the worth of its practice.

Increasingly, other professional groups have adopted concepts and methods that duplicate what has traditionally been occupational therapy practice. Claims to traditional professional territory will not win the day in asserting that occupational therapy offers a unique service. If occupational therapy wishes to stake out its professional territory, it must do so with clearly articulated theory, well-developed methods to apply that theory, and research demonstrating the validity of the theory and the efficacy of the methods.

Fields that are successful in creating powerful explanations of human problems and how to solve them and that have research evidence that their methods work will have a distinct advantage in the next century. Those that do not will have a difficult time surviving. More than ever in its history, occupational therapy should be asking how the profession can best create synergies between theory, practice, and research.

At this moment in history, occupational therapy finds itself in competition with other disciplines to provide solutions to the problems of incapacity. Society, beset with the massive costs, complexities, and challenges of disability, is seeking demonstrably sure and efficient methods of solving the problems of incapacity in daily life. Therefore, generating knowledge in the service of occupational therapy's problem-solving capacities is of paramount concern.

Certainly, occupational science must define its own parameters and the nature of its inquiry.* Whether or not occupational therapy is complemented by an occupational science that may "provide an especially handsome payoff to the profession,"[2] the fact remains that occupational therapy must go about the business of internally developing its own knowledge base. Occupational therapy must create a vision of what the profession is, and it must develop, apply, and test theory that is specifically designed to guide practice. In short, the profession of occupational therapy and no other entity must be the keeper of its own conceptual foundations—that is, the ongoing conversation about its paradigmatic constructs, viewpoint, and values; and the development, refinement, application, and testing of its conceptual practice models.

References

1. Burke, JP: A clinical perspective on motivation: Pawn versus origin. Am J Occup Ther 4:254, 1977.
2. Carlson, M, and Dunlea, A: Further thoughts on the pitfalls of partition: A response to Mosey. Am J Occup Ther, 49:73, 1995.
3. Clark, F, Parham, D, Carlson, M, Frank, G, Jackson, J, Pierce, D, Wolfe, R, and Zemke, R: Occupational science: Academic innovation in the service of occupational therapy's future. Am J Occup Ther 45:300, 1991.
4. Clark, F, Zemke, R, Frank, G, Parham, D, Neville-Jan, A, Hedricks, C, Carson, M, Fazio, L, and Abreu, B: Dangers inherent in the partition of occupational therapy and occupational science. Am J Occup Ther 47:185, 1993.
5. Clark, F: Occupation embedded in a real life: Interweaving occupational science and occupational therapy. Am J Occup Ther 47:1067, 1993.
6. Csikszentmihalyi, M: Foreword. Occupational Therapy in Health Care 6:xv, 1989.
7. Heard, C: Occupational role acquisition. Am J Occup Ther 31:243, 1977.
8. Henderson, A, et al: Occupational science is multidimensional. Am J Occup Ther 45:370, 1991.
9. Jackson, J: En route to adulthood: A high school transition program for adolescents with disabilities. Occupational Therapy in Health Care 6:33, 1989.
10. Kielhofner, G: Understanding adaptation: The evolution of knowledge in occupational therapy. Master's thesis. University of Southern California, Los Angeles, 1975.
11. Kielhofner, G: Temporal adaptation: A conceptual framework for occupational therapy. Am J Occup Ther 31:235, 1977.
12. Kielhofner, G: A heritage of activity: Development of theory. Am J Occup Ther 36:727, 1982.
13. Kielhofner, G: Health through Occupation: Theory and Practice in Occupational Therapy. FA Davis, Philadelphia, 1983.
14. Kielhofner, G: Occupation. In Hopkins, HL, and Smith, ND (eds): Willard and Spackman's Occupational Therapy, ed 6. JB Lippincott, Philadelphia, 1983, p 31.

---

*My main purpose here is to focus on the issue of occupational therapy's conceptual foundations. To the extent that occupational science has declared itself a separate academic discipline, it is not directly related to this topic. However, since occupational science has stated a desire to maintain a close relationship with occupational therapy, members of the profession must have some concern with how occupational science is judged by its peer disciplines. Mosey legitimately points out that occupational science is less likely to be readily recognized as a legitimate academic discipline if it blurs its boundaries with occupational therapy.

15. Kielhofner, G: A Model of Human Occupation. Williams & Wilkins, Baltimore, 1985.
16. Kielhofner, G, and Barris, R: Organization of knowledge in occupational therapy: A proposal and a survey of the literature. Occupational Therapy Journal of Research 6:67, 1986.
17. Kielhofner, G, and Burke JP: Occupational therapy after 60 years: An account of changing identity and knowledge. Am J Occup Ther 31:675, 1977.
18. Kielhofner, G: Conceptual Foundations of Occupational Therapy. FA Davis, Philadelphia, 1992.
19. Kuhn, T: The Structure of Scientific Revolutions, ed 2. University of Chicago Press, Chicago, 1970.
20. Mosey, AC: Occupational Therapy: Configuration of a Profession. Raven Press, New York, 1981, pp 50, 129.
21. Mosey, AC: Eleanor Clark Slagle Lecture. A monistic or a pluralistic approach to professional identity? Am J Occup Ther 8:504, 1985.
22. Mosey, AC: Psychosocial Components of Occupational Therapy. Raven Press, New York, 1986.
23. Mosey, AC: The proper focus of scientific inquiry in occupational therapy: Frames of reference. Occupational Therapy Journal of Research 9:195, 1989.
24. Mosey, AC: Applied Scientific Inquiry in the Health Professions: An Epistemological Orientation. American Occupational Therapy Association: Rockville, MD, 1992.
25. Mosey, AC: Partition of Occupational Science and Occupational Therapy. Am J Occup Ther 46:851, 1992.
26. Mosey, AC: The Issue Is: Partition of occupational science and occupational therapy: Sorting out some issues. Am J Occup Ther, 47:752, 753, 1993.
27. Primeau, LA, Clark, F, and Pierce, D: Occupational therapy alone has looked upon occupation: Future applications of occupational science to pediatric occupational therapy. Occupational Therapy in Health Care 6:19, 1989.
28. Reilly, M: Occupational therapy can be one of the great ideas of 20th century medicine. Am J Occup Ther 16:1, 1962.
29. Reilly, M: The educational process. Am J Occup Ther 23:299, 1969.
30. Reilly, M: Play as Exploratory Learning. Sage Publications, Beverly Hills, CA, 1973.
31. Yerxa, EJ, Clarle, F, Frank, G, Jackson, J, Parham, D, Pierce, D, Stein, C, and Zemke, R: An introduction to occupational science: A foundation for occupational therapy in the 21st century. Occupational Therapy in Health Care 6:1–18, 1989.
32. Zemke, R, and Clark, F: Occupational Science: The Evolving Discipline. FA Davis, Philadelphia, 1996, pp vii, 4.

GLOSSARY

activity analysis Detailed examination of a task to determine what is required to do the task (e.g., movements performed, steps involved) as well as the possible psychological meaning of the task.

affective Pertaining to emotions.

Alzheimer's disease A dementia (deterioration of one's mental state) resulting from organic brain disorder.

amyotropic lateral sclerosis A chronic progressive disease of unknown etiology involving deterioration of motor neurons in the cortex, medulla, and spinal cord. Symptoms may include hyperreflexia, spasticity, muscle weakness, and atrophy—beginning in the upper extremities.

arthritis Disease involving joint inflammation.

atrophy A wasting or decrease in size of an organ or tissue.

cardiopulmonary system The heart, circulatory vessels, and lungs.

catheterization Use or passage of a tube (catheter) through the body for evacuating or injecting fluids into body cavities.

caudal Relating to the spine's distal part (i.e., part farthest from the head).

caudocephally Referring to the course of development of motor functions from foot to head.

central nervous system The brain, spinal cord, spinal nerves, and their end organs.

cephalocaudally Referring to the course of development of motor functions from head to foot.

cerebral aneurysm Localized abnormal dilation of a blood vessel, usually in an artery, occurring in the cerebrum, which is due to congenital defect or weakness of the wall of the vessel.

cerebral cortex The thin, convoluted surface layer of gray matter of the cerebral hemispheres, consisting principally of cell bodies of neurons arranged in five layers.

cerebral palsy A disorder of motor functioning resulting from a nonprogressive lesion or defect in the brain at birth.

cerebrovascular accident (CVA) The occurrence of brain damage due either to interrupted blood flow or bleeding in the brain's blood vessels (commonly referred to as a stroke).

cognition Mental processing thought processes (e.g., memory, planning procedure solving).

cognitive Pertaining to thought processes (e.g., to memory, planning, problem solving).

compensation Making allowances for or adapting to permanent limitations of ability through the use of alternative behaviors or assistive devices.

compensatory techniques Methods of adapting to a limitation of ability by using alternative behaviors or assistive devices.

cortical Relating to the cortex of the brain, or to higher-level behaviors controlled by the cortex.

dementia Deterioration of one's mental state as a result of organic brain disease (i.e., memory loss, confusion).

demoralization Deprivation of spirit and courage.

disability An individual's limitation in or lack of the ability to participate in one or more of major life activities.

disciplinary knowledge Theories, facts, and technology unique to a profession or a discipline.

edema Increased fluid in the tissues that produces swelling.

efferent Referring to neural pathways that carry commands from the central nervous system to the muscles.

empirical Referring to the process of supporting or discounting theories by experimentation or observation (i.e., gathering evidence about the accuracy or "truth" of theories).

enervation Decrease in or lack of nervous strength or energy; nerve removal or resection.

engrams The change in neural tissue left by stimulation that allows experience to be stored biologically.

flaccidity Lack of muscle tone or tension.

functional performance Ability to complete tasks and functions needed for daily living.

gustatory Pertaining to sense of taste.

health care system The interrelated institutions and professions involved in providing health care.

hemiplegia Paralysis of one side of the body.

hierarchy The arrangement of parts of a system into interconnected lower and higher components in which higher components command lower ones and lower ones constrain the higher.

holistic Relating the functional relationship of parts and wholes to stress. In health care, holistic thinking considers the person's life circumstances and not just the disease or trauma.

hypertrophied Increased in size, generally in bulk and not the number of cells or tissue elements, of an organ or structure that does not involve tumor formation.

hypothesis (plural, hypotheses) Statement of theory that can be tested through research.

hypotonicity Subaverage muscle tone.

impairment Abnormally or loss in the function or structure of an individual's anatomy, physiology, or psychological status.

integumentary system The organ system made up of the tissue that covers the body, including the skin, hair, and nails.

intrapsychic Within the mind or soul; related to unconscious thoughts and feelings.

kinematics The study of motion.

kinesiology The study of functions and structures of the musculoskeletal system.

kinesthetic Regarding sensations of movement and tension from the joints, muscles, and tendons.

kinetics Regarding or involving motion.

learning disability Difficulty in learning in children with normal intelligence.

life roles The positions and/or statuses held by individuals in various parts of society (e.g., student, father, worker, retiree).

medical model Medicine's body of knowledge and beliefs regarding the role of the doctor and treatment. The medical model focuses on detecting disease and eliminating its causes and/or consequences. The medical model emphasizes the expert knowledge of the physician and the action of the physician upon the patient.

mental status State of the mind's functioning. Normally refers to whether a person's emotional and cognitive processes are functionally normal.

meta-analysis A statistical method for analyzing the results of many studies together.

motor Pertaining to the production of movement in the human body.

multiple sclerosis A chronic, slowly progressive disease of the central nervous system characterized by development of plaques (disseminated demyelinated glial patches).

musculoskeletal system The organization of muscles and bones in the body.

narrative The use of stories in human life as ways of thinking and sharing information with others.

neurological Pertaining to the study of nervous diseases.

neurons The nerve cells (found in the brain, spinal cord, and peripheral nerves).

neurophysiology The study of the biochemical functions of the nervous system.

neuroplasticity The nervous system's capacity for change and self-repair.

neuropsychology A branch of psychology that examines cognitive and perceptual functioning (i.e., intelligence, memory, visual sequencing).

neuroscience Any of the areas of science concerned with the nervous system.

occupational choice process The process by which an individual selects a career or occupation. This process ordinarily begins in childhood and culminates in entry into an adult occupation. It may be repeated when the individual changes careers or replaces work with leisure occupations upon retirement.

olfactory Pertaining to smell.

Parkinson's disease A chronic nervous disease characterized by a fine, slowly spreading tremor, muscular weakness and rigidity, and a peculiar gait.

participant observation Collecting research data while taking part in the activities of those studied.

perceptual Pertaining to the conscious identification and interpretation of sensory stimulation.

peripheral nervous system The nerves and ganglia that are not in the spinal cord or brain.

phenomenon (plural, phenomena) An event or a fact that can be observed.

phenomenological Referring to the experience of an event or process; referring to theory or research that emphasizes what a person experiences as basic to what a person does.

physical agents Therapeutic modalities, such as electricity, water, heat or cold, and light or sound administered for the treatment of soft tissue.

physiotherapist Treatment with physical and mechanical means, as massage or electricity.

presuppositions Beliefs that are not questioned and on which other beliefs are based.

proprioception The awareness of posture, movement, and changes in equilibrium and the knowledge of position, weight, and resistance of objects in relation to the body.

propositional Pertaining to logical relations between ideas.

proximal Closer to the trunk, center, or place of attachment.

psychic Regarding the psyche (i.e., emotions and thoughts).

psychodynamic Regarding the development of the mind and the mind's forces; usually refers to unconscious processes.

psychotherapeutic Related to the treatment of emotional disorders by exploring and altering the unconscious mind.

psychotropic Medicine given to improve psychic functioning (i.e., medications that influence thought processes or moods).

range of motion Amount of movement possible at a joint.

reductionism The study of phenomena by examining their constituent parts and the cause-and-effect relations between the parts.

reliability Refers to assessment or measurement procedures—specifically to the property of being consistent when used in different situations, by different persons.

remediate/remedial To provide a remedy for a problem, to achieve improvement.

residual limitations Remaining or continuing restrictions in function following disease or injury.

schizophrenia A less than well understood group of mental disorders usually representing a deterioration from a previous level of function. The onset is prior to age 45 and is characterized by delusions, hallucinations, or thought disturbances.

social darwinism A social movement that applied Darwin's evolutionary principle of the survival of the fittest to social relations; it valued self-reliance over mutual concern.

socialization The process through which individuals learn how to live in their social environment (i.e., "learning the ropes" in a new job).

sociocultural Referring to the beliefs and practices of groups of persons and to the organization of relationships between members of groups.

soft tissues Nonbony tissue affecting joint function; includes the tendons and skin that surround the joints.

spasticity Increased muscle tone or contractions (due to a lesion in the upper motor neuron) resulting in awkward and stiff movements.

spina bifida A congenital defect in which the laminae of the vertebrae fail to unite; may result in paralysis and other problems.

splinter skills Any trained, developed, or learned skill that is unrelated to any variety or integration of skills a person possesses and is acquired in an intermittent or inconsistent pattern.

subcortical Relating to the lower areas of the brain below the cortex; referring to nonconscious processes determined by these areas of the brain.

sublimate To divert instinctual impulses into socially acceptable ways of expression.

taxonomy System for classifying (e.g., categorization of animals into mammals, amphibians, etc.).

tendon Connective tissue that attaches the muscle to the bone.

tenodesis The surgical fixation of a tendon, which usually involves the transfer of the tendon from its initial point of origin to a new origin to restore muscle balance to a joint, restore lost function, or increase active power of joint motion.

topographical orientation The ability to find one's way from one place to another.

unilateral neglect Disregard for one side of the body.

valid Refers to the property of an assessment or measure—specifically pertains to whether the instrument or procedure measures what it is supposed to measure.

vestibular Referring to the sense of one's body in relation to gravity. This sense is regulated in the inner ear.

visuospatial Referring to the cognitive use of spatial data obtained by sight (e.g., distance and relative placement of objects).

INDEX

A "t" following a page number indicates a table; an "f" indicates a figure; an "n" indicates a footnote.